Lecture Notes in Computer Sc

Commenced Publication in 1973
Founding and Former Series Editors:
Gerhard Goos, Juris Hartmanis, and Jan van Leeuw

Hiroyuki Yoshida   Georgios Sakas
Marius George Linguraru (Eds.)

Abdominal Imaging

Computational and Clinical Applications

Third International Workshop
Held in Conjunction with MICCAI 2011
Toronto, ON, Canada, September 18, 2011
Revised Selected Papers

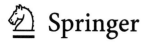 Springer

Volume Editors

Hiroyuki Yoshida
Massachusetts General Hospital, Department of Radiology
25 New Chardon Street, Suite 400C, Boston, MA 02114, USA
E-mail: yoshida.hiro@mgh.harvard.edu

Georgios Sakas
Fraunhofer-Institut für Graphische Datenverarbeitung (IGD)
Abteilung Cognitive Computing and Medical Imaging
Fraunhoferstraße 5, 64283 Darmstadt, Germany
E-mail: georgios.sakas@igd.fraunhofer.de

Marius George Linguraru
Sheikh Zayed Institute for Pediatric Surgical Innovation
Children's National Medical Center
111 Michigan Avenue, NW, Washington, DC 20010-2916, USA
E-mail: mlingura@cnmc.com

ISSN 0302-9743   e-ISSN 1611-3349
ISBN 978-3-642-28556-1   e-ISBN 978-3-642-28557-8
DOI 10.1007/978-3-642-28557-8
Springer Heidelberg Dordrecht London New York

Library of Congress Control Number: 2012931867

CR Subject Classification (1998): J.3, I.4, H.5.2, I.5, I.2.10, I.3.5, I.4

LNCS Sublibrary: SL 6 – Image Processing, Computer Vision, Pattern Recognition,
and Graphics

Typesetting: Camera-ready by author, data conversion by Scientific Publishing Services, Chennai, India

Printed on acid-free paper

Springer is part of Springer Science+Business Media (www.springer.com)

Preface

The Third International Workshop on Computational and Clinical Applications in Abdominal Imaging was held in conjunction with the 14th International Conference on Medical Image Computing and Computer-Assisted Intervention (MICCAI) on September 18, 2011, in Toronto, Canada.

In the abdomen, organs and disease appearances are complex and subtle, and thus the development of computational models that are useful in clinical practice are challenging. Nevertheless, diagnosis often relies on the quantitative measures of organs and lesions because their volumes and shapes are strong indicators of disorders. Given the complexity and high variability of abdominal organs, the identification of distinct computational challenges for integrative models of organs and abnormalities is essential for understanding anatomy and disease, evaluating treatment, and planning intervention.

The third international workshop focused on three areas in computational abdominal imaging: virtual colonoscopy and computer-aided diagnosis, abdominal intervention, and computational abdominal anatomy. The workshop aimed to bring together leading researchers and clinicians active in these fields around the world to discuss emerging techniques and clinical challenges in computational and clinical applications in abdominal imaging.

In response to the call for papers, a total of 40 papers were initially submitted to the workshop. These papers underwent a rigorous, double-blinded peer-review process, with each paper being reviewed by a minimum of two expert reviewers from the Scientific Review Committee. Based on the review results, 33 papers were accepted by the workshop. With additional three plenary lectures, the workshop accommodated a total of 26 oral presentations and 10 poster presentations.

The workshop successfully formulated a forum among participants for the dissemination of the state-of-the-art research and technologies, the exchange of emerging ideas, the initiation of collaborations, and the exploration of new clinical applications for diagnostic and interventional procedures in abdominal imaging. All of the 33 papers presented at the workshop were revised by incorporating the discussions at the workshop and re-submitted by the authors as post-conference proceedings papers to be included in this proceedings volume.

We would like to express our sincere appreciation to the authors whose contributions to this proceedings book have required considerable commitments of time and effort. We also thank the members of the Workshop Committee and Program Committee for their excellent work in reviewing the submitted manuscripts under a tight schedule. Special thanks go to the following individuals: Wenli Cai, the Program Chair, for his outstanding job in organizing the workshop program and in preparing the on-site abstract book; Janne Näppi, a member of the Workshop Committee and the Proceedings Editorial Board, for his excellent job in arranging and editing the proceedings papers; and June-Goo Lee, a member of the Workshop Committee and Proceedings Editorial Board, for his excellent work on developing the website for the workshop.

November 2011

Hiroyuki Yoshida
Georgios Sakas
Marius George Linguraru

Workshop Organization

Organizing Committee

Marius George Linguraru   Children's National Medical Center, USA
Georgios Sakas   Technische Universität Darmstadt / Fraunhofer Institute for Computer Graphics Research IGD, Germany
Hiroyuki Yoshida   Massachusetts General Hospital / Harvard Medical School, USA

Workshop Committee

Klaus Drechsler   Fraunhofer Institute for Computer Graphics Research IGD, Germany
Marius Erdt   Fraunhofer Institute for Computer Graphics Research IGD, Germany
David Hawkes   University College London, UK
David Holmes   Mayo Clinic / Mayo Medical School, USA
Lakhmi C. Jain   University of South Australia, USA
Jong Hyo Kim   Seoul National University, Korea
Honbing Lu   Fourth Military Medical University, China
June-Goo Lee   Massachusetts General Hospital / Harvard Medical School, USA
Sandy Napel   Stanford University, USA
Janne Näppi   Massachusetts General Hospital / Harvard Medical School, USA
Cristina Oyarzun Laura   Fraunhofer Institute for Computer Graphics Research IGD, Germany
Kazunori Okada   San Francisco State University, USA
Yoshinobu Sato   Osaka University Graduate School of Medicine, Japan
Akinobu Shimizu   Tokyo University of Agriculture and Technology, Japan
Frans Voss   Delft University of Technology / Academic Medical Center Amsterdam, The Netherlands
Stefan Wesarg   Technische Universität Darmstadt, Germany

Program Chair

Wenli Cai   Massachusetts General Hospital / Harvard Medical School, USA

Program Committee

Dean Barratt	University College London, UK
Miguel A. Gonzalez Ballester	Alma IT Systems, Spain
Yufei Chen	Tongji University, China
Jan Egger	University Hospital of Marburg, Germany
Karl Fritscher	Health and Life Sciences University Hall/Tyrol, Austria
Fredeqique Frouin	Pierre and Marie Curie School of Medicine, France
Hiroshi Fujita	Gifu University, Japan
Tobias Heimann	German Cancer Research Center, Germany
Kenneth R. Hoffmann	University at Buffalo, USA
Mingxing Hu	University College London, UK
Holger Reinhard Roth	University College London, UK
Shoji Kido	Yamaguichi University, Japan
Ron Kikinis	Brigham Women's Hospital / Harvard Medical School, USA
Andrew Laine	Columbia University, USA
Hans Lamaeker	Zuse Institute Berlin, Germany
Boudewijn Lelieveldt	Delft University of Technology, The Netherlands
Yoshitaka Masutani	Tokyo University, Japan
Kensaku Mori	Nagoya University, Japan
Yuichi Motai	Virginia Commonwealth University, USA
Stephane Nicolau	IRCAD, France
Toshiyuki Okada	Osaka University, Japan
Iván Macía Oliver	Vicomtech, Spain
Cornelis Roel Oost	Tokyo University of Agriculture and Technology, Japan
Hyunjin Park	Gachon University of Medicine and Science, South Korea
Matthias Raspe	SOVAmed GmbH, Germany
Mauricio Reyes	University of Bern, Switzerland
Greg Slabaugh	MedicSight Inc., UK
Ronald M. Summers	National Institutes of Health, USA
Kenji Suzuki	University of Chicago, USA
Fei Wang	IBM Almaden Research Center, USA
Thomas Wittenberg	Fraunhofer IIS, Germany
Xiang Zhou	Siemens Medical Solutions, USA
Hongbin Zhu	State Unviersity of New York at Stony Brook, USA
Stephan Zidowitz	Fraunhofer MEVIS, Germany

Proceedings Editors

Hiroyuki Yoshida	Massachusetts General Hospital / Harvard Medical School, USA
Georgios Sakas	Technische Universität Darmstadt / Fraunhofer Institute for Computer Graphics Research IGD, Germany
Marius George Linguraru	Children's National Medical Center, USA

Proceedings Editorial Board

Janne Näppi	Massachusetts General Hospital / Harvard Medical School, USA
June-Goo Lee	Massachusetts General Hospital / Harvard Medical School, USA
Wenli Cai	Massachusetts General Hospital / Harvard Medical School, USA

Table of Contents

Virtual Colonoscopy and CAD

Abdominal Intervention

Computational Abdominal Anatomy

Inverse Consistency Error in the Registration of Prone and Supine Images in CT Colonography

Holger R. Roth[1], Thomas E. Hampshire[1], Jamie R. McClelland[1],
Mingxing Hu[1], Darren J. Boone[2], Greg G. Slabaugh[3],
Steve Halligan[2], and David J. Hawkes[1]

[1] Centre for Medical Image Computing, University College London, UK
[2] Department of Specialist Radiology, University College Hospital, London, UK
[3] Medicsight PLC, London, UK
h.roth@ucl.ac.uk

Abstract. Robust registration between prone and supine data acquisitions for CT colonography is pivotal for medical interpretation but a challenging problem. One measure when evaluating non-rigid registration algorithms over the whole of the deformation field is the inverse consistency error, which suggests improved registration quality when the inverse deformation is consistent with the forward deformation. We show that using computed landmark displacements to initialise an intensity based registration reduces the inverse consistency error when using a state-of-the-art non-rigid b-spline registration method. This method aligns prone and supine 2D images derived from CT colonography acquisitions in a cylindrical domain. Furthermore, we demonstrate that using the same initialisation also improves registration accuracy for a set of manually identified reference points in cases exhibiting local luminal collapse.

Keywords: CT colonography, image registration, computer aided diagnosis and interventions.

1 Introduction

Recently, Roth et al. [6] presented a method for establishing spatial correspondence between prone and supine colonic surfaces derived from computed tomographic (CT) colonography (CTC) data. This method involves the conformal mapping of both endoluminal surfaces derived from colon segmentations to cylindrical 2D domains, in order to simplify this challenging 3D registration problem. This is followed by a non-rigid cylindrical registration based on the well-accepted b-spline registration method [7,5]. The similarity metric used to drive the cylindrical registration is the sum-of-squared differences (SSD) of the shape index (SI). Shape index [4] has also been used for detection of colonic polyps by computer-aided detection (CAD) methods also applied to CT colonography data [9]. The SI values are computed on the original surface meshes which describe the endoluminal colon surface with the patient in the prone and supine

H. Yoshida et al. (Eds.): Abdominal Imaging 2011, LNCS 7029, pp. 1–7, 2012.
© Springer-Verlag Berlin Heidelberg 2012

positions. Regions of possible local colonic collapse can be ignored during computation of the similarity measure when performing this cylindrical registration. This is important since luminal collapse is commonly encountered during clinical interpretation.

The registration method promises good accuracy in regions where the colon is well-distended in both orientations and when no segmentation errors are present. The reported mean ($\pm$ std. dev.) registration error of 13 polyps was 5.7 (± 3.4) mm when tested in 13 validation cases. However, the method might be less accurate if marked differences in distension or segmentation between prone and supine acquisitions are encountered, since this can precipitate marked dissimilarities in derived surface features: similar feature patterns for driving the registration are required to align both surfaces accurately.

Hampshire et al. [3] show that landmark features (e.g. haustral folds) matched robustly between prone and supine acquisitions can further improve algorithm accuracy by providing an initialisation for the cylindrical registration along the length of the colon. Registration accuracy improved significantly from 9.7 ($\pm$ 8.7) mm to 7.7 ($\pm$ 7.1) mm in cases exhibiting local luminal collapse. The registration error was unchanged at 6.6 mm for 8 cases where the colon was already adequately distended.

The present paper aims to further investigate the effect of this initialisation on the registration, via evaluation of the inverse consistency error (ICE). The ICE was proposed by Christensen et al. [1] as an important criterion for evaluation of non-rigid registration methods.

2   Inverse Consistency Error

The cylindrical registration can be computed in two directions: prone to supine and supine to prone. We arbitrarily denote the prone to supine direction as the forward transformation T_{ps}, e.g. prone as source and supine as target image. Supine as source and prone as target is denoted as the inverse (supine to prone) transformation T_{sp}. The standard b-spline registration method is not inverse consistent, with the result that registration can result in different solutions depending on the transformation direction; i.e. prone to supine or supine to prone. The inverse consistency error ICE measures this inconsistency as follows [2]: any point p on the prone surface S_p can be transformed to the supine surface S_s using the forward transformation T_{ps}. The inverse transformation T_{sp} is then applied to map the transformed point back to p' on S_p. The Euclidean distance $\|\cdot\|$ between point p and p' in 3D space gives the value of ICE for any point p. This principle is illustrated in Fig. 1 for a point p in the transverse colon and can be formulated as

$$ICE = \|p' - p\| = \|T_{sp}(T_{ps}(p)) - p\|. \tag{1}$$

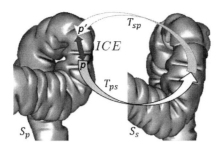

Fig. 1. Computing the inverse consistency error (ICE)

3   Evaluation of Inverse Consistency

3.1   Data

For the following experiments, we used anonymised CTC data acquired during normal clinical practice and following generally-accepted recommendations for CTC data acquisition [8]. These data consist of a total of 13 validation cases of which 5 exhibited local luminal collapse in at least one patient orientation. A radiologist (experienced in over 400 validated colonography studies) manually identified haustral folds of confident correspondence. This was achieved using cylindrical image representations and virtual 3D fly-through renderings for navigation through the prone and supine acquisitions. This procedure resulted in a total of 1175 pairs of corresponding landmarks with an average of 90 pairs of haustral folds per case.

3.2   Inverse Consistency without Feature Initialisation

Accuracy of registration can only be evaluated where corresponding features have been manually identified. This is only feasible when there are easily identifiable corresponding features (e.g. polyps) in both acquisitions (i.e. where the registration is more likely to give a good result). In contrast, the ICE can be calculated anywhere on the cylindrical representations and does not require manually identified landmarks, thus simultaneously eliminating any error due to landmark mismatching.

The ICE values can vary for different regions of the images. Large ICE values often occur where the surface features in the two acquisitions appear very different, since the registration algorithm is unable to align the different features successfully. Figure 2 illustrates the ICE computed for each pixel of the cylindrical images and mapped back to the endoluminal colon surface in Fig. 3. The total mean ICE for all 13 validation patients is 3.7 mm. The mean ICE is slightly higher in the 5 collapsed cases; 4.9 mm as opposed to the mean ICE of 3.0 mm for the 8 well insufflated cases.

We propose that areas of high ICE precipitate more uncertainty in both images regarding which features need to be aligned with which. Therefore, registration does not necessarily converge towards the same solution in forward and inverse directions. However, a registration result with low ICE does not necessarily suggest good correspondence between two images [1]; further evaluation of registration accuracy is necessary. The manual selected fold correspondences can be used to establish a fold registration error (FRE) which measures misalignment of reference points in 3D after cylindrical non-rigid registration as an index of accuracy, resulting in a mean ($\pm$ std. dev.) FRE of 7.7 ($\pm$7.4) mm for all 13 cases. The 5 cases exhibiting local colonic collapse have a higher FRE : 9.7 ($\pm$8.7) mm compared to 6.6 ($\pm$6.3) mm for the 8 well insufflated cases.

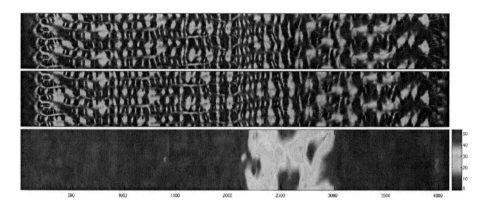

Fig. 2. Difference between forward (top) and inverse (middle) registrations for patient 4. The registration results are shown using a false colour scheme which displays source features as blue and target features as red. After non-rigid alignment, overlapping features are displayed in grey. The forward (top) and inverse (middle) registrations show areas of inconsistency, especially around 2500 pixels in x-direction (along the colon). This is reflected in the ICE values in these areas (bottom).

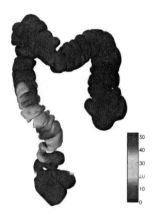

Fig. 3. ICE values for patient 4 mapped onto the colon surface

3.3 Inverse Consistency after Feature Initialisation

Hampshire et al. [3] show that an initialisation of the registration method using robustly matched features (e.g. haustral folds) can improve the registration accuracy. Using a good initialisation can roughly align the correct folds of the cylindrical images leading to convergence to the correct solution in the subsequent b-spline registration. A significant improvement from 9.7 ($\pm$ 8.7) mm to 7.7 ($\pm$ 7.1) mm was reported in the cases where the dissimilarity of features is higher (e.g. the 5 cases exhibiting local colonic collapses) while it stays unchanged at 6.6 mm in 8 well-distended cases.

This improvement in registration accuracy suggests the method is more robust when initialisation is good. Increased accuracy is also reflected in the ICE metric. Figure 4 shows the reduction of an area of high ICE after initialisation for patient 4. The mean ICE for this patient is reduced from 7.6 mm to 2.2 mm. Another example is shown in Fig. 5 and confirms this assumption for patient 12 in which a short section of colon is collapsed. The mean ICE for this patient is reduced from 8.2 mm to 3.9 mm. The total mean ICE for all 13 validation patients is reduced from 3.7 mm to 2.6 mm. Table 1 lists the mean FRE and mean ICE before and after using a feature-based initialisation for each patient. In all but two cases (patient 6 and 13) a reduction of mean ICE can be observed after feature-based initialisation. Here, the ICE was low before initialisation and the increase of the ICE is negligible (0.2 mm and 0.1 mm respectively).

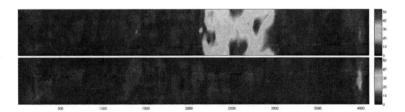

Fig. 4. The inverse difference metric (ICE) before (top) and after (bottom) initialisation using feature correspondences for patient 4

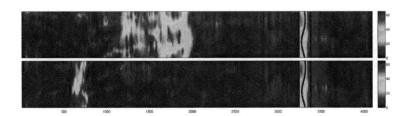

Fig. 5. The inverse difference metric (ICE) before (top) and after (bottom) initialisation using feature correspondences for a collapsed case (patient 12)

Table 1. The mean fold registration error $\overline{FRE}$ and mean inverse consistency error ($\overline{ICE}$) in mm for 13 patients used for validation before ($_1$) and after ($_2$) using a feature-based initialisation. The locations of where the colon is collapsed are given (DC: descending colon, SC: sigmod colon).

Patient	Collapse in prone	Collapse in supine	FRE_1 [mm]	FRE_2 [mm]	ICE_1 [mm]	ICE_2 [mm]
1	none	none	11.5	11.5	2.9	2.6
2	none	none	8.6	7.2	3.4	2.6
3	none	none	5.3	5.5	2.0	1.9
4	none	none	5.7	5.7	7.6	2.2
5	none	none	5.5	5.8	2.1	2.0
6	none	none	5.2	5.5	1.7	1.9
7	none	none	5.8	6.1	2.1	2.0
8	none	none	6.7	6.9	2.3	2.3
9	none	1 x DC	9.6	9.1	4.1	2.3
10	none	1 x SC	7.8	7.8	5.6	3.4
11	1 x DC	1 x DC	6.5	5.8	3.3	3.2
12	3 x (DC, SC)	none	13.5	8.7	8.2	3.9
13	1 x DC	1 x DC	12.2	7.9	2.9	3.0
Total [mm]			7.7	7.0	3.7	2.6

4   Conclusion

We show that a robust initialisation can improve the inverse consistency of the cylindrical b-spline registration method. While improved inverse consistency alone does not guarantee good correspondence, concomitant improvement in registration accuracy suggests that registration is more robust when using a feature-based initialisation.

Further improvement might be achieved by implementing an inverse-consistent non-rigid registration method. This might help optimise registration in cases where false local minima in the similarity function that is being optimised are present. Information from both forward and inverse direction may enforce convergence towards the correct solution.

References

1. Christensen, G., Geng, X., Kuhl, J., Bruss, J., Grabowski, T., Pirwani, I., Vannier, M., Allen, J., Damasio, H.: Introduction to the non-rigid image registration evaluation project (nirep). Biomedical Image Registration, 128–135 (2006)
2. Christensen, G., Johnson, H.: Consistent image registration. IEEE Transactions on Medical Imaging 20(7), 568–582 (2001)
3. Hampshire, T., Roth, H., Hu, M., Boone, D., Slabaugh, G., Punwani, S., Halligan, S., Hawkes, D.: Automatic Prone to Supine Haustral Fold Matching in CT Colonography Using a Markov Random Field Model. In: Fichtinger, G., Martel, A., Peters, T. (eds.) MICCAI 2011, Part I. LNCS, vol. 6891, pp. 508–515. Springer, Heidelberg (2011)

4. Koenderink, J.: Solid shape. MIT Press, Cambridge (1990)
5. Modat, M., Ridgway, G., Taylor, Z., Lehmann, M., Barnes, J., Hawkes, D., Fox, N., Ourselin, S.: Fast free-form deformation using graphics processing units. Comput. Meth. Prog. Bio. 98(3), 278–284 (2010)
6. Roth, H.R., McClelland, J.R., Boone, D.J., Modat, M., Cardoso, M.J., Hampshire, T.E., Hu, M., Punwani, S., Ourselin, S., Slabaugh, G.G., Halligan, S., Hawkes, D.J.: Registration of the endoluminal surfaces of the colon derived from prone and supine ct colonography. Medical Physics 38(6), 3077–3089 (2011)
7. Rueckert, D., Sonoda, L., Hayes, C., Hill, D., Leach, M., Hawkes, D.: Nonrigid registration using free-form deformations: Application to breast mr images. IEEE Trans. Med. Imaging 18(8), 712–721 (1999)
8. Taylor, S., Laghi, A., Lefere, P., Halligan, S., Stoker, J.: European Society of Gastrointestinal and Abdominal Radiology (ESGAR): Consensus statement on CT colonography. European Radiology 17(2), 575–579 (2007)
9. Yoshida, H., Nappi, J.: Three-dimensional computer-aided diagnosis scheme for detection of colonic polyps. IEEE Trans. Med. Imaging 20(12), 1261–1274 (2002)

Dual-Energy Electronic Cleansing
for Artifact-Free Visualization of the Colon
in Fecal-Tagging CT Colonography

Wenli Cai[1], June-Goo Lee[1], Se Hyung Kim[2], and Hiroyuki Yoshida[1]

[1] Massachusetts General Hospital and Harvard Medical School, Boston, 02114, USA
[2] Seoul National University College of Medicine, Seoul, South Korea
{cai.wenli,yoshida.hiro}@mgh.harvard.edu

Abstract. The partial volume effect (PVE) is one of the major causes of the artifacts in electronic cleansing (EC) for fecal-tagging CT colonography (CTC). In this study, we developed a novel dual-energy EC (DC-EC) scheme for minimizing the EC artifacts caused by the PVE. In our approach, the colonic lumen, including air and tagged fecal materials, was first marked by a dual-energy index (DEI). The high DEI value of air and tagged fecal materials provides a means to efficiently differentiate the voxels at the boundary between air and tagged materials from those of the soft-tissue structures that have the DEI value of around zero. As a result, the colonic lumen, including air and tagged materials, could be accurately segmented based on their high DEI values. Our DE-EC scheme was shown to provide an electronically cleansed colon that is free from artifacts caused by the PVE at the air-tagging boundary.

Keywords: computer-aided diagnosis (CAD), dual-energy CT, electronic cleansing, fecal-tagging CT colonography.

1   Introduction

Tagging of feces by an oral contrast agent (iodine or barium) is a promising method for differentiating residual feces from colonic soft-tissue structures in CT colonography (CTC). The orally administered contrast agent is opaque to X-rays, and thus it opacifies residual solid stool and fluid in the colon. Electronic cleansing (EC) is an emerging method for segmentation of the tagged fecal material, subtracting it from the CTC images for generation of digitally cleansed images of the colon.

Due to the partial volume effect (PVE), voxels at the boundary between the lumen and tagged materials, called the air-tagging boundary (AT-boundary), not only have CT values that are close to those of soft-tissue structures, but also have gradient values that are similar to a thin soft tissue structure that is sandwiched between the tagged region and the lumen, which we call the air-tissue-tagging layer (ATT-layer). Both the AT-boundary and the ATT-layer are generated by the PVE, a mixture of multiple materials at one voxel. EC requires the subtraction of both the AT-boundary and tagged regions.

H. Yoshida et al. (Eds.): Abdominal Imaging 2011, LNCS 7029, pp. 8–17, 2012.

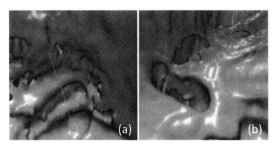

Fig. 1. Demonstrations of EC artifacts. (a) Pseudo-soft-tissue structures caused by the uncleansed air-tagging boundary (AT-boundary). (b) False fistula caused by the over-cleansed air-tissue-tagging layer (ATT-layer).

Existing EC methods tend to use gradient-based approaches to detect an AT-boundary; however, such methods tend erroneously to remove a part or the entire thin soft-tissue structure within an ATT-layer, or preserve a part or the entire AT-boundary. The former causes the degradation of the thin colonic wall and folds, and the latter creates pseudo-soft-tissue structures, as demonstrated in Figure 1. For addressing this issue, advanced methods such as the local roughness analysis method [1] and the statistical classification method [2] have been proposed. However, these solutions are heuristic and incomplete, especially for non-cathartic CTC.

Because the aforementioned EC artifacts are caused by the PVE, a mixture of CT numbers (attenuation values) of multiple materials in a single voxel, it is an ill-posed condition in single-energy CTC images. It cannot be completely solved when conventional single-energy CT scanning is used.

Dual-energy CT (DE-CT), which recently became widely available in clinical practice, provides a theoretical means of solving the PVE of a material mixture by its multi-spectral material differentiation capability [3, 4]. By an analysis of two attenuation values acquired simultaneously at two photon energies (such as 80 kVp and 140 kVp), DE-CT offers spectral information for estimation of material composition [3, 5], which works especially well in materials with large atomic numbers such as iodine that has a k-edge energy close to the mean value of the diagnostic energy range [6, 7]. Iodine is one of the commonly used contrast agents in fecal-tagging CTC, and it is generally known to have strong enhancement on CT images acquired at a low tube voltage. Applying DE-CT to fecal-tagging CTC image acquisition, denoted as dual-energy CTC (DE-CTC), provides a solution for solving the above material mixture problem.

In this study, we developed a novel dual-energy EC (DC-EC) scheme for minimizing the EC artifacts caused by the PVE. This approach employed the dual-energy index (DEI), which is calculated from the DE-CTC images, and we used the higher DEI values of air and tagged materials to differentiate them from the soft-tissue structures, which have the DEI value of around zero. As a result, the colonic lumen, including air and tagged materials, was segmented based on its high DEI values. Our DE-EC scheme provides a cleansed colon that is free from artifacts caused by the PVE at the air-tagging boundary.

2   Methods

2.1   Dual-Energy Index

By definition, the Hounsfield unit (HU) is computed by use of the attenuation coefficient of water as the reference. The HU of water is set to be 0 and it remains unchanged at different energy levels. The behavior of the HU of any material depends on three factors: (a) photon energy, (b) atomic number (Z), and (c) material density.

At different energy levels, the change of HU values of any material depends on its effective atomic number compared to that of water. If the effective Z of a material is higher than that of water (Z_{water}), its HU value increases as the energy level decreases (e.g., bone, iodine, etc.), whereas the HU value decreases as the energy level decreases if the effective Z of a material is lower than Z_{water} (e.g., fat).

The dual-energy index (DEI), defined as $(HU_i^{80} - HU_i^{140})/(HU_i^{80} + HU_i^{140} + 2000)$ [8], represents the ratio of the relative change of the HU values of a material of two different photon energies, such as 80 kVp and 140 kVp. By definition of the HU, the DEI value of water is 0, i.e., the HU values of water stay identical at two energy levels. Table 1 lists the effective Z and the theoretical DEI values of several materials commonly seen in CTC images.

In general, water-like materials (Z ~ 7.5) show only modest variation in HU at different photon energies in CT, as depicted by the near-zero DEI values in Table 1. In addition, we notice that the DEI values of air and CO_2 are positive due to their slightly higher effective Z values compared to Z_{water}, although the attenuation coefficients, i.e., the HU values of air and CO_2, are very low (around -1000 HU in single-energy CT) because of their low material densities. The positive DEI value of air and CO_2 indicates that the HU value of the coloic lumen decreases as the photo energy increases in CTC images, and it has the same trend as that of iodine.

Table 1. Effective atomic numbers (Z) and dual-energy index (DEI) of several commonly seen materials obtained at 80 kVp and 140 kVp

Material	Effective Z	DEI
Water	7.42	0.0000
Fat	6.3	-0.0194
Soft tissue	7.22	-0.0052
Muscle	7.56	0.0021
Bone	13.8	0.1148
Iodine (20 mg/ml)	53	0.1414
Air	7.64	0.0049
CO_2	7.55	0.0020

2.2   Virtual Lumen Tagging by Dual-Energy Index

For a dual-source CT scanner, there are two tubes (A, B) and two detectors (A, B). The expected intensity at pixel (x,y) of a detector (e.g., A) can be expressed by:

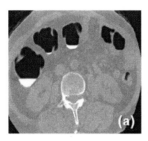 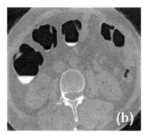 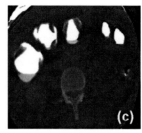

Fig. 2. Illustration of dual-energy CT colonography and the dual-energy-index image. (a) One axial image at low energy (80 kVp). (b) One axial image at high energy (140 kVp). (c) DEI image for all voxels ≥-990HU in a mixed image.

$$I^A(x,y) = I_p^{A,A}(x,y) + I_{fs}^{A,A}(x,y) + I_{cs}^{B,A}(x,y) \ , \tag{1}$$

which shows that the detected signal consists of the photoelectric intensity $I_p^{A,A}$ that originates from tube A and registered at detector A, the forward-scatter intensity $I_{fs}^{A,A}$ from tube A, and the cross-scatter $I_{cs}^{B,A}$ generated by the photons emitted by tube B and scattered to detector A.

Both forward scattering and cross scattering are "Compton scattering," which is energy-dependent and material-dependent. In general, materials of higher atomic number are more likely to absorb photons, and high-energy photons are more likely to be scattered. Thus, the artifacts caused by the cross-scattering in low-energy detector and in low-atomic-number materials are more severe than that in a high-energy detector and in high-atomic-number materials.

The cross-scattering contribution, originated from the x-ray from the high-energy tube received at a low-energy detector, may cause "pseudo beam hardening" in the low-energy projection data. This triggers the beam-hardening correction process that is built in the image reconstruction process in the scanner. Therefore, in fecal-tagging CTC, luminal air may be affected more severely by the cross-scattering in low-energy images than in high-energy images.

Figure 2 demonstrates a fecal-tagging DE-CTC case. As expected, the tagged regions have high and positive DEI values. However, we also observed that the DEI values of luminal air were unexpectedly higher than that of tagged regions, which is caused by the cross-scattering and is different from the theoretical values shown in Table 1. We observed that the actual DEI value of air was substantially higher than its theoretical value. The DEI image in Figure 2(c) also demonstrates this phenomenon. This high DEI value provides the ability to mark the entire coloic lumen, including both the lumen air and tagged fecal materials, which we call "virtual lumen tagging" of the colon.

We selected 10 patients who underwent DE-CTC (80 kVp and 140 kVp) examinations with reduced cathartic bowel preparation and with orally administered iodine-based fecal tagging. Twenty volume-of-interest (VOIs) were selected from luminal air, abdominal soft tissue, or tagged fecal materials. The mean CT value was measured in each VOI, and its DEI was calculated. The resulting DEI values were 0.456±0.024, -0.017±0.006, and 0.146±0.011 for luminal air, abdominal soft tissue, and tagged fecal materials, respectively.

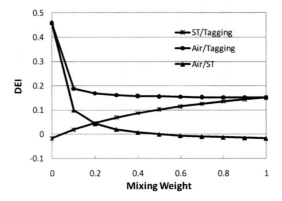

Fig. 3. DEI curves for three mixture types: soft tissue and tagged fecal materials (ST/Tagging), air and tagged fecal materials (Air/Tagging), and air and soft tissue (Air/ST). The Air/Tagging curve is located substantially above the value of soft-tissue. The plot indicates that the DEI is an efficient index for differentiation of soft tissue from the mixture of air and tagged materials, although their CT values are overlapped.

The ambiguity between soft tissue and the AT-boundary caused by the PVE can be solved efficiently by DEI. Because air has the highest DEI value and soft tissue has the lowest DEI value, the DEI value of air-tagging boundary is substantially higher than that of soft tissue, as illustrated in Figure 3. The DEI curve of the air/tagging mixture is clearly above the DEI value of soft tissue, which is around 0. Thus, the high DEI value of air provides a useful index for differentiating the air-tagging boundary from soft tissue, although the CT values of the Air/Tagging mixture range from -800 HU to 600 HU and overlap significantly with that of the soft-tissue structures.

In addition, "virtual lumen tagging" by DEI value can remove the air bubbles submerged in the tagged materials, which is commonly seen in non-cathartic fecal-tagging CTC. Figure 4 demonstrates the "virtual lumen tagging" in a non-cathartic fecal-tagging phantom study. Air bubbles are marked, as are the AT-boundaries. The inhomogeneity of the tagged materials is reduced substantially.

2.3   Hessian Response of DEI Field

We applied the structure-analysis EC scheme (SA-Cleansing) [9-11] for cleansing of the virtually tagged coloic lumen. The SA-Cleansing scheme uses the local morphologic information to classify the submerged soft-tissue structures while removing the tagged materials. Specifically, in the DE-CTC cases, we used the eigenvalue signatures of a Hessian matrix [12, 13] of the DEI values to enhance fold-like and polyp-like structures, whereas other structures were de-enhanced and thus subtracted from the CTC images.

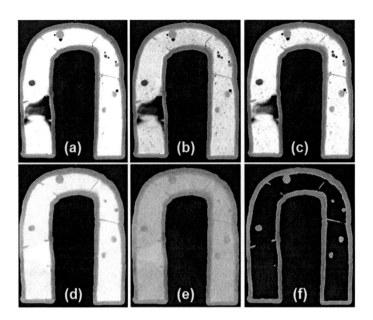

Fig. 4. Illustration of virtual lumen tagging of the colon by DEI in the phantom study. (a) Coronal image of the phantom at low energy (80 kVp). (b) Coronal image at high energy (140 kVp). (c) Weighted average images (30% 80 kVp mixed with 70% 140 kVp). (d) DEI image from (a) and (b). Both air bubbles in the tagged fecal materials and air-tagging boundaries are virtually tagged. (e) The voxels marked by green color are those of DEI ≥ 0.1. (f) The marked voxels in (e) were subtracted by thresholding, which results in a cleansed image of (c).

Morphologically, folds and polyps submerged in the DEI field present rut like (concave ridge) and cup-like (concave cap) shapes because the surrounding air and tagged materials have higher DEI values than do those for soft-tissue structures. Based on the eigenvalue signatures that are characteristic of folds and polyps, a cup-enhancement function (F_{cup}) and a rut-enhancement function (F_{rut}) were formulated [10], so that their product had a high response from submerged polyps and folds.

Figure 5 demonstrates the Hessian response field of the DEI field by use of the cup- and rut-enhancement functions. The submerged polyps and folds are well enhanced, whereas the neighboring tagged materials, including noise, are de-enhanced. Comparing Figure 5(b) with Figure 4(a), we observed that the Hessian response field could preserve the submerged folds and polyps well.

2.4   DE-EC Scheme

Our DE-EC process consists of the following five steps: (1) initial segmentation of the colon, (2) virtual tagging of the colon by using DEI field, (3) computation of the Hessian response field in virtual-tagged images, (4) segmentation of tagged regions based on the level set method, and (5) replacement of the tagged regions that are segmented in step (4) with air, followed by reconstruction of the colonic wall submerged in tagged regions.

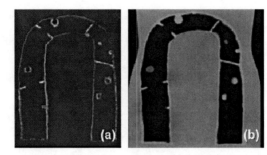

Fig. 5. (a) Hessian response field of DEI volume shown in Figure 4(d). (b) Cleansed CTC images of Figure 4 using Hessian response field. Compared to Figure 4(f), Hessian response filed preserves the folds and polyps well.

To segment the tagged materials precisely and subsequently remove (cleanse) them from the colonic lumen, we employed a level-set method combined with the gradient field (G) and the Hessian response field (H) based on the DEI. The level-set front is initialized by the classified tagged regions, and it is evolved by use of the partial differential equation shown below:

$$\partial \Phi / \partial t = -(F_H(X) + F_G(X) + F_S)|\nabla \Phi|; \qquad (2)$$

Here, X is the point on the level-set front, and F is a speed function, for which we employ a conventional threshold speed function [14]. This evolution equation has two speed functions from images: the speed function of image gradients, $F_G(X)$, and the speed function of the Hessian response field, $F_H(X)$. These speed functions are balanced with F_S, which is a smoothing term of the shape of the level-set front that is proportional to the mean curvature flow, $F_S \propto \nabla(\nabla \Phi / |\nabla \Phi|)$, and which ensures the numerical stability of the forward-in-time, centered-in-space solution of the partial differential equation [14]. With use of these speed functions, the level-set front becomes sensitive to soft-tissue structures, whereas it is insensitive to the air-tagging boundary and tagged regions. Thus, tagged regions are segmented and removed with the air-tagging boundaries, whereas the soft-tissue structures are preserved.

3   Results

Twenty-three patients underwent a 24-hour bowel preparation with a low-fiber, low-residue diet, oral administration of 50 ml non-ionic iodine (300 mg/ml concentration of Omnipaque iohexol, GE Healthcare, Milwaukee, WI). DE-CT scanning (SOMATON Definition, Siemens Healthcare, Germany) was performed at tube voltages of 140 kVp and 80 kVp in both supine and prone positions with Auto mA. For both supine and prone scanning, we used the soft-tissue reconstruction algorithm and a 0.625 mm slice reconstruction interval. In total, there were 48 pathology-confirmed polyps ≥ 6 mm, of which 7 polyps were submerged in the tagged materials.

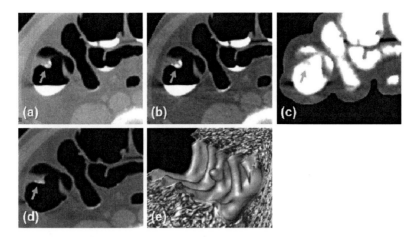

Fig. 6. A 12 mm pathology-confirmed adenomatous polyp in a 47 year-old male patient. (a,b) Axial DE-CTC image at 140 kVp (a) and 80 kVp (b). The submerged polyp is marked by the orange arrow. (c) The virtual-lumen-tagging image by DEI. The air, tagged fecal materials, and the AT-boundaries are clearly marked by their high DEI values, whereas soft tissues are marked by the low values of the DEI. (d) Same axial image of (a) and (b) after the application of the DE-EC scheme. (e) Volume-rendering image of the cleansed DE-CTC images.

After the application of proposed DE-EC scheme, initial evaluation showed the EC artifacts were significantly reduced. We observed 0-1 minor EC artifacts per case compared to the 5-6 significant EC artifacts in single energy EC methods. In addition, all submerged polyps were clearly visualized without EC artifacts.

Figure 6 demonstrates the effectiveness of the virtual lumen tagging by DEI and the DE-EC scheme in one example of a DE-CTC case. After the virtual lumen tagging based on DEI, the air, tagged fecal materials, and the air-tagging boundaries caused by PVE are clearly marked by their high DEI values, whereas the submerged polyp is preserved because of its low DEI values. After the application of the DE-EC scheme, tagged fecal materials and air-tagging boundaries were removed without any major artifacts, as shown in the 3D volume-rendering image in Figure 6(e).

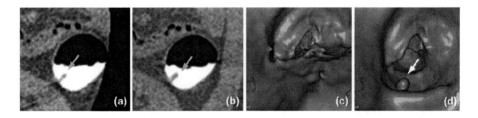

Fig. 7. Example of fecal-tagging DE-CTC images. (a,b) One axial DE-CTC image at 140 kVp (a) and 80 kVp (b). The submerged polyp is marked by orange arrows. (c,d) virtual colonoscopic images before (c) and after (d) the application of DE-EC scheme.

Figure 7 demonstrates another example of a DE-CTC case. A submerged polyp was clearly visualized after the application of the DE-EC scheme. The uneven air-tagging boundary is accurately and precisely removed by the comparison between the virtual colonoscopic images before and after the application of the DE-EC scheme.

4   Conclusions

In our study, we observed that the DEI value of colonic luminal air were substantial higher than its theoretical value in clinical fecal-tagging CTC cases. This finding provides an effective means for the removal of the EC artifacts caused by the PVE between air and tagged fecal materials, based on which we developed our DE-EC scheme. Preliminary evaluation of the results based on the phantom and on clinical cases showed that our DE-EC method can effectively differentiate soft tissues from air and tagged materials. Thus, the DE-EC method has the potential to provide an artifact-free visualization of the colonic lumen for fecal-tagging CTC.

Acknowledgements. The project described was partly supported by Research Scholar Grant RSG-11-076-01-CCE from the American Cancer Society, and by Grant Numbers R01CA095279 and R01CA131718 from National Cancer Institute (NCI).

References

1. Cai, W., Yoshida, H., Zalis, M.E., Näppi, J.: Delineation of Tagged Region by Use of Local Iso-Surface Roughness in Electronic Cleansing for CT Colonography. In: Proc. SPIE Medical Imaging: Computer-Aided Diagnosis, pp. 65141–65149 (2007)
2. Wang, Z., Liang, Z., Li, X., et al.: An Improved Electronic Colon Cleansing Method for Detection of Colonic Polyps by Virtual Colonoscopy. IEEE Trans. Biomed. Eng. 53, 1635–1646 (2006)
3. Bazalova, M., Carrier, J., Beaulieu, L., Verhaegen, F.: Dual-Energy CT-Based Material Extraction for Tissue Segmentation in Monte Carlo Dose Calculations. Phys. Med. Biol. 53, 2439–2456 (2008)
4. Johnson, T.R., Krauss, B., Sedlmair, M., et al.: Material Differentiation by Dual Energy CT: Initial Experience. Eur. Radiol. 17, 1510–1517 (2007)
5. Cai, W., Zalis, M., Näppi, J., Harris, G., Yoshida, H.: Structure-Based Digital Bowel Cleansing for Computer-Aided Detection of Polyps in CT Colonography. Int. J. Comput. Assist. Radiol. Surg. 4(suppl. 1), S184–S185 (2009)
6. Roessl, E., Proksa, R.: K-Edge Imaging in X-Ray Computed Tomography Using Multi-Bin Photon Counting Detectors. Phys. Med. Biol. 52, 4679–4696 (2007)
7. Schlomka, J.P., Roessl, E., Dorscheid, R., et al.: Experimental Feasibility of Multi-Energy Photon-Counting K-Edge Imaging in Pre-Clinical Computed Tomography. Phys. Med. Biol. 53, 4031–4047 (2008)
8. Graser, A., Johnson, T.R.C., Bader, M., et al.: Dual Energy CT Characterization of Urinary Calculi: Initial In Vitro and Clinical Experience. Invest. Radiol. 43, 112–119 (2008)
9. Cai, W., Näppi, J., Zalis, M.E., Harris, G.J., Yoshida, H.: Digital Bowel Cleansing for Computer-Aided Detection of Polyps in Fecal-Tagging CT Colonography. In: Proc. SPIE Medical Imaging 6144, pp. 221–229 (2006)

10. Cai, W., Zalis, M.E., Näppi, J., Harris, G.J., Yoshida, H.: Structure-Analysis Method for Electronic Cleansing in Cathartic and Noncathartic CT Colonography. Med. Phys. 35, 3259–3277 (2008)
11. Cai, W., Zalis, M.E., Näppi, J., Harris, G.J., Yoshida, H.: Structure-Based Digital Bowel Cleansing for Computer-Aided Detection of Polyps in CT Colonography. Int. J. Comput. Assist. Radiol. Surg. 1(S1), 369–371 (2006)
12. Sato, Y., Nakajima, S., Shiraga, N., et al.: Three-Dimensional Multi-Scale Line Filter for Segmentation and Visualization of Curvilinear Structures in Medical Images. Med. Image Anal. 2, 143–168 (1998)
13. Frangi, A.F., Niessen, W.J., Hoogeveen, R.M., van Walsum, T., Viergever, M.A.: Model-Based Quantitation of 3-D Magnetic Resonance Angiographic Images. IEEE Trans. Med. Imaging 18, 946–956 (1999)
14. Ho, S., Bullitt, E., Gerig, G.: Level Set Evolution with Region Competition: Automatic 3-D Segmentation of Brain Tumors. In: Proceedings of 16th International Conference on Pattern Recognition, pp. 532–535 (2002)

Computer-Aided Polyp Detection
for Laxative-Free CT Colonography

Neil Panjwani[1], Marius George Linguraru[1],
Joel G. Fletcher[2], and Ronald M. Summers[1]

[1] Imaging Biomarkers and Computer-Aided Diagnosis Laboratory, Radiology and Imaging
Sciences, Clinical Center, National Institutes of Health, Bethesda, MD
[2] Department of Radiology, Mayo Clinic, Rochester, MN
{paniwani,mglinguraru}@gmail.com

Abstract. Image-based colon cleansing performed on fecal-tagged CT
colonography (CTC) allows the laxative-free detection of colon polyps, unlike
optical colonoscopy (OC), the preferred screening method. Compared to OC,
CTC increases the patient comfort and compliance with colon cancer screening.
However, laxative-free CTC introduces many challenges and imaging artifacts,
such as poorly and heterogeneously tagged stool, thin stool close to the colon
walls, pseudoenhancement of colon tissue, and partial volume effect. We
propose an automated algorithm to subtract stool prior to the computer aided
detection of colonic polyps. The method is locally adaptive and combines
intensity, shape and texture analysis with probabilistic optimization. Results
show stool removal accuracy on data with various bowel preparations. The
automatic detection of polyps using our CAD system on cathartic-free data
improves significantly from 70% to 85% true positive rate at 5.75 false
positives/scan.

Keywords: CTC, colon cancer, laxative-free, cleansing, heterogeneous stool,
polyp detection.

1   Introduction

With the advent of large screening programs for colon cancer, computed tomography
colonography (CTC) has become a viable tool for the noninvasive detection of polyps
and a complement or alternative to optical colonoscopy (OC) [1,2]. While OC can
provide better visual confirmation of colon polyps, it has a few downsides compared
to CTC, such as the inability to detect polyps hidden behind folds, stool, or fluid and
the discomfort and risks of the colonoscope. In addition, studies have demonstrated
that a large portion (72%) of the patients would prefer CTC instead of OC [3].
Furthermore, in CTC stool can be enhanced with tagging agents such as barium or
iodine, as opposed to the use of a laxative. The automated and reliable removal of
tagged feces remains challenging due to high variability in contrast intake that leads

H. Yoshida et al. (Eds.): Abdominal Imaging 2011, LNCS 7029, pp. 18–26, 2012.

to poorly and heterogeneously tagged stool, thin stool close to the colon walls, pseudoenhancement of colon tissue, and partial volume effect.

In recent years, several studies have been developed for image-based colon cleansing, which perform well on fully homogeneously tagged stool [4,5,8]. Fewer publications addressed the cleansing of heterogeneously tagged stool. In [9], shape analysis and mosaics contributed to the removal of heterogeneous stool, but the added value for polyp detection was not shown. Alternatively, in [7] level sets and minimum variance were employed to cleanse CTC data in a parametric and empirical method associated with the computer aided detection (CAD) of polyps.

We present an automated algorithm for the removal of stool with tagging variability from cases with various colonic preparations. The method is locally adaptive to adjust for inconsistent tagging and combines intensity, shape and texture analysis with probabilistic optimization. The detection of colon polyps is significantly improved by removing false positive candidates related to heterogeneous stool.

2   Materials and Methods

Thirty-eight CTC data (19 patients with matched prone/supine scans) from patients that underwent cathartic-free bowel preparation were acquired on LightSpeed Ultra and Pro:16 scanners (GE Healthcare). Cases underwent various colonic preparations of barium or Gastroview. The dataset was selected from an original set of 50 to include only those cases high in polyps, in which at least 90% of the solid stool was visually estimated to be tagged, and each colonic segment was distended in either the prone or supine view.   There were a total of 44 confirmed polyps (22 unique polyps) detected by an experienced radiologist. All polyps selected in the dataset were 10mm or larger; polyps smaller than 10mm were ignored for this experiment. The data were split into 18 training cases (9 patients/ 18 polyps) and 20 testing cases (10 patients/ 26 polyps). An outline of the method can be found in Fig 1.

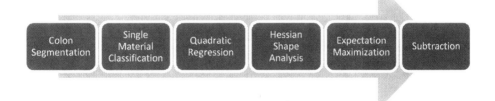

Fig. 1. Methodology Flow Chart

2.1   Colon Segmentation

The first step in our algorithm segments the colon by locating the colonic air and identifying the adjacent tissue and tagged materials. Colonic air is identified by thresholding at -600 HU and eliminating the components which border the image in the transverse plane and superior position. The stool tagged regions are identified by thresholding at 250 HU and removing the spine and ribs via region growing from high intensity seeds automatically placed in a superior position. After joining the colonic air and tagged materials, a morphological dilation is performed to include any surrounding tissue. A median filter is applied to reduce noise while preserving edges.

2.2   Adaptive Thresholding and Single Material Classification

We aim to conservatively classify each voxel into one material type (air, tissue, stool, or unclassified) by utilizing image intensity, I, gradient magnitude, GM, and texture, T. In [4], material classes were detected via hard thresholds. The adaptive intensity threshold (I_o) in Table 1 is computed by applying Otsu's method [10] to the histograms of each local stool region. Regions are selected by locating each set of connected voxels with intensity higher than 200 HU, performing a morphological opening to remove weak, thin connections, and including the rectangular bounding box of each set, with a padding of 5 voxels. These regions allow a unique I_o for each large, distinct stool region while providing significant information to the adaptive histogram computation.

To isolate heterogeneous stool via texture, we locally compute Haralick's Correlation [12], which is a derivation of the 14 classic texture features proposed by Haralick (originally used to classify satellite imagery). Because T shows a strong response to heterogeneity and sharp intensity contrast, higher measures of T are indicative of stool. We compare the value of T computed at a particular voxel to the maximum global texture response, T_{max}, to normalize the texture measure. T is computed at every non-air voxel as follows, where $g(i,j)$ is the element in cell i, j of a normalized grey level co-occurrence matrix (μ_t and σ_t are the mean and standard deviation of the row sums):

$$T = \frac{\sum_{i,j}(i,j)g(i,j) - \mu_t}{\sigma_t} \tag{1}$$

Table 1. Single material adaptive threshold values

Classes	Thresholds
Air	$I \leq -700$
Tissue	$I \leq I_o$ and $I \geq -250$ and $GM \leq 300$ and $T < 0.75T_{max}$
Stool	$I \geq I_o$ and $GM < 0.8*I$ or $I > 1000$
Unclassified	Everything else

2.3   Quadratic Regression

To address material boundaries, a slightly modified version of the quadratic regression (QR) algorithm published in [4] was applied. Unclassified voxels are assigned a material transition by finding the shortest orthogonal distance from a set of points in the I vs. GM graph to the parabolic curves modeling tissue-air, stool-tissue, and stool-air transitions. Because the intensities for tissue and air are relatively constant in comparison to the variably tagged stool, the tissue-air parabola is unvarying. However, the stool-tissue and stool-air parabolas are defined by a local stool maximum (S_{max}), which is computed across the image by minimizing the least-squares estimate of the stool-air parabola only. We found that computing separate local stool maxima for stool-air and stool-tissue was counter-intuitive and produced unpredictable results. We also utilized a morphological distance transform to classify any stool-related voxel into thin-stool if its maximum distance to the nearest non-stool voxel was less than or equal to 2.5mm. After classification, the partial probabilities of air, tissue, and stool were computed for each voxel based on intensity and S_{max}.

2.4   Hessian Shape Analysis

To address the pseudoenhancement of colonic folds, we studied local concavity by computing the Hessian matrix at every voxel. The polarity of the eigenvalues ($\lambda_1 \geq \lambda_2 \geq \lambda_3$) of the Hessian matrix indicates local extrema, while particular combinations of the eigenvalue magnitudes can be used to discriminate various shapes. We followed the formulation set forth by Sato et al [11] to identify dark sheets in order to enhance submerged folds surrounded by brightly tagged materials. The Hessian response, S_σ was computed as the maximum across scales to selectively enhance both thin and medium-sized folds:

$$w(\lambda_s, \lambda_t) = \begin{cases} \left(1 - \frac{\lambda_t}{|\lambda_s|}\right)^\gamma, & \lambda_s \geq \lambda_t \geq 0 \\ \left(1 - \alpha \frac{\lambda_t}{|\lambda_s|}\right)^\gamma, & \frac{-|\lambda_s|}{\alpha} < \lambda_t < 0 \\ 0, & else \end{cases} \quad (2)$$

$$S_\sigma = \begin{cases} |\lambda_1| w(\lambda_1, \lambda_2) w(\lambda_1, \lambda_3), & \lambda_1 > 0 \\ 0, & else \end{cases} \quad (3)$$

where $\alpha = 0.25$ to restrict the response from negative eigenvalues and $\gamma = 1$ to sharpen the response within a limited range. Pseudoenhanced tissue was classified by applying a median filter to the histogram of S_σ and selecting voxels with responses higher than 30% of the maximum value. Because submerged folds represent local minima within stool, the partial tissue probability, pt_h, was recalculated by comparing the intensity at a voxel, I, to the maximum local intensity, HS_{max}, as follows:

$$pt_h = 1 - \left(\frac{I}{HS_{max}}\right) \quad (4)$$

2.5   Expectation Maximization and Subtraction

After the partial probabilities were computed, a Gaussian mixture model expectation maximization algorithm was used to update the probabilities on the basis of intensity and neighboring probabilities. The probability, $P_{j,i}^{t+1}$, of voxel i being in class j at time $t+1$ time step is:

$$P_{j,i}^{t+1} = \frac{W_i^t}{2\pi \sqrt{\sigma_j^t \rho_{j,i}^t}} exp\left[-\frac{\left(I_i - \mu_j^t\right)^2}{2\sigma_j^t} - \frac{\left(P_{j,i}^t - \lambda_{j,i}^t\right)^2}{2\rho_{j,i}^t} \right], \tag{5}$$

where I_i is the intensity for voxel i, μ_j^t, σ_j^t, and W_i^t are the mean, variance and weight for class j at time step t, $P_{j,i}^t$ is the probability of class j for voxel i at time t, and lastly $\rho_{j,i}^t$ and $\lambda_{j,i}^t$ are the mean and variance of the probability for class j on the first order neighbors around voxel i. We utilized the neighborhood values to reduce the effect of noise and discontinuities. The EM was run for 5 iterations.

Given the updated partial probabilities, a connected component was performed joining voxels with high probability of tissue under the knowledge that all tissue should be connected. The input intensity was then rescaled into the range [-1000, $I_{original}$] according to its probability of tissue, pt, value as follows:

$$I_{new} = pt\left(I_{original} + 1000\right) - 1000 \tag{6}$$

Thus, tagged materials disconnected from the colon wall were removed while identified stool with a low probability of tissue were set to the intensity of air. Gaussian smoothing of $\sigma = 0.7$ mm was performed at the air edges to ease the transition of subtracted stool into tissue.

2.6   Colonic Polyp CAD

For the automated deception of colonic polyps, the CAD tool presented in [2] was used on the CTC database with and without colon cleansing. Results are compared using free-response operator characteristic (FROC) analysis.

3   Results

The intermediate results of the automated method for stool subtraction can be found in Fig. 2. The algorithm removed heterogeneous stool (Fig. 3,4,5), thin stool linings (Fig. 3), and weakly tagged stool (Fig. 4), while preserving polyps (Fig. 5) and colonic tissue.

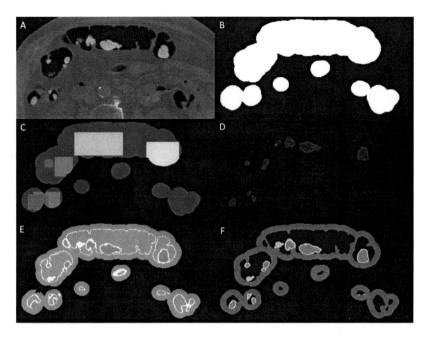

Fig. 2. The original CT (A) processed after colon segmentation (B), adaptive thresholding (C), texture computation (D), single material classification (E), and quadratic regression (F). In (C), the blocks represent regions of locally computed intensity thresholds. Brighter colors represent higher values in figures (C) and (D). Figure (E) depicts the classification of air (blue), tissue (orange), stool (green), and unclassified (white). Figure (F) illustrates the classification of air (dark blue), tissue (light blue), stool (green), tissue-air (orange), stool-air (yellow), tissue-stool (purple), and thin stool (white).

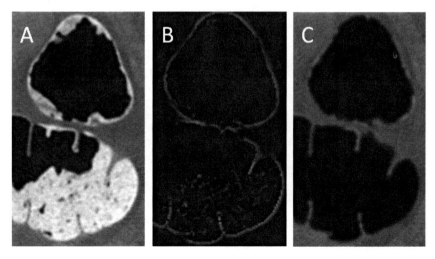

Fig. 3. (A) Original CT. (B) After Hessian shape analysis enhancement of submerged folds. (C) Final subtracted result.

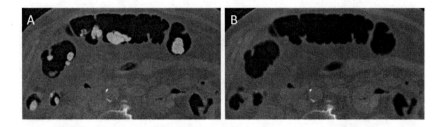

Fig. 4. The original CT (A) from Figure 2A and the result of our stool removal algorithm (B)

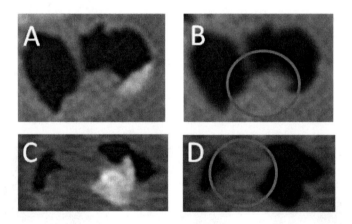

Fig. 5. CT images with polyps (green circles) before (A and C) and after (B and D) cleansing. The CAD system was run on the CTC scans with and without the new module for stool subtraction. The comparative FROC curves are presented in Fig. 7. As expected, the automatic detection of polyps is hampered by the presence of stool in the scans, as heterogeneous stool represents a prevailing source of false positives (FP). The FROC curve improves significantly after stool subtraction from 70% to 85% true positive (TP) rate at 5.75 FP/scan (p = 0.007). The statistical significance was computed using ROCKIT.

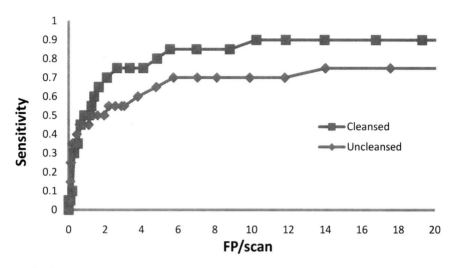

Fig. 6. FROC curves of the performance of the CAD system before and after cleansing

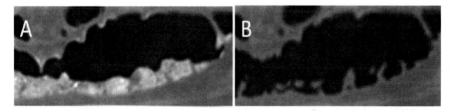

Fig. 7. (A) CT image depicting poorly tagged heterogeneous stool. (B) Erroneous subtraction.

4   Discussion

We presented a method to automatically subtract tagged stool from cathartic-free CT data to aid in the detection of colorectal cancer. The stool subtraction algorithm was particularly designed to address the challenges of local variability in tagging, pseudoenhancement of submerged colon tissue, and the heterogeneity of stool enhancement. The results are robust on fine details around folds, thin stool linings on the colonic wall, near polyps and in large fluid pools. The method adaptively adjusts to variable patient data and tagging conditions. However, the method relies on adequate stool tagging to work properly, as depicted in Fig. 7.

The runtime for our cleansing algorithm averages 5 min per case, while the CAD system approaches 15 min per case. We noticed, however, that the CAD system runtime decreased to roughly 10 min per case after cleansing due to the elimination of several false detections. The CAD system detected colonic polyps with sufficient accuracy on data with cathartic-free bowel preparation without employing the cleansing algorithm. However, the performance of the CAD system improved significantly after the cleansing module was applied, with results appropriate for routine clinical use.

Future work will address specific artifacts brought on by air bubbles within the stool and weak or no stool tagging. Cases with polyps under 10mm should be examined. We also hope to reduce tagging variability by utilizing a single improved type of bowel preparation.

Acknowledgments. This work was supported in part by the Intramural Research Program of the National Institutes of Health, Clinical Center.

References

1. Cotton, P.B., et al.: Computed Tomographic Colonography (Virtual Colonoscopy): A Multicenter Comparison with Standard Colonoscopy for Detection of Colorectal Neoplasia. Jama 291(14), 1713–1719 (2004)
2. Summers, R.M., et al.: Computed Tomographic Virtual Colonoscopy Computer-Aided Polyp Detection in a Screening Population. Gastroenterology 129(6), 1832–1844 (2005)
3. Gluecker, T.M., et al.: Colorectal Cancer Screening with CT Colonography, Colonoscopy, and Double-Contrast Barium Enema Examination: Prospective Assessment of Patient Perceptions and Preferences. Radiology 227(2), 378–384 (2003)
4. Carston, M., Manduca, A., Johnson, C.D.: Electronic Stool Subtraction Using Quadratic Regression, Morphological Operations, and Distance Transforms. In: Proceedings of SPIE 6511 (Part 1), 65110W (2007)
5. Wang, Z., et al.: An Improved Electronic Colon Cleansing Method for Detection of Colonic Polyps by Virtual Colonoscopy. IEEE Trans. Biomed. Eng. 53(8), 1635–1646 (2006)
6. McLachlan, G.J., Krishnan, T.: The EM Algorithm and Extensions. Wiley Series in Probability and Statistics. Applied Probability and Statistics. Wiley, New York (1997)
7. Linguraru, M.G., et al.: Heterogeneous Stool Removal for Laxative-Free Diagnosis of Colon Cancer – FROC Study. In: MICCAI Workshop on Virtual Colonoscopy, pp. 85–90 (2008)
8. Cai, W., et al.: Structure-Analysis Method for Electronic Cleansing in Cathartic and Noncathartic CT Colonography. Med. Phys. 35(7), 3259–3277 (2008)
9. Cai, W., et al.: Mosaic Decomposition: An Electronic Cleansing Method for Inhomogeneously Tagged Regions in Noncathartic CT Colonography. IEEE Trans. Med. Imaging 30(3), 559–574 (2011)
10. Otsu, N.: A Threshold Selection Method from Gray Level Histograms. IEEE Trans. Syst. Man Cybern. 9, 62–66 (1979)
11. Sato, Y., et al.: 3D Multi-Scale Line Filter for Segmentation and Visualization of Curvilinear Structures in Medical Images. In: Troccaz, J., Mösges, R., Grimson, W.E.L. (eds.) CVRMed-MRCAS 1997, CVRMed 1997, and MRCAS 1997. LNCS, vol. 1205, pp. 213–222. Springer, Heidelberg (1997)
12. Haralick, R.M., Shanmugam, K.: Dinstein, Its'Hak: Textural Features for Image Classification. IEEE Trans. Syst. Man Cybern. 3(6), 610–621 (1973)

Comparative Performance of Random Forest and Support Vector Machine Classifiers for Detection of Colorectal Lesions in CT Colonography

Janne J. Näppi[1], Daniele Regge[2], and Hiroyuki Yoshida[1]

[1] Department of Radiology,
Massachusetts General Hospital and Harvard Medical School,
25 New Chardon Street, Suite 400C, Boston, MA 02114, USA
`jnappi@partners.org, yoshida.hiro@mgh.harvard.edu`
[2] Institute for Cancer Research and Treatment,
Candiolo Str. Prov. 142, IT-10060, Turin, Italy

Abstract. A major problem of computer-aided detection (CAD) for computed tomographic colonography (CTC) is that CAD systems display large numbers of false-positive detections, thereby distracting users. Support vector machine (SVM) classifiers have been a popular choice for reducing false-positive detections in CAD systems. Recently, random forests (RF) have emerged as a novel type of highly accurate classifier. We compared the relative performance of RF and SVM classifiers in automated detection of colorectal lesions in CTC. The CAD system was trained with the CTC data of 123 patients and tested with an independent set of 737 patients. The results indicate that the performance of an RF classifier compares favorably with that of an SVM classifier in CTC.

Keywords: computer-aided detection, CAD, random forest, flat lesions, support vector machine, x-ray tomography, virtual colonoscopy.

1   Introduction

Computer-aided detection (CAD) systems for computed tomographic colonography (CTC) display large numbers of false-positive (FP) detections. This distracts CAD users who are often experienced radiologists who have low tolerance for routine display of obvious false positives, it increases the recall rate, and it may also impair true-positive (TP) detections [1]. Therefore, improving the detection specificity of CAD remains an important challenge in CTC.

Many CAD systems for CTC reduce FP CAD detections by use of a support vector machine (SVM) [2] that is seen as a state-of-the-art classifier. The SVM classifiers have become popular because of their flexible methodology and robust optimization. However, SVM classifiers have a number of limitations, such as high computational cost and difficulties with model selection.

Recently, random forest (RF) classifiers have emerged as a novel type of classifier that has several advantages over conventional classifiers [3]. The RF classifiers

H. Yoshida et al. (Eds.): Abdominal Imaging 2011, LNCS 7029, pp. 27–34, 2012.

do not overfit, they run efficiently on large databases, they are highly paralleliz-able, and they can handle thousands of input variables without variable deletion. They can also provide unbiased estimates of classification error or the relative importance of input features for classification.

Our purpose in this study was to compare the performance of an RF classifier with that of a conventional SVM classifier in the detection of colorectal lesions in CTC. The results are potentially useful for improving the detection accuracy of CAD in CTC.

2   Methods

2.1   Support Vector Machine

An SVM classifier maps input samples into a high-dimensional feature space H. Let $D = \{(x_i, y_i)|x_i \in R^p\}_{i=1}^n$ represent input training data, where $y_i = \pm 1$ indicates the correct class of input sample x_i. Given a projection $\phi : X \rightarrow H$, the feature space can be defined by a kernel function

$$k(x, x') = < \phi(x), \phi(x') > . \tag{1}$$

The use of a kernel function is computationally simpler than explicitly projecting data points into the feature space. The samples are separated by a hyperplane

$$< w, \phi(x) > + b = 0 \tag{2}$$

corresponding to a decision function

$$f(x) = sign(< w, \phi(x) > + b). \tag{3}$$

The training of the SVM involves determining a hyper-plane that maximizes the margin of separation between input classes [4] (Fig. 1). It can be constructed by solving of a constrained quadratic optimization problem. In the case of the L_2-norm soft-margin classification, the optimization minimizes

$$t(w, \xi) = \frac{1}{2}||w||^2 + \frac{C}{m} \sum_{i=1}^{m} \xi_i, \tag{4}$$

where

$$y_i(< \phi(x_i), w > + b) \geq 1 - \xi_i. \tag{5}$$

Here, m is the number of training patterns, and $x_i \geq 0$ $(i = 1, .., m)$. The solution has an expansion

$$w = \sum_{i=1}^{m} \alpha_i y_i \phi(x_i), \tag{6}$$

where non-zero coefficients (called the support vectors, see Fig. 1) occur when a data point (x_i, y_i) meets the constraint. The coefficients α_i can be found by maximizing

$$W(\alpha) = \sum_{i=1}^{m} \alpha_i - \frac{1}{2} \sum_{i,j=1}^{m} \alpha_i \alpha_j y_i y_j k(x_i, x_j), \tag{7}$$

where $0 \leq \alpha_i \leq \frac{C}{m}$ $(i = 1, .., m)$ and $\sum_{i=1}^{m} \alpha_i y_i = 0$. The cost parameter C controls the penalty of misclassification: a high cost value forces the SVM to create a complex prediction function that misclassifies as few training points as possible, whereas a low cost value creates a simple prediction function with a potentially large training error.

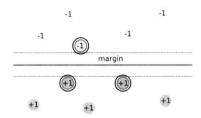

Fig. 1. The support vectors (indicated by black circles) of an SVM are training samples that define the margin of hyper-plane (indicated by the black line) separating TP and FP training samples

2.2 Random Forests

An RF classifier is an ensemble of decision trees. Let T denote the set of all trees, C the set of input classes (TP or FP), and L the leaves of a tree. For each tree $t \in T$, the input data are subsampled by use of out-of-bag bootstrapping. Suppose D_t denotes bootstrapped input data of t. At the root node, child nodes l and r are created that divide the input data into disjoint subsets $D_t = D_l \cup D_r$ $(D_l \cap D_r = \emptyset)$. This division is based on a node test, where the feature is chosen from a randomly sampled subset of all input features. Each candidate node is scored by use of the Shannon entropy as

$$E_f = -\Sigma_i \frac{|D_i|}{|D_t|} E(D_i), \tag{8}$$

where D_i are the partitions of input data as determined by the node test, and $E(D_i) = -\sum_{j=1}^{N} p_j \log_2(p_j)$ is entropy, with p_j denoting the proportion of samples in D_i belonging to class j. The posterior probability $P_{t,l}(Y(x) = c)$ of each class $c \in C$ at each leaf $l \in L$ is the ratio of the number of input samples that reach l in the tree. This is repeated recursively with D_l and D_r, until further subdivision becomes impossible.

The node tests can be interpreted as hyperplanes dividing the feature space into disjoint regions (Fig. 2). Each decision leaf corresponds to a hyperrectangle, where the union of all hyperrectangles is the complete feature space.

For an unseen sample, the RF classifier is tested by propagation of the sample through each tree. The predictions by the trees are aggregated into an RF prediction by majority vote.

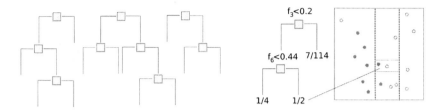

Fig. 2. An RF classifier is a collection of decision trees (on the left) that divide the feature space into hyperrectangles (on the right)

2.3   The CAD System

The CAD system is fully automated. A thick region encompassing the colonic mucosa is extracted automatically from input CTC data [5]. Volumetric shape features are calculated within the extracted region, and lesion candidates are detected by hysteresis thresholding of the shape features [6]. Complete regions of the detections are extracted by use of a dedicated segmentation algorithm [7]. Several shape and texture features are calculated from the detected regions [8]. Based upon the feature values, a classifier separates TP detections from FP detections to determine the final output of the CAD system [9].

2.4   Materials

The training population contained 123 abnormal patients from 15 institutions (Fig. 3). There were 162 lesions $\geq$6 mm. These data were collected primarily from two large multi-center CTC screening trials [10,11]. The patients were prepared with cathartic bowel preparation. Orally administered positive-contrast tagging was used for labeling of residual fluid and feces in 41 patients.

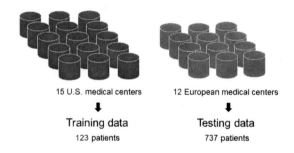

15 U.S. medical centers   12 European medical centers

Training data   Testing data

123 patients   737 patients

Fig. 3. The materials included 860 patients from 27 medical centers divided into independent training and testing sets

The testing population contained 737 patients from 12 institutions that were completely different from those of the training population [12] (Fig. 3). The patients were prepared with cathartic bowel preparation. Orally administered positive-contrast tagging was performed for opacifying residual bowel materials in CTC images with hydrosoluble iodine alone or in combination with barium sulfate in 34% of the patients. The CTC was performed in supine and prone positions with 120 kVp, $\leq$50 mAs, and a section thickness of $\leq$2.5 mm. Expert radiologists correlated the locations of same-day colonoscopy-confirmed lesions with the CTC image data. There were 262 adenomas or carcinomas (hereafter called "advanced" lesions) $\geq$6 mm in maximum diameter, including 30 advanced flat lesions.

2.5   Evaluation Methods

The TP lesion candidates detected by CAD were identified as those located within the radius of a known lesion in CTC data. All other CAD detections were labeled as FP detections, including multiple detections within the same region.

For determination of optimal input features for the classifiers, a recursive backward feature selection algorithm [13] was used. First, the CAD system characterized the detected regions by use of 20 volumetric shape and texture features [8]. Next, the input data of the training population were boostrapped, the classifiers were trained with the bootstrap data by use of all available features, and each feature was ranked for its importance in the training. Then, the classifier performance was reassessed in this manner with decreasing numbers of top-ranking features. The top-ranking feature combination with the best performance was recorded. The bootstrapping and feature selection steps were repeated 10 times for identifying and excluding outlier features, and the final features were selected by use of consensus ranking over the iterations. The optimal feature combinations of the SVM and RF classifiers contained 17 and 20 features, respectively.

To build optimal classifiers for the training population, we performed parameter tuning by use of 10-fold cross-validation with bootstrapping. At each iteration, the training data were bootstrapped into separate training-testing sets. The SVM was used with a Gaussian radial basis function involving parameter tuning of the cost parameter C and the spread of the basis function. The RF was used with 500 decision trees involving parameter tuning of the number of sampled features at each decision node.

The detection performances of the trained RF and SVM classifiers were compared by use of a paired-sample randomization test on the independent testing population. The figure of merit (FOM) was the partial area under the fitted free-response receiver-operating characteristic (FROC) curve [14]. It was calculated as the trapezoidal area under the FROC curve limited by γ, where γ is the smaller number of false positives generated by either classifier at its maximum detection sensitivity [14]. The randomization test yields the distribution of the FOM under the null hypothesis by rearranging the class labels of bootstrapped input data [15].

The per-lesion detection performance was assessed for all advanced lesions and for advanced polypoid (sessile and pedunculated) and flat lesions. Lesions with polypoid morphology are the most common type of colorectal lesion, and unaided trained radiologists can detect most of these types of lesions at high sensitivity. Flat lesions are less common than polypoid lesions, but they tend to be more advanced and more challenging to detect than polypoid lesions [16].

3 Results

The results are the testing results on the testing population after the classifiers had first been trained with the training population (see Section 2.5). The FOM is the average fitted area under the FROC curve normalized to the value range of $[0, 1]$. The indicated 95% confidence intervals were obtained by use of bootstrapping.

Table 1 shows the per-lesion detection accuracy of the RF and SVM classifiers for advanced lesions ≥ 6 mm (n=262). The RF classifier outperformed the SVM classifier both for large lesions (≥ 10 mm) and for moderate-size lesions (6 – 9 mm). The improvement was statistically significant.

Table 1. Per-lesion detection accuracy between the RF and SVM classifiers. Brackets indicate 95% confidence intervals.

	RF	SVM	p-value
≥ 10 mm	0.83 [0.827, 0.833]	0.81 [0.806, 0.814]	<0.000001
6 – 9 mm	0.71 [0.702, 0.712]	0.65 [0.650, 0.660]	<0.000001

Table 2 shows the per-lesion detection accuracy for advanced lesions with polypoid morphology (n=232). Again, the RF classifier outperformed the SVM classifier with statistically significant improvement.

Table 2. Per-lesion detection accuracy between the RF and SVM classifiers for advanced polypoid lesions. Brackets indicate 95% confidence intervals.

	RF	SVM	p-value
≥ 10 mm	0.82 [0.818, 0.831]	0.80 [0.789, 0.804]	<0.000001
6 – 9 mm	0.69 [0.689, 0.700]	0.65 [0.643, 0.656]	<0.000001

Table 3 shows the per-lesion detection performance for advanced flat lesions (n=30). In the detection of moderate-size flat lesions (6 – 9 mm), the RF classifier outperformed the SVM classifier with statistically significant improvement. However, for large flat lesions, the detection performance was similar.

Table 3. Per-lesion detection accuracy between the RF and SVM classifiers for advanced flat lesions. Brackets indicate 95% confidence intervals.

	RF	SVM	p-value
≥ 10 mm	0.81 [0.800, 0.814]	0.81 [0.800, 0.815]	0.98
$6 - 9$ mm	0.70 [0.688, 0.718]	0.60 [0.582, 0.609]	<0.000001

4 Discussion

The results indicate that the RF classifier outperforms the SVM classifier significantly in the detection of most colorectal lesions. For large flat lesions, the detection performance was similar. This could be explained by the relatively small number of large flat lesions in the training data. On the other hand, the largest relative gain with the application of RF was obtained for small flat lesions, where the FOM increased from 0.6 to 0.7. Because small flat lesions are often distorted by partial-volume artifacts due to their small size and flatness, the outperformance of the RF classifier suggests that it may have a more robust performance than the SVM classifiers in the presence of image noise and artifacts.

We performed the classifier comparison by use of a large and heterogeneous patient population. Most CAD studies have used much smaller numbers of cases, even though studies on validation methodologies have recommended using several hundreds of cases for credible CAD evaluation studies [14]. We also used truly independent multi-center populations for training and testing: the patients in the training and testing sets represented different hospitals and different bowel preparations, and the testing data were collected after the training data. In contrast, previous CAD studies have suffered from positive biases because they generally used single-center cases or mixed multi-center populations in training and testing.

5 Conclusion

We compared the performance of RF and SVM classifiers in the detection of colorectal lesions in CAD for CTC by using large, independent multi-center CTC patient populations. The results indicate that the performance of the RF classifier compares favorably with that of the popular SVM classifier in the detection of advanced lesions in CTC. Therefore, RF classifiers may be useful in improving the detection accuracy of CAD in CTC.

Acknowledgments. The project described was partly supported by a grant from the Prevent Cancer Foundation and Grant Numbers R21CA140934, R03CA139600, R01CA095279, and R01CA131718 from National Cancer Institute (NCI). We thank Dr. Richard Choi (Virtual Colonoscopy Center, Walter Reed Army Medical Center, Washington, DC, USA) for providing CTC cases for this study. We also thank Partners Research Computing for providing high-performance computing services.

References

1. Näppi, J., Nagata, K.: Sources of False Positives in Computer-Assisted CT Colonography. Abdom. Imaging 36, 153–164 (2011)
2. Schölkopf, B., Burges, C.J.C., Smola, A.J. (eds.): Advances in Kernel Methods: Support Vector Learning. MIT Press, Cambridge (1999)
3. Breiman, L.: Random Forests. Machine Learning 45, 5–32 (2001)
4. Vapnik, V.: Statistical Learning Theory. Wiley, New York (1998)
5. Näppi, J., Yoshida, H.: Fully Automated Three-Dimensional Detection of Polyps in Fecal-Tagging CT Colonography. Acad. Radiol. 14, 287–300 (2007)
6. Yoshida, H., Näppi, J.: Three-Dimensional Computer-Aided Diagnosis Scheme for Detection of Colonic Polyps. IEEE Trans. Med. Imaging 20, 1261–1274 (2001)
7. Näppi, J., Yoshida, H.: Feature-Guided Analysis for Reduction of False Positives in CAD of Polyps for Computed Tomographic Colonography. Med. Phys. 30, 1592–1601 (2003)
8. Näppi, J., Yoshida, H.: Automated Detection of Polyps with CT Colonography: Evaluation of Volumetric Features for Reduction of False-Positive Findings. Acad. Radiol. 9, 386–397 (2002)
9. Yoshida, H., Näppi, J., MacEneaney, P., Rubin, D.T., Dachman, A.H.: Computer-Aided Diagnosis Scheme for Detection of Polyps at CT Colonography. Radiographics 22, 963–979 (2002)
10. Pickhardt, P.J., Choi, J.R., Hwang, I., et al.: Computed Tomographic Virtual Colonoscopy to Screen for Colorectal Neoplasia in Asymptomatic Adults. N. Engl. J. Med. 349, 2191–2200 (2003)
11. Rockey, D.C., Paulson, E., Niedzwiecki, D., et al.: Analysis of Air Contrast Barium Enema, Computed Tomographic Colonography, and Colonoscopy: Prospective Comparison. Lancet 365, 305–311 (2005)
12. Regge, D., Laudi, C., Galatola, G., et al.: Diagnostic Accuracy of Computed Tomographic Colonography for the Detection of Advanced Neoplasia in Individuals at Increased Risk of Colorectal Cancer. JAMA 301, 2458–2461 (2009)
13. Ambroise, C., McLachlan, J.H.: Selection Bias in Gene Extraction on the Basis of Microarray Gene-Expression Data. PNAS 99, 6562–6566 (2002)
14. Chakraborty, D.P.: Validation and Statistical Power Comparison of Methods for Analyzing Free-Response Observer Performance Studies. Acad. Radiol. 15, 1554–1566 (2008)
15. Noreen, E.W.: Computer-Intensive Methods for Testing Hypotheses: an Introduction. John Wiley & Sons, New York (1989)
16. Fidler, J., Johnson, C.: Flat Polyps of the Colon: Accuracy of Detection by CT Colonography and Histologic Significance. Abdom. Imaging 34, 157–171 (2009)

Image-Enhanced Capsule Endoscopy Preserving the Original Color Tones

Hai Vu[1], Tomio Echigo[2], Keiko Yagi[3], Hirotoshi Okazaki[4], Yasuhiro Fujiwara[4], Yasushi Yagi[1], and Tetsuo Arakawa[4]

[1] The Institute of Scientific and Industrial Research, Osaka University
[2] Osaka Electro-Communication University
[3] Kobe Pharmaceutical University
[4] Graduate School of Medicine, Osaka City University
vhai@am.sanken.osaka-u.ac.jp

Abstract. This paper describes a technique to enhance a region-of-interest (ROI) in a capsule endoscopy (CE) image. Our aim is to improve distinguishing suspicious regions from normal ones without over-enhancing the image. Given a ROI by physicians, the proposed technique enhances the ROI so that the enhanced region remains as natural as possible. To achieve this, we utilize image features relating to a specific color space dedicated to gastrointestinal (GI) wall regions. The proposed approach starts by utilizing a self-organizing map to handle GI wall color components. The goal of preserving the original color tones is obtainable by using a histogram equalization technique in the proposed color space. As a result, the enhanced images only contain color components inferred from the color gamut of the human small bowel. The results of the proposed method are judged in terms of visual appearance by comparison with images obtained by the conventional enhancement technique.

Keywords: capsule endoscopy, self-organizing map.

1 Introduction

Capsule endoscopy (CE) technology [7] is used to locate obscure bleeding regions in the human small bowel [14]. However, since the lesions from bleeding, angioectasia, and erythema disease are often poorly visible on the acquired images, the physicians may have difficulty in analyzing them [14,1]. Approaches for enhancing the images help differentiate abnormal tissues from normal ones. Conventional image-enhanced endoscopy (IEE) techniques such as Fuji Intelligent Chromo Endoscopy (FICE), Narrow Band Imaging (NBI) [1] usually depict the original images with false-color expressions. In terms of reading video capsule endoscopy (VCE), a report in [2] states that FICE images identify more abnormal lesions than standard CE images. However, the same report also points out a high false-positive rate with FICE images. Because FICE images are often unable to be interpreted without appropriate training, many physicians do not use them in clinical practice. To avoid over-diagnostic or undesirable effects of the

H. Yoshida et al. (Eds.): Abdominal Imaging 2011, LNCS 7029, pp. 35–43, 2012.

enhanced image, physicians require the colors and texture of the inner wall near the abnormality to be preserved. To satisfy these requirements, we introduce a method to enhance CE images that takes proper care of the enhanced regions. The proposed technique attempts to retain the natural color tones of the ROI as far as possible. Consequently, the enhanced image appears very similar to the natural image, which is clearly different from the false-color expressions of conventional IEE techniques. This is useful for physicians not only to confirm suspicious regions, but also to explain clearly to patients the different conditions of normal/abnormal regions when observed simultaneously in a natural form.

To preserve the color tones of the original ROIs, the most common approaches [3,13,11] involve controlling and manipulating the intensity and saturation components of color, while the hue is left unchanged. However, these approaches often lead to a gamut problem in which the image data exceed the normal range when they are re-transformed to RGB data for display [12]. Recently, in the approach by Li et al. [10,9], forward and backward anisotropic diffusion functions are constructed in a contrast space to enhance the CE images. Because the diffusion procedure encourages intra-region smoothing, while inhibiting inter-region smoothing, it can produce an enhanced version with a natural appearance. However, the diffusion procedure needs the set of parameters to be determined beforehand. Without appropriate values, increasing the Gaussian kernel size σ, for example, can lead to stronger blurring of large homogenous regions, and may even cause the ROI to no longer be observable in the diffused image.

In this paper, we propose a new method that enhances a ROI by preserving the natural tones based on the color characteristics of the wall regions of the gastrointestinal (GI) tract. The color gamut of the human small bowel is generally restricted to a subspace of the original color space (e.g., 24 bit RGB), which is more specific than that of the natural images. Theoretically, an image is considered to be more informative if its histogram resembles a uniform distribution over a color space. Additionally, our goal requires eliminating the distorted colors in the enhanced image. To achieve this, the proposed technique is deployed in a subspace containing only suggestive components of the GI wall regions. In this sense, a ROI is enhanced through a spatial transformation. The transformation attempts to assign new color values to the original color points so that the new colors are almost uniformly spread over the available color levels. The proposed method starts with a learning scheme based on a self-organizing map (SOM) to handle the GI color components. Their features are extracted to define a specific color space, called the GI color space. Histogram equalization is applied to the ROI's image data in the proposed GI color space. Consequently, by merging the enhanced version of the ROI with the original image, the proposed method generates a full enhanced image that preserves the natural tones.

2   Constructing the GI Color Space

The GI color space was first mentioned in [15]. Based on common appearances of CE images, the approach in [15] separated color components belonging the GI wall from non-wall groups (e.g, areas including dark lumen, water bubbles, gas,

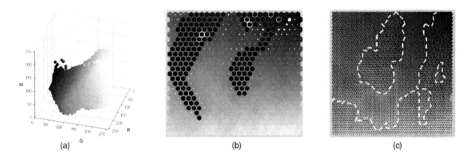

(a)   (b)   (c)

Fig. 1. Color components classification. (a) Distribution of the color components in RGB space. (b) A coarse SOM map with 25×25 nodes. Blue nodes are manually assigned as GI wall components. (c) A fine SOM with 60×60 nodes. The white contours depict regions of GI wall components.

and food). Using a large set of CE images, Vu et al. [15] observed the probability P(.) of the color components. This probability P(.) was then compared with thresholds for the classification task. However, to avoid ambiguous selections of the threshold values, we use a self-organizing map (SOM) [8] in a learning scheme to handle GI wall color components.

Let us denote a color component c_i belonging to a set of random variables $\{c_i \in x | c_i = [R, G, B]\}$. Fig. 1(a) shows the distribution x in RGB color space, as indexed in the work by Vu et al. [15]. Given an input x, the SOM in an unsupervised manner generates a 2-D map for clustering the color components c_i. An advantage of the SOM is that the 2-D map provides a visualization to easily observe the color gamut of the GI wall (i.e., c_i ranges from pinkish to yellowish). In this study, the SOM technique is deployed as a two-stage scheme. The first stage is to construct a coarse map in order to label groups of c_i easily. Fig. 1(b) shows a coarse map (25×25 nodes), of which the blue nodes are manually assigned to be GI wall regions. Results of the first stage provide the training data set containing a small number of the

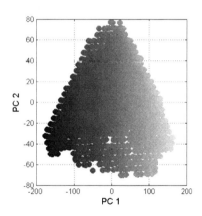

Fig. 2. Distribution of the GI wall colors components based on two principal components

labeled color components. In the second stage, the coarse map is fine-tuned by increasing the size of the map. To assign labels to the new map, the K-Nearest-Neighbors (K-NN) algorithm is deployed. A label is assigned to a new node based on the majority votes of the K objects found on the coarse map. Fig. 1(c) shows the color components of the GI wall within the white boundary regions (denoted as Ω regions) of a fine 2-D map (60×60 nodes).

Let us denote wall color components extracted from the 2-D map in Fig. 1(c) as the set $\Theta = \{c_i : c_i \in \Omega\}$. Θ forms a subspace of the full RGB space, called the GI color space. To maximize the trace of features, principle component analysis (PCA) is applied to the data set Θ. Fig. 2 shows the distribution of Θ along its two main components (pc_1, pc_2). The optimal mapping obtained by PCA is identified by eigenvectors (ν_Θ) of Θ's covariance matrix and mean values (μ_Θ). Hence, a c_i color belonginging to the wall region is projected onto the GI color space by linear transformation ζ: $c_i \rightarrow c_{pc1,pc2,pc3} = \nu_\Theta^T(c_i - \mu_\Theta)$.

3   CE Image Enhancement Algorithms

The proposed method begins with the region-of-interest (ROI) identified by a physician. Given a ROI, our enhancement algorithm is designed to retain the natural color tones as far as possible. To achieve this, we deploy a histogram equalization (HE) technique [6] in the proposed GI color space. Theoretically, the HE technique is well founded based on the criterion of maximal entropy. However, with a wide color range of the RGB color space (i.e., 24-bit color) the HE technique produces distorted colors on enhanced images. Using the proposed GI color space, the HE technique can be applied without color distortion because the GI color space presents only the color gamut of the GI wall. Given image data $I(pc_1, pc_2, pc_3)$ of a ROI, the available color levels in the GI color space are collected by:

$$L_i = \{c_i : (min(I_i) - \Delta) \le c_i \le (max(I_i) + \Delta)\} \tag{1}$$

where $i \in (pc_1, pc_2, pc_3)$, $c_i \in \Theta$, and Δ is an adjustable threshold to expand the color ranges in case the ROI is very small. The HE algorithm aims to re-distribute the colors as uniformly as possible over these color ranges. Because the color variance is intended to be uncorrelated between each color channel in the GI color space, spreading the histogram across single channels (pc_1, pc_2, and pc_3) is an acceptable solution that does not greatly impact inter-channel correlations. A readily available procedure for redistributing the pixels is the histogram matching technique [6]. For image data on each axis, a white-noise one-dimensional signal is generated. The normalized cumulative histograms of the white-noise signal and the original image data are used to map pixel data with the new color levels used in the enhancement. Fig. 3 compares the enhance-ment results of the original ROI of size 128×128 pixels (Fig. 3(a)). Fig. 3(b) shows the result using the HE deployed with the full RGB color space. Here, the abnormal region has been obscured and the colors are distorted in the normal regions. After applying the proposed method, the abnormal region in Fig. 3(c) is more clearly visualized in the enhanced image, which also preserves the natural color tones around the abnormal regions.

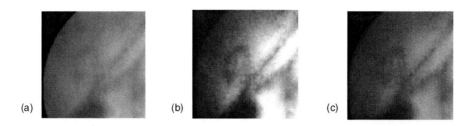

Fig. 3. Histogram equalization results. (a) Original image. (b) HE results applied to individual RGB channels. (c) Results of HE using the GI color space.

4   Experimental Results

To validate the proposed method, we set up evaluations with clinical involvement. Our results were compared with images generated by the FICE images, which is the current enhancement technique supported by VCE reader software (RapidReader Ver. 6, [5]). First, the ROIs including abnormalities were extracted from the original images with a fixed window size of 128×128 pixels. For the evaluation, 60 images were prepared containing different types of abnormalities such as angiodysplasia, erosion, ulcers, and polyps. Four physicians, with rich experience in CE image analysis, were asked to assess the enhanced images according to two criteria:

- Acceptable rate v: determines whether the enhanced images are useful in clinical practice. Several acceptable images can be selected in an evaluation.
- The most preferred rate ρ: is the preferred image in the opinion of the evaluator. Only one enhanced image can be chosen in an evaluation.

Figure 4 shows four cases of the 60 evaluations. In each row, besides the original image (a), the results of the proposed method (b) are visually compared with different FICE images ((c) -(f)). The evaluation results of an expert are given on the top of each case. The acceptable rate v in all evaluations is given in Fig. 5(a). On average, the proposed method achieved 86% acceptable cases, whereas the results of the FICE images are: 79% for FICE_2, 69% for FICE_3, and 5% for FICE_4. The FICE_1 images did not obtain any positive assessment in the evaluations. For images containing bleeding regions, FICE_2 and FICE_3 results were competitive in the evaluations, because they were designed to deeply absorb the red/reddish color of the abnormal regions. However, with other types of abnormalities, as shown in Fig. 4 Case 2 (erosion) and Case 4 (polyp), parameter v deteriorated with FICE images.

Results of the most preferred rate ρ are given in Fig. 5(b). MD.D was clearly biased towards images generated by FICE_3; MD.B preferred FICE_2 images, whereas MD.A and MD.C gave positive evaluations to the results of the proposed method. Obviously, this criterion depends on the experience (or familiarity) of the physicians with respect to each type of enhanced image. Inter-observer agreement (e.g, using the Kappa statistic) is not expected to be a good measurement.

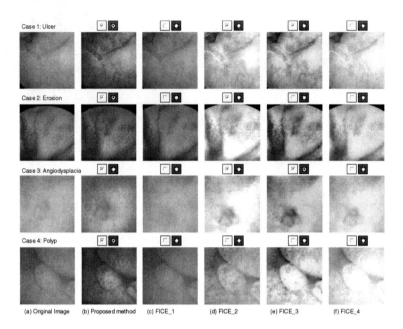

Fig. 4. Comparative results with four different types of abnormal regions. Images from left to right: (a) Original image. (b) The proposed method. (c)-(f) FICE images. On the top of each row, the evaluation results of an expert are given. Yellow buttons are to select the acceptable images, while red buttons are to select the most preferred image.

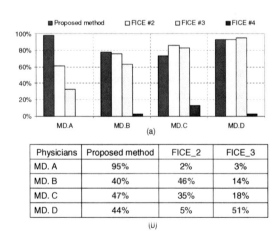

Physicians	Proposed method	FICE_2	FICE_3
MD. A	95%	2%	3%
MD. B	40%	46%	14%
MD. C	47%	35%	18%
MD. D	44%	5%	51%

(b)

Fig. 5. Evaluation Results. (a) Acceptable rate results. (b) The most preferred rate.

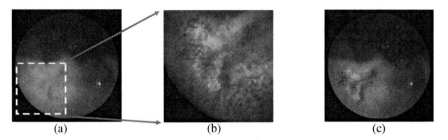

Fig. 6. Applying the proposed method to full images. (a) Original image with the ROI manually demarcated with a white rectangle. (b) The enhanced result of the ROI. (c) The enhanced image after merging (b) into the original image.

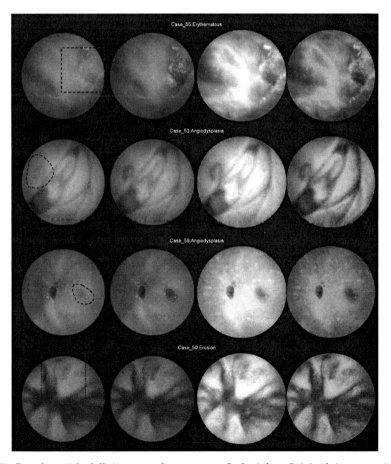

Fig. 7. Results with full image enhancement. Left-right: Original image, with the boundaries of the suspicious regions manually demarcated by blue dotted-lines; Results of the proposed method; FICE_2 and FICE_3 images

In other words, voting for the most preferred enhanced mode (e.g, based on the average of ρ) is ill-considered. Generally, ρ is more stable with the proposed method, even in the case of MD.B or MD.D, who preferred the FICE_2 or FICE_3 images. The lowest ρ was $\approx 40\%$ for these physicians, which is much higher than the corresponding values of the FICE images ($\approx 3\%$).

Finally, we applied the proposed approach to full images as shown in Fig. 6. A ROI was manually demarcated by a simple shape such as a rectangle of size 128×128 pixels. The enhanced regions were then merged into the original image without seams between them by using a Laplacian pyramid rendering algorithm [4]. Additionally, Fig. 7 shows the full image enhancement with ROIs marked in different situations (e.g., closed curves). Compared visually with the FICE images, the results of the proposed method shown in Fig. 7 not only help physicians confirm suspicious regions, but also help explain clearly to patients the differential conditions of the normal/abnormal regions when they are observed simultaneously in a natural form. Furthermore, in the practical clinics, physicians usually mark the suspicious regions using simple markings such as a circle and arrow markers (i.e. RapidReader Ver. 6 [5]). The operator for marking ROIs required in the proposed method is feasible and easily deployed.

5 Conclusion

We have proposed a novel region-based enhancement method for CE images. The significant advantage of this procedure is that the endoscopist can more clearly observe abnormal regions, without the need for any special training to interpret the enhanced images. To retain natural color tones in the enhanced image, the proposed enhancement technique uses a specific color space, designed for the GI wall. Evaluations with clinical involvement were used to validate the performance of the proposed method. Because the proposed approach requires physicians to identify a region-of-interest beforehand, a limitation is that it is not able to be applied to image sequences. The current limitation motivates us to automatically identify suspicious regions before enhancing the image.

References

1. American Gastroenterological Association: Assessment on image-enhanced endoscopy. GastroEnterology 134, 327–340 (2008)
2. Aschmoneit, I., Schumann, S., et al.: Fice enhanced video capsule endoscopy in patients with suspected small bowel bleeding: A randomized prospective pilot study. In: Proceeding of 18th United European Gastroenterology Week (October 2010)
3. Bockstein, I.: Color equalization method and its application to color image processing. Journal of Optical Society American A 3(5), 735–737 (1986)
4. Burt, P., Adelson, E.: A multiresolution spline with application to image mosaics. ACM Transaction on Graphics 2(4), 217–236 (1983)
5. Given Imaging Ltd.: RAPID Reader 6.0, http://www.givenimaging.com
6. Heckbert, P.: Color image quantization for frame buffer display. Computer Graphics 16(3) (1982)

7. Iddan, G., Meron, G., et al.: Wireless capsule endoscope. Nature 405, 417 (2000)
8. Kohonen, T.: Self-Organizing Maps, 3rd edn. Springer, Heidelberg (2001)
9. Li, B., Meng, M.: Wireless capsule endoscopy images enhancement by tensor based diffusion. In: Proceeding of 26th EMBS (August 2006)
10. Li, B., Meng, M.: Wireless CE images enhancement using contrast driven forward and backward anisotropic diffusion. In: Proceeding of ICIP, pp. 437–440 (2007)
11. Mlsna, P.A., Zhang, Q., Rodriguez, J.: 3-d histogram modification of color images. In: Proceeding of ICIP, vol. 3, pp. 1015–1018 (1996)
12. Naik, S., Murthy, C.: Hue-preserving color image enhancement without gamut problem. IEEE Transactions on Image Processing 12(12), 1591–1598 (2003)
13. Pitas, I., Kinikilis, P.: Multichannel techniques in color image enhancement and modeling. IEEE Trans. Image Processing 5(1), 168–171 (1996)
14. Swain, P.: Wireless capsule endoscopy. GUT 52, 48–50 (2003)
15. Vu, H., Echigo, T., Yagi, K., et al.: Color analysis for segmenting digestive organs in video capsule endoscopy. In: Proceeding of 20th ICPR, pp. 2468–2471 (August 2010)

3D Non-rigid Motion Correction
of Free-Breathing Abdominal DCE-MRI Data

Zhang Li[1], Matthan W.A. Caan[2], Manon L. Ziech[2], Japp Stoker[2],
Lucas J. van Vliet[1], and Frans M. Vos[1,2]

[1] Quantitative Imaging Group, Delft University of Technology, The Netherlands
[2] Department of Radiology, Academic Medical Center, The Netherlands
z.li-1@tudelft.nl

Abstract. Inflammatory bowel diseases (IBD) constitute one of the largest healthcare problems in the Western World. Grading of the disease severity is important to determine treatment strategy and to quantify the response to treatment. The Time Injection Curves (TICs) after injecting a contrast agent contain important information on the degree of inflammation of the bowel wall. However, respiratory and peristaltic motions complicate an easy analysis of such curves since spatial correspondence over time is lost. We propose a gated, 3D non-rigid motion correction method that robustly extracts time intensity curves from bowel segments in free-breathing abdominal DCE-MRI data. It is shown that the mean TICs in small bowel segments could be robustly computed and contained   less fluctuations than prior to the registration.

Keywords: Inflammatory bowel disease, small bowel, DCE-MRI, motion correction, time intensity curves.

1   Introduction

Inflammatory bowel diseases (IBD) constitute one of the largest healthcare problems in the Western World. It affects over 1 million European citizens alone, 700,000 of who suffer from Crohn's disease. Grading of Crohn's disease severity is important to determine treatment strategy and to quantify the response to treatment.

Colonoscopy in combination with the assessment of biopsy samples is considered the reference standard for diagnosis and assessment of all IBD. However, the procedure is invasive and requires extensive bowel preparation, which is considered very burdensome by most patients. Moreover, it only gives information on superficial abnormalities.

The project called VIGOR++, in which the research presented in this paper is performed, aims to create a noninvasive procedure for improving grading of Crohn's disease severity by means of magnetic resonance imaging (MRI).

Specifically, in Dynamic Contrast Enhanced MRI (DCE-MRI), the Time Injection Curves (TICs) after injecting a contrast agent are expected to contain important information on the degree of inflammation of the bowel wall. The advent of high temporal resolution scanning protocols has opened the way to TIC-measurements over

H. Yoshida et al. (Eds.): Abdominal Imaging 2011, LNCS 7029, pp. 44–50, 2012.
© Springer-Verlag Berlin Heidelberg 2012

longer time intervals during free breathing. However, respiratory and peristaltic motions complicate an easy analysis of such curves since spatial correspondence over time is lost.

Therefore, the data analysis should comprise a 3D motion correction procedure. Previous work included motion tracking in rats [1] and 2D non-rigid registration of cardiac data [2].

We propose a 3D non-rigid motion correction method that robustly extracts time intensity curves from bowel segments in free-breathing abdominal DCE-MRI data.

2   Methods

2.1   Data Acquisition

DCE-MRI data were acquired during free-breathing of 7 consenting subjects on a 3.0T Philips Intera scanner using a 3D spoiled gradient echo sequence. The scan parameters were: scan matrix 200x200, in plane resolution 2x2 mm, 14 coronal slices, slice thickness 2.5 mm, TE/TR =1.0/2.2 ms, flip angle $6°$, temporal resolution 0.8 s, total scanning time 6.1 minutes. Buscopan was administered to the subjects to minimize bowel movement. A contrast agent (Gadovist) was injected (0.1 ml/kg) after the 10th image volume was acquired. As such 450 3D image volumes were acquired capturing the inflow and outflow of the contrast medium. Fig.1 demonstrates the high spatial and temporal resolution of our data (notice the small bowel segments and the effects of the respiratory cycle).

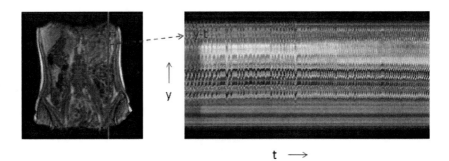

Fig. 1. Illustration of the high spatial and temporal resolution of data. The left image is one randomly selected coronal slice. The right image shows the intensity along the red line(vertically) over time (horizontally).

2.2   Respiratory Gating

The focus of our interest is the varying contrast uptake that is reflected in the MRI signal value. During contrast uptake there is respiratory and bowel movement. Unfortunately, a simple motion correction by means of registration cannot be applied. This is because susceptibility effects influence the MRI signal values. These susceptibility effects make that the image intensity varies as a function of position in the scanner. What is more, the respiration imposes a discontinuous deformation to the bowel structures which is usually not incorporated in a non-rigid deformation models.

We hypothesize that retrospective gating to one phase of the respiratory cycle reduces the abovementioned effects to a large extent. Accordingly, we computed in each patient the Sum of Squared Differences (SSD) of all dynamically acquired 3D volumes to a selected dynamic (here we simply chose middle dynamic, i.e. number 225):

$$D_n = \sum_i (f_n(X_i) - f_{middle}(X_i))^2 \tag{1}$$

in which $f_n(X_i)$ is the intensity of each voxel of dynamic n and D_n is the SSD of volume n to the middle dynamic. The oscillatory behavior of D_n (reflecting the breathing cycle) is shown in Fig.2.

Subsequently, we selected those 3D images that corresponded to the local minima of the oscillatory curve based on the Gaussian-weighted second-order derivative. This delivers a gated subset of the original data, representing volumes in the same phase of respiratory cycle. However, the images are not well registered, particularly due to bowel motion.

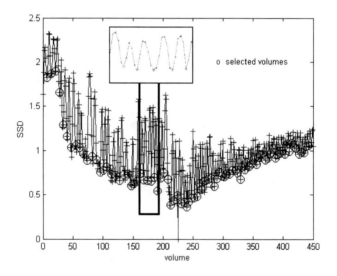

Fig. 2. Illustration of the oscillatory of D_n. The black rounds correspond to the selected subset of images that are in the same breathing phase.

2.3   Image Registration

A non-rigid registration procedure was adopted to compensate for the remaining misalignment. Thereby, we first selected a reference dynamic from the subset of images that are in the same respiratory phase. We chose as a reference the one dynamic with the lowest accumulated SSD with respect to the other dynamics within the subset:

$$D_s = \sum_i \sum_j (f_s(\boldsymbol{X}_i) - f_j(\boldsymbol{X}_i))^2 \tag{2}$$

$$f_{ref} = f_{\min D_s} \tag{3}$$

Here D_s is the accumulated SSD for dynamic s to the other volumes in the subset.

Now, the next step is to non-rigidly register the subset of images to the reference image from (3). To do so, we adopted a Discrete Cosine Transformation (DCT) model [3] with two successive cut-off values applied to the DCT basis functions of 50 and 25 mm. The first cut-off value serves to achieve global registration and particularly corrects for any remaining displacement due to breathing (predominantly taking place in the x-y plane). The second, smaller cut-off was chosen to correct for smaller movement like peristalsis.

The DCT model we used here is a nonlinear spatial transformation. The transformation is defined in 3D as follows:

$$x_i' = x_i + \sum_{j=1}^{J} p_{xj} b_{1j}(\boldsymbol{X}) \quad y_i' = y_i + \sum_{j=1}^{J} p_{yj} b_{2j}(\boldsymbol{X}) \quad z_i' = z_i + \sum_{j=1}^{J} p_{zj} b_{3j}(\boldsymbol{X})$$

where x_i, y_i, z_i are the coordinates of a voxel $\boldsymbol{X}$ in the image that needs to be transformed and x_i', y_i', z_i' are the new coordinates after transformation. Furthermore, p_{xj}, p_{yj}, p_{zj}, are the jth coefficient of the cosine functions for each spatial dimension and J is number of basic functions. $b_{1j}(\boldsymbol{X})$, $b_{2j}(\boldsymbol{X})$, $b_{3j}(\boldsymbol{X})$ represent the jth cosine function at position $\boldsymbol{X}$ defined as follows:

$$b_{mj}(\boldsymbol{X}) = \sqrt{\frac{1}{J}} \quad J = 1, m = 1 \dots M \tag{4}$$

$$b_{mj}(\boldsymbol{X}) = \sqrt{\frac{2}{J}} \cos\left(\frac{\pi(2m-1)(j-1)}{2J}\right) \quad j = 2 \dots J, m = 1 \dots M \tag{5}$$

In fact, the transformation is based on a linear combination of low spatial frequency cosine basis functions to reduce the number of coefficients.

2.4   ROI Annotation and Segmentation

The effectiveness of the registration procedure was evaluated by assessment of the TIC curves in three ROIs (region of interests). These three ROIs were manually annotated in 3D by an expert in small parts of the bowel wall in various locations in the abdomen, using ITK-SNAP software (itksnap.org). The ROIs were drawn in the reference image delivered by Equation 3 (see also Fig.4, inset, dark blue color). A simple segmentation procedure based on isodata thresholding [4] was applied to discard the voxels relating to the bowel lumen from each ROI and retain the bowel wall voxels (which is the focus of our interest, Fig.4, inset, bright blue color).

3 Experimental Results

Notice that each patient initially delivers 450 dynamically acquired 3D images consisting of 224x224x14 voxels(The images were interpolated in the in- plane area. The inplane resolution was changed from 2.0*2.0mm to 1.8*1.8mm). The gated subset (see Section 2.2) contained 80-120 volumes (range over the 7 included patients). Fig. 3 shows the initial time-averaged image as well as this same image after registration procedure. It demonstrates the increase in anatomical detail, for example at the bowel walls. The average TICs in the ROIs in the original and processed dataset are compared in Fig. 4 (notice the reduced number of volumes in the gated dataset). ROI #3 (red) is of relatively large size and contains negligible motion due to its location in the lower abdomen. ROIs #2 (green) and #1 (blue) have smaller sizes and are positioned more proximate to the lungs. Clearly, a dramatic increase in contrast in the processed dataset is visible in the latter areas.

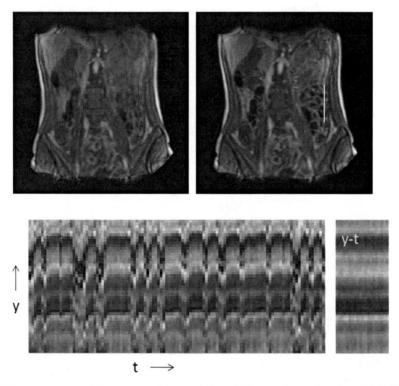

Fig. 3. Top: comparison of time-averaged images before (left) and after registration (right). These mean images are calculated over the 7 included patients. Bottom: intensity (vertically) over time for the profiles indicated in the top images from one patient, i.e. before (left) and after registration (right). Notice that the bottom right image is taken from the gated subset, which is why the bottom two images have different scale.

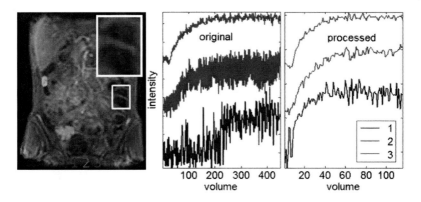

Fig. 4. Left: Three ROIs are annotated in 3D and processed to segment the bowel wall, c.q. remove lumen and air (dark/bright blue, inset). Right: Mean Time Intensity Curves (TICs) over the ROIs in the original and processed datasets are plotted.

4   Discussion

We have presented a method to correct for motion in free-breathing DCE-MRI data. The mean TICs in small bowel segments could be robustly computed and contained less fluctuations than prior to the registration. We aim to proceed now to a voxel-based TIC reconstruction. For that, contrast change modeling [2] and time-constrained registration may be beneficial. Also, we have found that the linear model underlying the DCT transform is not flexible enough for some situations. Fig.5 shows misalignment around the bowel wall after registration. It demonstrates that the bowel wall is hardly warped in the annotated rectangles. In fact, a more flexible transforms such as B-spline transform may yield a better registration result. Moreover, the SSD similarity does not account for the contrast variation that is inherently present in images. Therefore mutual information might be a better metric [5].

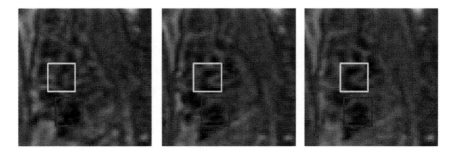

Fig. 5. Left: reference volume (t=225). Middle: volume (t=128) before registration. Right: volume after registration.

Acknowledgement. The research leading to these results has received funding from the European Community's Seventh Framework Programme (FP7/2007-2013) of the VIGOR++ Project under grant agreement nr. 270379.

References

1. Ailiani, A.C., Neuberger, T., Brasseur, J.G., Branco, G., Wang, Y., Smith, N.B., Webb, A.G.: Quantitative Analysis of Peristaltic and Segmental Motion in Vivo in the Rat Small Intestine Using Dynamic MRI. Magn. Reson. Med. 62, 116–126 (2009)
2. Filipovic, M., Vuissoz, P.A., Codreanu, A., Claudon, M., Felblinger, J.: Motion Compensated Generalized Reconstruction for Free-Breathing Dynamic Contrast-Enhanced MRI. Magn. Reson. Med. 65, 812–822 (2011)
3. Ashburner, J., Friston, K.J.: Nonlinear Spatial Normalization Using Basis Functions. Hum. Brain Mapp. 7, 254–266 (1999)
4. Velasco, F.R.D.: Thresholding Using the ISODATA Clustering Algorithm. IEEE Trans. Syst. Man, and Cybern. 10, 771–774 (1980)
5. Pluim, J.P.W.: Mutual Information based Registration of Medical Images. University Medical Center Utrecht, Utrecht (2000)

Segmentation of Liver Tumor Using Efficient Global Optimal Tree Metrics Graph Cuts

Ruogu Fang[1], Ramin Zabih[2], Ashish Raj[3], and Tsuhan Chen[1]

[1] Department of Electrical and Computer Engineering, Cornell University, Ithaca, NY, USA
`rf294@cornell.edu, asr2004@med.cornell.edu`
[2] Department of Computer Science, Cornell University, Ithaca, NY. 14850, USA
`rdz@cs.cornell.edu`
[3] Department of Radiology, Cornell University, New York City, NY. 10021, USA
`tsuhan@ece.cornell.edu`

Abstract. We propose a novel approach that applies global optimal tree-metrics graph cuts algorithm on multi-phase contrast enhanced contrast enhanced MRI for liver tumor segmentation. To address the difficulties caused by low contrasted boundaries and high variability in liver tumor segmentation, we first extract a set of features in multi-phase contrast enhanced MRI data and use color-space mapping to reveal spatial-temporal information invisible in MRI intensity images. Then we apply efficient tree-metrics graph cut algorithm on multi-phase contrast enhanced MRI data to obtain global optimal labeling in an unsupervised framework. Finally we use tree-pruning method to reduce the number of available labels for liver tumor segmentation. Experiments on real-world clinical data show encouraging results. This approach can be applied to various medical imaging modalities and organs.

Keywords: multi-phase contrast enhanced MRI, tree-metrics graph cuts, liver tumor segmentation, color-space mapping, global optimal labeling.

1 Introduction

In the United States, liver tumor (or hepatocellular carcinoma) is one of the most common malignancies leading to an estimated one million deaths annually, and it has become the fastest growing cancer up to date [1]. Liver tumors segmentation is an important prerequisite for surgical interventions planning. The major difficulty in liver tumor segmentation is low contrasted boundaries and a large variability of shapes, sizes and locations presented by the tumor in the liver. Local intensity or intensity gradient feature based techniques are proved to be inadequate to differentiate between liver tissue and healthy structures. High performance segmentation methods should be capable to deal with the high variation in shape and gray value of the liver.

In order to alleviate this problem, multi-phase contrast enhanced MRI is used in clinical practice to characterize tumor response to contrast agent, yet most of the current methods still lack maturity in terms of quantifying tumor burden and viability. We propose to extract a set of features in multi-phase contrast enhanced MRI images,

H. Yoshida et al. (Eds.): Abdominal Imaging 2011, LNCS 7029, pp. 51–59, 2012.

and apply an efficient tree-metrics graph cuts algorithm in computer vision to segment the tumor in the liver. In this manner, we design a classifier for semi-automatic diagnosis of hepatocellular carcinoma.

The contributions and novel aspects of our proposed approach include:

1. **New Framework for Global Optimal Multi-label Segmentation in Medical Image Data.**

    This framework is based on directly clustering the available labels (intensity values or dynamic features) in medical image data, and use efficient tree-metrics graph cuts to find the global optimal labeling, while previous approaches have focused on conventional methods as active contours [2], level-sets [3], as well as machine learning [4]. The advantages of this new framework are discussed below in Section 2.2.

2. **Specific Focus on Multi-phase Contrast Enhanced MRI of Liver Tumor.**

    In contrast to the works previously [5][6], our work on tree-metrics graph cuts segmentation focuses on multi-phase contrast enhanced MRI of liver tumor, which has not been explored to the best of our knowledge.

3. **Evaluation on Real-World Clinical Data with Many Applications.**

    Our experiments employ segmentation problems of liver tumor and compared with the state-of-art work. The proposed method is also applicable to multiple image modalities, such as dynamic contrast enhanced MRI, CT perfusion.

2   Method

To find the segmentation boundary of tumor in low contrast multi-phase contrast enhanced MRI of liver tumor images, we propose a set of novel features along with the computational approaches to obtain them, and detail our framework of tree-metrics graph-cut (TM) algorithm. Finally we propose a tree-cutting approach to interpret the labeling returned by the TM algorithm for tumor segmentation in the multi-phase contrast enhanced MRI liver data.

2.1   Dynamic Feature Extraction

Here we describe the general protocol for multi-phase contrast enhanced MRI. In multi-phase contrast enhanced MRI a bolus injection of a contrast agent, usually gadolinium-DTPA (Gd) is given to the subject (patients or animals). A set of T_1-weighted MRI volumes are acquired a few seconds (pre-contrast time) before the injection and at several time points after the injection (arterial phase, portal-venous phase and delayed phase), to first obtain a baseline or pre-contrast MRI, as well as the time-varying MRI with the contrast agent. As the contrast bolus perfuses through the vasculature, the time-course of the contrast at a given voxel, indicating the MRI signal, can be characterized from the plot. The specific time points for the data collection vary for different MRI settings, and the detailed time points in our experiments are illustrated in Section 3.1.

We denote a voxel in the volume as v_i indexed by the set of voxels $i \in I$. The associated time-course curve is denoted as $y_i(t)$ where t indexes the time points in the multi-phase contrast enhanced MRI scan. The total number of voxels in the volume is $|I|$. Healthy tissue in general is less enhanced by the contrast agent than the enhancing carcinomas, but more than necrotic tissue, which basically does not enhance apparently.

The dynamic features that we extract from the time-series signals include: baseline (pre-contrast) MR signal (BL), peak enhancement (PE), and area under the enhancement curve (AUC), rise time (RT), and arrival time (AT), as depicted in Figure 1. For the coarse time-scale curves, the first three dynamic features are used, as depicted in Fig. 1(a). For more high resolution time-course curves, additional detailed dynamic features are extracted, as shown in Fig. 1(b). Our work uses both models, depending on the availability of the temporal resolution of the data.

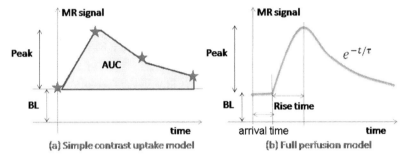

Fig. 1. Dynamic feature extracted from time-course curves of the MR signals. (a) A simple model where three features are used. (b) Full model where richer dynamic features are used.

In the multi-phase contrast enhanced images, the first three features (BL, PE and AUC) are mapped in pseudocolor onto RGB color space for better visualization. Figure 2 visualizes the baseline MR image, along with the dynamic feature-enhanced image and pseudo-color mapped image. The feature-space mapping conveys additional information unavailable in any single MRI intensity image.

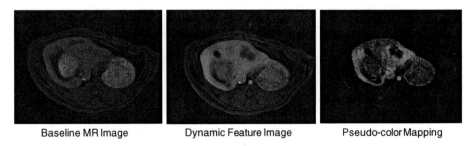

Baseline MR Image   Dynamic Feature Image   Pseudo-color Mapping

Fig. 2. Dynamic feature extraction and mapping. Left: Baseline MR image without dynamic feature extraction. Middle: MR image after using dynamic feature extraction method. Right: Pseudo-color image after feature-spacing mapping onto RGB color space.

2.2   Liver Tumor Segmentation as Metric Labeling

The liver tumor segmentation problem can be interpreted as an instance of metric labeling; specifically an instance of spatially coherent clustering, where the observations are labels and we want to assign the voxels with new label. The new labels are gray-scale intensity levels, and further tree-pruning step will generate the actual segmentation for the liver tumor in multi-phase contrast enhanced MRI. Each of the new values should be close to the observed one in the original liver tumor multi-phase contrast enhanced MRI image, and the values of nearby voxels should be similar. Spatially coherently clustering has been addressed by several papers recently [7, 8, 9, 10]. All of them rely on iterative techniques without provable error bounds. In this paper, we propose to use tree-metrics graph cuts [6] which computes a global minimum solution of an energy function, to liver tumor segmentation in smulti-phase contrast enhanced MRI. The tree-metrics graph cuts algorithm applies graph cuts [11] on a tree of labels for distance measure.

Let the dynamic features extracted from the liver multi-phase contrast enhanced MRI image be represented as an undirected weighted graph $G = (V, E)$, where vertices V correspond to voxels and E are edges between neighboring voxels. Let L be the set of labels, and let $f : V \rightarrow L$ be a labeling. Furthermore, let $d(o(v), f(v))$ be the cost for giving label $f(v)$ to object v, where $o(v)$ is the observed label and $d(a, b)$ is a distance on L. Let $d(f(u), f(v))$ be the cost for giving label $f(u)$ to object u and $f(v)$ to object v, where u and v are the neighboring voxels. The goal is to find a labeling f that minimizes the cost function

$$Q(f) = \sum_{v \in V} d(o(v), f(v)) + \sum_{(u,v) \in E} \lambda \cdot d(f(u), f(v)) \qquad (1)$$

We refer to the first summation in $Q(f)$ as the "data term" and the second summation in $Q(f)$ as the "prior term" (or "smoothness term"). As our prior, we want objects connected by an edge in E to have similar labels. The weights λ decides the relative importance of the data terms and the smoothness terms. The larger the value of λ, the more smooth the output labeling. The choice of the parameter λ is detailed in the experiments in Section 3.1.

2.3   Tree-Metrics Graph Cuts

To apply the tree-metrics graph cuts (TM) algorithm [6] on multi-phase contrast enhanced MRI liver tumor segmentation, we perform a pre-processing step to create suitable inputs to the TM algorithm, and a post-processing step on the output segmentation returned by the TM algorithm to create the final segmentation.

The TM algorithm takes three things as input: a multi-phase contrast enhanced MRI liver image, a tree of labels, and a smoothness parameter $\lambda \geq 0$. We generate a tree of labels with agglomerative clustering based on the extracted dynamic features from multi-phase contrast enhanced MRI data.

Each stage of our approach – tree generation, sweep and pruning – is detailed in the sections followed.

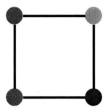

Fig. 3. An examples of tree generation. Left: A synthetic image with tree colors as input. Middle: Binary tree of labels generated from the synthetic image. Right: Graph structure of the image.

2.2.1   Tree Generation

We apply agglomerative hierarchical clustering to create a tree of labels. Closest pairs of clusters (or labels) in the feature space are repeatedly merged. We cluster all the available colors from the image based on Ward's variance criteria [12]. Fig. 3 illustrates the agglomerative clustering on a synthetic image of three colors. For multi-phase contrast enhanced MRI liver image, we perform agglomerative hierarchical clustering on the pseudo-color mapped image from dynamic features. In practice, the agglomerative hierarchical clustering is implemented in phases, and k-nearest neighbors (measured in Euclidean distance) are used as the candidate clusters and merged. Approximate nearest neighbors [13] are used when the number of clusters are very large. The stopping criterion is when the maximum variance becomes greater than two times of the minimum variance.

2.2.2   Sweep Algorithm

The tree of labels generated from the multi-phase contrast enhanced MRI pseudo-color mapped image represents the tree-metrics distance function d. Now we apply the TM algorithm to the multi-phase contrast enhanced MRI liver image, with the tree of labels and a smoothness parameter $\lambda \geq 0$. The TM algorithm will minimize the cost function for a distance d and labeling f:

$$Q(f) = \sum_{v \in V} d(o(v), f(v)) + \lambda \sum_{(u,v) \in E} d(f(u), f(v)) \tag{2}$$

We use graph cuts [11] to optimize the objective function $Q(f)$ in Equation (2), and use tree-metric distance to measure the cost in both the data term and the smoothness term. Compared with conventional graph cuts where the distance function is the Euclidean distance, the upmost advantages of using tree-metrics graph cuts are the global optimality and the efficiency. The TM algorithm computes the globally optimal labeling f for the cost function Q(f) in Equation (2) in $O(\log(k)(g(n)+k))$ time for n voxels and k labels, where g(n) is the running time of the min-cut algorithm on graph with n nodes.

2.2.3   Tree Cutting

The labeling returned by TM algorithm is usually more than the required number of segments in the multi-phase contrast enhanced MRI liver image. Therefore we need to interpret the labels returned from the TM algorithm to find the exact tumor boundary in the liver. To reduce the number of labels, we "cut" the binary tree of labels at depth

d; for each node at depth d (where the root node is depth 0), their child subtrees now map to the same label as their ancestor node at depth d). By cutting the tree at depth d, we are left with N labels, where $N = \sum_{n=0}^{d} 2^n$. Finally, we use an interactive interface to ask radiologist to pick the segment (or label) of the tumor in the liver.

3   Experimental Results

Significant experimental work has been completed towards a new framework for liver tumor segmentation using tree-metrics graph-cuts in multi-phase contrast enhanced MRI.

3.1   Liver Tumor Segmentation in Rabbit HCC Model

Our method was developed and tested on data from a pre-existing study at John Hopkins University involving hepatocellular carcinoma (HCC) grown in a rabbit model. It has been shown that rabbit model demonstrates a physiology similarity to that of humans. The multi-phase contrast enhanced MRI exams were obtained using a standard T1-weighted MR acquisition sequence, with the following timed phases: pre-contrast phase (0s), arterial phase (20s), portal-venous phase (60) and delayed phase (120s). Tumor size was determined through pathologic dissection in all animals. Dissections were performed by pathologists under guidelines and techniques that ensure accurate and reproducible measurement of tumor size. This pathology data served as the gold standard. A novel liver-specific Gadolinium-based contrast agent Gadoxetate Disodium (Eovist®) was intravenously injected. In our experiment, 11 rabbit liver multi-phase contrast enhanced MRI volumetric data were used.

In the energy minimization problem in Equation 2, the smoothness parameter λ decides the level of smoothness in the output segmentation. We experimented with different λs for the rabbit HCC 4-phase multi-phase contrast enhanced MRI data and found that the proper range of λ is between 2 to 10, depending on the specific dataset. In our experiment, we fixed λ to be 5 for all the 11 rabbit multi-phase contrast enhanced MRI volumetric data.

Fig. 4 shows one frame of the segmentation results on 3D volumetric multi-phase contrast enhanced MRI liver tumor data. Using feature-space mapping and tree-metrics graph cuts, the segmentation results on rabbit liver tumor is promising. We have designed an interactive interface for radiologists to actively choose the tumor region by clicking on the segment and the algorithm eases the task of liver tumor segmentation by performing an initial segmentation of the tumor and other tissue types.

We also compared our tumor segmentation results with a recent work on liver tumor segmentation [14]. In their work, Raj et.al. also applies the dynamic feature mapping method to improve the contrast between the tumor and the other tissue types. However, after the dynamic feature extraction, they use K-means to cluster the voxels and segment out the tumor. K means algorithm takes $O(n^{dk+1} \log n)$ for running time, where n is the number of entities to be clustered, k is the number of clusters and d is the distance measure, compared to $O(\log(k)(g(n)+k))$ of our method. Moreover K-means clustering does not give the globally optimal labeling. A comparison of the liver tumor segmentation result using our method and [14] is shown in Fig. 5.

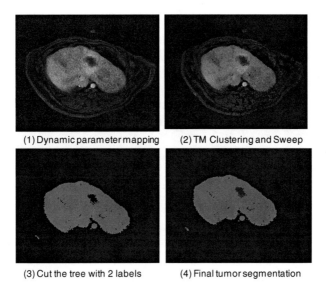

(1) Dynamic parameter mapping   (2) TM Clustering and Sweep

(3) Cut the tree with 2 labels   (4) Final tumor segmentation

Fig. 4. Experiment results of rabbit liver tumor segmentation using tree-metrics graph cuts. The parameters are λ=5, $d = 2$.

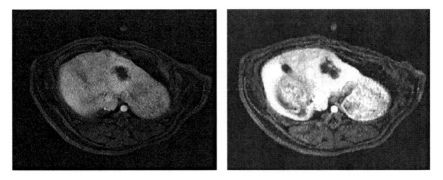

Fig. 5. Comparison of our algorithm (left) with [14] (right) on rabbit liver. The dark blue region in the right image is the final tumor segmentation using methods in [14].

Quantitative evaluation of our method is conducted by correlating the liver tumor size using our method (DPM+TM) with the gold standard, and compare with the segmentation results of [14] (DPM+K-means) on the same dataset. We use our proposed method to segment the liver tumor on 11 rabbit liver multi-phase contrast enhanced MRI 3D volumetric data and Fig. 6 shows the regression between our method and the gold standard, compared with that of [14] on the same dataset. The figure demonstrates that our method correlates with the dissections of pathologists with higher accuracy, while the volume size of the segmented tumor using [14] deviates from the gold standard at higher variation.

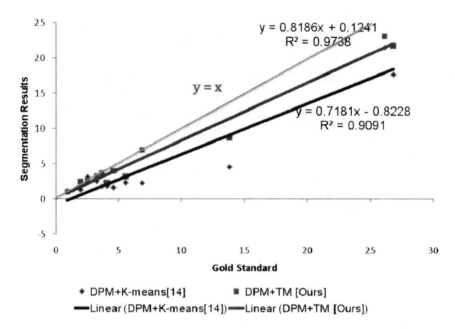

Fig. 6. Comparison of our method with [14] on the regression plot with gold standard

4   Conclusion

In this paper, we present a novel approach to apply dynamic feature mapping and tree-metrics graph cuts with tree pruning to the liver tumor segmentation in dynamic enhanced abdominal MRI data and compare our results with the state-of-art method. Our approach, which is efficient in computation and globally optimized in the tree-metrics labeling, performs better than the conventional existing approaches in terms of qualitative visualization, quantitative tumor size measure, and avoids iterated method which is computational intense.

There are several interesting directions for future work on this problem. To learn the proper structure of the tree, for instance, the optimal degree of the tree and the clustering criterion, will improve the segmentation result for arbitrary number of segments in the output. To find the accurate segmentation of the liver tumor from the initial segmentation of TM algorithm, an active learning approach can be adopted to determine the optimal smoothing parameter in the sweep stage and pruning depth in the cutting stage.

References

1. Fong, I.L., Schoenfield, L.J.: Hepatocellular Carcinoma (Liver Cancer),
    http://www.medicinenet.com
2. Lu, R., Marziliano, P., Thng, C.H.: Liver Tumor Volume Estimation by Semi-Automatic Segmentation Method. In: Proceedings of the 2005 IEEE Engineering in Medicine and Biology 27th Annual Conference, pp. 3297–3299 (2005)

3. Popa, T., Ibanez, L., Levy, E., White, A., Bruno, J., Cleary, K.: Tumor Volume Measurement and Volume Measurement Comparison Plug-Ins for Volview Using Itk. In: Proceedings of the SPIE: The International Society for Optical Engineering, vol. 6141, pp. 395–402 (2006)

4. Li, Y., Hara, S., Shimura, K.: A Machine Learning Approach for Locating Boundaries of Liver Tumors in CT Images. In: Proceedings of the 18th International Conference on Pattern Recognition, pp. 400–403 (2006)

5. Fang, R., Chen, Y.H., Zabih, R., Chen, T.: Tree-Metrics Graph Cuts For Brain MRI Segmentation With Tree Cutting. In: IEEE Western New York Image Processing Workshop. IEEE Press (2010)

6. Felzenszwalb, P., Pap, G., Tardos, E., Zabih, R.: Globally Optimal Pixel Labeling Algorithms for Tree Metrics. In: IEEE Conference on Computer Vision and Pattern Recognition. IEEE Press (2010)

7. Zabih, R., Kolmogorov, V.: Spatially coherent clustering using graph cuts. In: CVPR, pages II: 437–444 (2004)

8. Figueiredo, M., Cheng, D., Murino, V.: Clustering under prior knowledge with application to image segmentation. In: NIPS (2007)

9. Ishikawa, H., Geiger, D.: Segmentation by grouping junctions. In: CVPR, pp. 125–131 (1998)

10. Sfikas, G., Nikou, C., Galatsanos, N.: Edge preserving spatially varying mixtures for image segmentation. In: CVPR, pp. 1–7 (2008)

11. Boykov, Y., Veksler, O., Zabih, R.: Fast approximate energy minimization via graph cuts. PAMI 23(11), 1222–1239 (2001)

12. Ward Jr., J.: Hierarchical grouping to optimize an objective function. Journal of the American Statistical Association 58(301), 236–244 (1963)

13. Arya, S., Mount, D., Netanyahu, N., Silverman, R., Wu, A.S.: An optimal algorithm for approximate nearest neighbor searching fixed dimensions. JACM 45(6), 891–923 (1998)

14. Raj, A., Juluru, K.: Visualization and segmentation of liver tumors using dynamic contrast MRI. In: Conf. Proc. IEEE Eng. Med. Biol. Soc., pp. 6985–6989 (2009)

Ensemble Detection of Colorectal Lesions for CT Colonography

Janne J. Näppi[1], Daniele Regge[2], and Hiroyuki Yoshida[1]

[1] Department of Radiology,
Massachusetts General Hospital and Harvard Medical School,
25 New Chardon Street, Suite 400C, Boston, MA 02114, USA
jnappi@partners.org, yoshida.hiro@mgh.harvard.edu
[2] Institute for Cancer Research and Treatment,
Candiolo Str. Prov. 142, IT-10060, Turin, Italy

Abstract. Even though different computer-aided detection (CAD) systems for computed tomographic colonography (CTC) have similar overall detection accuracies, they are known to detect different types of lesions and false positives. We implemented an ensemble CAD scheme for merging the detection results of different CAD systems in CTC. After normalizing of the lesion-likelihood data between different systems, a Bayesian classifier was used for determining the final detections. For evaluation, we collected 218 abnormal patients with 263 lesions ≥6 mm. The detection accuracies of three CAD systems were compared with that of their ensemble CAD scheme by use of independent training and testing. The preliminary results indicate that the ensemble CAD scheme can yield a higher overall detection accuracy than can individual CAD systems. In particular, the ensemble scheme was able to detect flat lesions at high sensitivity without compromising a high polyp detection accuracy.

Keywords: computer-aided detection, ensemble detection, polyp detection, machine learning, virtual colonoscopy.

1 Introduction

Colorectal cancer would be largely preventable by early removal of its precursor lesions [1]. A practical minimally invasive population screening for colorectal cancer could be implemented by use of computed tomography colonography (CTC) [2]. With primary CTC screening, only patients with significant CTC findings would need to be subjected to invasive conventional colonoscopy.

Although expert radiologists are able to detect large polyps from CTC data at a sensitivity comparable to that of conventional colonoscopy [3], the interpretation of CTC data involves a number of pitfalls and requires dedicated training [4]. Computer-aided detection (CAD) could be used for improvement of the accuracy and consistency of radiologists' interpretation in CTC [5]. Although current CAD systems can detect polyps at a high detection sensitivity, they display large numbers of false-positive (FP) detections and miss flat lesions [6].

H. Yoshida et al. (Eds.): Abdominal Imaging 2011, LNCS 7029, pp. 60–67, 2012.

False positives are a problem, because their review increases radiologists' interpretation time and it may reduce the detection accuracy. Flat lesions are a problem, because they tend to be more advanced and more challenging to detect than are polypoid lesions.

The design of a CAD system for CTC involves several design decisions about image preprocessing, extraction of the colon region, detection of lesions, computation of discriminating features, and classification of detections [7]. Studies have shown that, although many CAD systems for CTC can yield a high detection accuracy, a specific system can detect quite different types of lesions and FPs than other systems [8,9]. Therefore, a combination of CAD systems that reflects different design decisions might be able to outperform a single CAD system.

The idea of combining several CAD methods is not new, but most studies have explored only ensembles of statistical classifiers [10]. Recently, approaches that combined the results of several complete CAD systems have emerged in the context of pulmonary nodule detection [11,12]. Significant increases in detection performance were observed when such ensembles of CAD systems were compared to individual CAD systems.

In this study, inspired by a previous approach used in pulmonary nodule detection [11], we implemented an ensemble CAD scheme for merging the detection results of different CAD systems in CTC. To assess the potential improvement in detection accuracy, we compared the performance of three individual CAD systems and that of their ensemble in detecting colorectal lesions in CTC.

2   Methods

2.1   Conventional CAD System

A conventional CAD system (Fig. 1) was developed for detection of polyps in CTC. The region of the colon is extracted automatically from CTC data [13]. Volumetric shape features are calculated for the extracted region of the colonic mucosa. Suspicious sites are detected by hysteresis thresholding of the shape features [14]. Candidate regions are extracted by use of a morphologic segmentation algorithm [15]. Additional shape and texture features are calculated from the extracted candidate regions and their surrounding regions [16], after which a classifier uses these features to differentiate between true-positive (TP) and FP detections [14]. The classifier calculates a lesion likelihood (LL) that a detected region represents a TP detection. The lesion candidates with the highest LL are reported as the final detections.

2.2   CAD Systems for Ensemble Detection

A CAD system can produce different detection results based on its parameter values. Let P_i denote the parameter values of a CAD system CAD_i, including values such as the CT-value thresholds for extracting the region of the colon from CTC data, the threshold values of shape features for initial detection, the

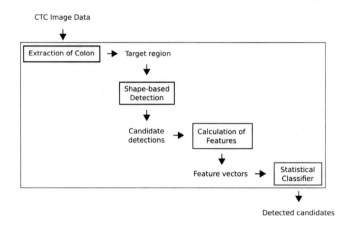

Fig. 1. Conventional CAD for CTC typically performs the steps of colon extraction, lesion detection, feature extraction and FP reduction, before displaying final detections

minimum size of detected candidate regions to consider, or the set of features used for FP reduction. We considered two sets of detection parameters, P_1 and P_2. The first set (P_1) was designed to detect conventional polypoid lesions, whereas the second set (P_2) was designed to detect subtler and smaller lesions than is possible with the first set. The input features were similar to those that we have described previously [16].

For the FP reduction step, we considered two types of classifiers. A Bayesian neural network (BNN) had been identified previously as an effective classifier for detection of colorectal lesions [13]. It maps an input feature vector to an output scalar value by use of a sigmoid activation function. The network weights are determined by use of a Bayesian algorithm [17].

The second classifier was a random forest (RF) classifier [18]. The RF is a collection of decision trees that is constructed by subsampling of the input data D with bootstrapping into input data sets D_t that are used to construct the trees t. Two nodes, l and r, of a decision tree divide their input recursively into disjoint subsets $D_t{}^{il} \cup D_t{}^{ir}$ ($D_t{}^{il} \cap D_t{}^{ir} = \emptyset$) by the best split provided by a random subsample of input features. The leaves of the decision trees represent estimates of the correct category of an input sample. For performing a prediction on an input sample, the decision trees vote for the correct category. The votes are aggregated into a single prediction by majority vote of the trees.

We implemented several CAD systems that were optimized to detect specific types of lesions. For this pilot study, we considered three CAD systems that are summarized in Table 1. The first column indicates the CAD system, and the other columns indicate design choices: the parameter set, the type of classifier that was used for FP reduction, and the types of lesions that the CAD system was designed to detect.

Table 1. Overview of the three CAD systems used in the study

CAD system	Parameters	Classifier	Target lesion
CAD-01	P1	BNN	any
CAD-21	P1	RF	flat 6 – 9 mm
CAD-41	P2	RF	6 – 9 mm

2.3   Ensemble Detection Scheme

The ensemble detection scheme combines the detection results of different CAD systems into a single unified scheme (Fig. 2). First, we identify the unique candidate lesions that were detected by any CAD system. Suppose that c_i and d_j are candidate detections of two CAD systems, CAD_i and CAD_j. These detections are considered to represent the same unique candidate u_{ij}, if the spatial distance between their mass centers is <5 mm. Otherwise, c_i and d_j are considered to be different unique detections with respect to CAD_i and CAD_j.

Let u_i $(i = 1, \cdots, n)$ denote the established set of unique candidates detected by the ensemble. The LLs calculated by each CAD system for each u_i are collected into likelihood vectors

$$\bar{P}(u_i) = (p_{i1}, \cdots, p_{in}), \tag{1}$$

where p_{ik} is the LL calculated by CAD_k. If CAD_k did not detect u_i, then $p_{ik} = 0$.

The LLs calculated by different CAD systems could be incompatible, because they have been calculated by different classifiers and with different types of input data. Therefore, the LLs are normalized by use of a cumulative scaling method [11]. Suppose that θ_k is the set of all unique LL values calculated by CAD_k for its candidate detections. If we threshold the LL values with the value $p \in \theta_k$, the thresholded detections will include T_p TP detections and F_p FP detections. Using this information, we construct a mapping $f : \theta_k \rightarrow P_k$, where for each $p_m \in \theta_k$,

$$f(p_m) = \frac{T_{pm}}{T_{pm} + F_{pm}}. \tag{2}$$

Here, T_{pm} and F_{pm} are the numbers of TP and FP detections, respectively, obtained by thresholding with p_m. The value of $f(p_m)$ approximates the probability that a lesion candidate with an LL value $\geq p_m$ is a TP detection.

For resolution of the final ensemble detections, the normalized likelihoods are analyzed by use of a Bayesian classifier. According to the Bayes' rule, we assign an input candidate u_i to category C_j (TP or FP), if

$$\frac{P(\bar{F}(u_i)|C_j)P(C_j)}{\sum_k P(\bar{F}(u_i)|C_k)P(C_k)} > \frac{P(\bar{F}(u_i)|C_m)P(C_m)}{\sum_k P(\bar{F}(u_i)|C_k)P(C_k)} \qquad \text{for all } j \neq m, \tag{3}$$

where $\bar{F}(u_i) = (f_{i1}, \cdots, f_{in})$ is the vector of normalized likelihoods.

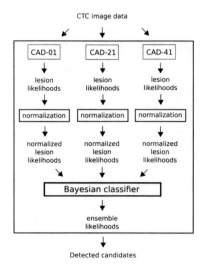

Fig. 2. Ensemble CAD for CTC normalizes the lesion-likelihood data of individual CAD systems and determines the final result by use of a Bayesian classifier

2.4   Materials

The study materials included the CTC data of 218 patients with abnormal findings, collected from 12 institutions. The patients were prepared for CTC with cathartic bowel preparation. Orally ingested iodine tagging alone or in combination with barium was used to opacify the residual bowel contents in 74 of the patients. The CTC was performed in supine and prone positions. The tube current was 20 – 50 mA with 120 kVp. The CT slice thickness was 1.0 – 2.5 mm.

For establishing a ground truth about the lesions, a same-day colonoscopy was performed after the CTC. Expert radiologists correlated the colonoscopy-confirmed lesions retrospectively with the CTC image data.

2.5   Evaluation

The patients were divided randomly into a training set and a testing set. In the training set, there were 109 patients who had 133 adenomas or carcinomas measuring ≥ 6 mm in their largest diameter: 81 were ≥ 10 mm, and 52 were 6 – 9 mm in size. There were 93 polypoid lesions, 17 flat lesions, and 23 lesions with other morphologies. The individual CAD systems were trained on the training set. Optimal input features for each CAD system were determined by use of a recursive backward feature-selection algorithm [19]. The ensemble CAD scheme was trained with the outputs of the individual CAD systems.

The testing set included 109 patients with 130 adenomas or carcinomas ≥ 6 mm in their largest diameter: 78 lesions were ≥ 10 mm and 52 were 6 – 9 mm in size. There were 107 polypoid lesions, 13 flat lesions, and 10 lesions with other morphologies. The trained CAD systems and their ensemble scheme were tested on the CTC data of the testing set.

Because it is not practical for a radiologist to review large numbers of CAD detections, each CAD system and their ensemble were allowed to display at most 15 detections per patient.

3   Results

Table 2 shows the detection accuracy of individual CAD systems (CAD-01, CAD-21, CAD-41) and their ensemble (ECAD) for adenomas and carcinomas. The results demonstrated the asymmetry of the detection performance between different CAD systems: CAD-01 yielded a high detection sensitivity for large ($\geq$10 mm) lesions, but a low detection sensitivity for small (6 – 9 mm) lesions, whereas CAD-41 yielded a high detection sensitivity for small lesions, but a relatively low detection sensitivity for large lesions. In contrast, ECAD yielded a high detection sensitivity for both large and small lesions.

Table 2. Per-lesion detection accuracy of the individual CAD systems and their ensemble. The number of CAD detections was limited to a maximum of 15 per patient. Abbreviations: FPs = median number of false positives per patient.

	$\geq$10 mm	FPs	6 – 9 mm	FPs
CAD-01	95%	8	71%	9
CAD-21	51%	13	71%	13
CAD-41	85%	13	81%	6
ECAD	95%	9	81%	7

Figure 3 represents the overall detection accuracy of ECAD and those of individual CAD systems for polypoid and flat lesions in terms of free-response receiver operating characteristic (FROC) curves. Importantly, for flat lesions (n=13), the detection sensitivity of ECAD was 92% with a median of 7 FP detections per patient, whereas CAD-01 detected 77% of the flat lesions with 8 FP detections, CAD-21 detected 54% with 13 FP detections, and CAD-41 detected 85% with 12 FP detections per patient.

4   Discussion

Our preliminary results indicate that an ensemble CAD scheme can indeed provide higher overall detection accuracy than that of individual CAD systems in CTC. In particular, an ensemble scheme may be used for improving the detection accuracy of CAD for subtle lesions such as flat lesions, without compromising the established high detection accuracy for polypoid lesions.

The computational burden for an ensemble CAD scheme is higher than that for conventional CAD, because it is necessary to calculate the results for multiple CAD systems. However, such computations are highly parallelizable, and high-performance computing solutions are becoming increasingly affordable. Therefore, the added computational burden is not likely to be a practical issue.

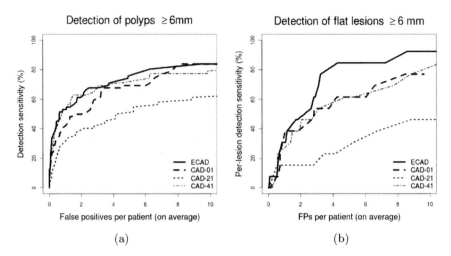

Fig. 3. Per-lesion detection accuracy of the ensemble scheme (black line) and individual CAD systems (dotted lines) for (a) polyps and (b) flat lesions

Another issue is how to select the CAD systems for the ensemble. In this study, we considered an ensemble of three CAD systems that were selected manually. For finding an optimal combination, it may be necessary to calculate the detection results for several CAD systems and to select a suitable combination by use of an optimization algorithm. This remains a topic for future study.

Acknowledgments. The project described was partly supported by a grant from the Prevent Cancer Foundation and Grant Numbers R21CA140934, R03CA139600, R01CA095279, and R01CA131718 from National Cancer Institute (NCI). We thank Partners Research Computing for providing high-performance computing services.

References

1. Winawer, S.J., Fletcher, R.H., Miller, L., et al.: Colorectal Cancer Screening: Clinical Guidelines and Rationale. Gastroenterology 112, 594–642 (1997)
2. Levin, B., Lieberman, D.A., McFarland, B., et al.: Screening and Surveillance for the Early Detection of Colorectal Cancer and Adenomatous Polyps, 2008: a Joint Guideline from the American Cancer Society, the US Multi-Society Task Force on Colorectal Cancer and the American College of Radiology. CA Cancer J. Clin. 58, 130–160 (2008)
3. Johnson, C.D., Chen, M.H., Toledano, A.Y., et al.: Accuracy of CT Colonography for Detection of Large Adenomas and Cancers. N. Engl. J. Med. 359, 1207–1217 (2008)
4. Pickhardt, P.J.: Differential Diagnosis of Polypoid Lesions seen at CT Colonography (Virtual Colonoscopy). Radiographics 24, 1535–1556 (2004)

5. Dachman, A.H., Obuschowski, N.A., Hoffmeister, J.W., et al.: Effect of Computer-Aided Detection for CT Colonography in a Multireader, Multicase Trial. Radiology 256, 827–835 (2010)
6. Lawrence, E.M., Pickhardt, P.J., Kim, D.H., Robbins, J.B.: Colorectal Polyps: Stand-Alone Performance of Computer-Aided Detection in a Large Asymptomatic Screening Population. Radiology 256, 791–798 (2010)
7. Yoshida, H., Näppi, J.: CAD in CT Colonography without and with Oral Contrast Agents: Progress and Challenges. Comput. Med. Imaging Graph 31, 267–284 (2007)
8. Hein, P.A., Krug, L.D., Romano, V.C., Kandel, S., Hamm, B., Rogalla, P.: Computer-Aided Detection in Computed Tomography Colonography with Full Fecal Tagging: Comparison of Standalone Performance of 3 Automated Polyp Detection Systems. Can Assoc. Radiol. J. 61, 102–108 (2010)
9. Park, H.S., Kim, S.H., Kim, J.H., et al.: Computer-Aided Polyp Detection on CT Colonography: Comparison of Three Systems in a High-Risk Human Population. Eur. J. Radiol. 75, 147–157 (2010)
10. Kuncheva, L.: Combining Pattern Classifiers: Methods and Algorithms. Wiley Interscience (2004)
11. Niemeijer, M., Loog, M., Abràmoff, M.D., Viergever, M.A., Prokop, M., van Ginneken, B.: On Combining Computer-Aided Detection Systems. IEEE Trans. Med. Imaging 30, 215–223 (2011)
12. van Ginneken, B., Armato III, S.G., de Hoop, B., et al.: Comparing and Combining Algorithms for Computer-Aided Detection of Pulmonary Nodules in Computed Tomography Scans: The ANODE09 Study. Med. Image Anal. 14, 707–722 (2010)
13. Näppi, J., Yoshida, H.: Fully Automated Three-Dimensional Detection of Polyps in Fecal-Tagging CT Colonography. Acad. Radiol. 14, 287–300 (2007)
14. Yoshida, H., Näppi, J.: Three-Dimensional Computer-Aided Diagnosis Scheme for Detection of Colonic Polyps. IEEE Trans. Med. Imaging 20, 1261–1274 (2001)
15. Näppi, J., Yoshida, H.: Feature-Guided Analysis for Reduction of False Positives in CAD of Polyps for Computed Tomographic Colonography. Med. Phys. 30, 1592–1601 (2003)
16. Näppi, J., Yoshida, H.: Automated Detection of Polyps with CT Colonography: Evaluation of Volumetric Features for Reduction of False-Positive Findings. Acad. Radiol. 9, 386–397 (2002)
17. Kupinski, M.A., Edwards, D.C., Giger, M.L., Metz, C.E.: Ideal Observer Approximation using Bayesian Classification Neural Networks. IEEE Trans. Med. Imaging 20, 886–899 (2001)
18. Breiman, L.: Random Forests. Machine Learning 45, 5–32 (2001)
19. Ambroise, C., McLachlan, J.H.: Selection Bias in Gene Extraction on the Basis of Microarray Gene-Expression Data. PNAS 99, 6562–6566 (2002)

Automated Detection of Colorectal Lesions in Non-cathartic CT Colonography

Janne J. Näppi[1], Stefan Gryspeerdt[2], Philippe Lefere[2],
Michael Zalis[1], and Hiroyuki Yoshida[1]

[1] Department of Radiology,
Massachusetts General Hospital and Harvard Medical School,
25 New Chardon Street, Suite 400C, Boston, MA 02114, USA
jnappi@partners.org, yoshida.hiro@mgh.harvard.edu
[2] Department of Radiology, Stedelijk Ziekenhuis,
Bruggesteenweg 90, 8800 Roeselare, Belgium

Abstract. Cathartic bowel preparation is a major barrier in implementing clinically feasible colorectal screening programs. We developed a fully automated computer-aided detection (CAD) scheme for non-cathartic computed tomographic colonography (CTC). In a pilot evaluation with an independent testing set of 46 clinical non-cathartic CTC cases, the CAD scheme detected 100% of large ≥ 10 mm lesions with 3.7 false-positive (FP) detections per patient and 90% of ≥ 6 mm lesions with 5.0 FP detections per patient, on average. The results indicate that CAD can detect colorectal lesions with high accuracy in non-cathartic CTC.

Keywords: computer-aided detection, noncathartic, cathartic-free, laxative-free, computed tomographic colonography, CT colonography, x-ray tomography, virtual colonoscopy.

1   Introduction

Although colorectal cancer is the second leading cause of cancer deaths in Western countries, it would be largely preventable. Most colorectal cancers develop from initially benign polyps: therefore, early removal of polyps can prevent later development of cancer.

A large-scale colorectal screening scheme could be implemented by use of computed tomographic colonography (CTC), followed optionally by therapeutic colonoscopy for removing significant CTC-detected lesions [1]. At present, patients need to be prepared for colorectal examination by CTC and colonoscopy with thorough cathartic bowel cleansing. This cathartic cleansing has been identified as the single most important reason why less than 40% of age-eligible adults participate in colorectal examinations [2,3]. Catharsis interrupts daily activities, it causes diarrhea and abdominal discomfort, and it may not be suitable for elderly or fragile patients. Thus, to maximize patient adherence to colorectal screening guidelines, bowel preparation should be minimized.

H. Yoshida et al. (Eds.): Abdominal Imaging 2011, LNCS 7029, pp. 68–75, 2012.
© Springer-Verlag Berlin Heidelberg 2012

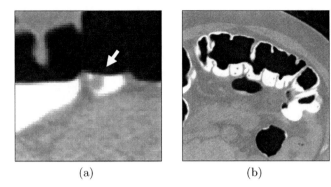

(a)   (b)

Fig. 1. (a) An example of cathartic CTC, where positive-contrast tagging was used to opacify fluid, thereby revealing a polyp (arrow) submerged in fluid. (b) An example of non-cathartic CTC, where residual materials appear not as fluid, but in solid forms.

Clinical studies have indicated that a non-cathartic CTC examination could be implemented by opacifying of residual feces in CTC images with an orally administered non-laxative positive-contrast tagging agent (Fig. 1) [4]. Then, only patients with clinically significant CTC findings (approximately 5% of patients) would need to undergo full catharsis in preparation for colonoscopy. However, the interpretation of non-cathartic CTC data is demanding, and computer-aided detection (CAD) schemes that have been developed for cathartic CTC tend to fail in non-cathartic CTC even if they have been designed to function in the presence of positive-contrast tagged fluid [5]. This is because, in non-cathartic CTC, residual materials appear in solid forms that tend to imitate the morphology of lesions (Fig. 1b). Furthermore, not all residual materials are tagged clearly and homogeneously, and tagging can also cause pseudo-enhancement that complicates the identification of soft-tissue materials in CTC [6].

In this study, we developed a fully automated CAD scheme for detecting colorectal lesions in non-cathartic CTC. Input CTC data are manipulated by use of a pseudo-enhancement correction, virtual tagging, and pseudo-subtraction methods. The region of the colon is extracted automatically from the CTC data, colorectal lesions are detected by use of volumetric shape features, and false positives are reduced by use of a neural network. The detection performance of the CAD scheme was evaluated by use of clinical non-cathartic CTC cases.

2   Methods

2.1   Correction of Pseudo-enhancement Artifacts

The positive-contrast tagging that is used for identifying residual fluid and feces in CTC can cause nearby lesions and normal structures to have unusually high

CT numbers that erroneously indicate that these materials are tagged. Thus, a high CT number can represent tagged material in one region, but a polyp in another region of the same colon [6].

To minimize pseudo-enhancement, we developed an iterative image-based correction method where pseudo-enhancement is modeled as an energy field distributed by tagged voxels [7]. A CT number v_p observed at voxel p is considered to have two components $v_p = \hat{v}_p + v_p^{\mathrm{PE}}$, where $\hat{v}_p$ is the actual radiodensity at the spatial location of voxel p, and v_p^{PE}, is the additive effect of pseudo-enhancement. To estimate v_p^{PE}, the initial pseudo-enhancement energy emitted by a nearby voxel q and received by voxel p is modeled as

$$r_q^0(p) = \frac{C}{\sqrt{2\pi}\sigma_1(v_q)} \exp(-\frac{1}{2}(\frac{D(p,q)}{\sigma_1(v_q)})^2), \tag{1}$$

where $\sigma_1(\bullet)$ is a parameter function to be optimized, $D(p,q)$ represents the spatial distance between the voxels q and p, and C is a scaling constant. At subsequent iterations, voxel p receives pseudo-enhancement energy from all surrounding voxels. The pseudo-enhancement energy is redistributed similarly to Eq. (1), except that, instead of $\sigma_1(\bullet)$, a second parameter function, $\sigma_2(\bullet)$ is used that causes the available energy to decrease [7]. The iteration terminates when the redistributable energy becomes negligible, after which the observed CT numbers are corrected by subtracting of the estimated (distributed) pseudo-enhancement energy from the CTC data.

The parameter functions $\sigma_1(\bullet)$ and $\sigma_2(\bullet)$ were optimized by comparison of unenhanced and corrected pseudo-enhanced CTC data at known tagging levels in a colon phantom [7]. After the pseudo-enhancement correction, the CT numbers represent materials in CTC data according to the standard Hounsfield unit (HU) scale (Fig. 2).

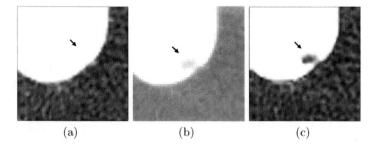

(a)   (b)   (c)

Fig. 2. (a) A pseudo-enhanced polyp (arrow) is invisible in a soft-tissue intensity display window. (b) The polyp can be seen in a wide intensity display window. (c) After pseudo-enhancement correction, the polyp is visible in the soft-tissue intensity display window.

2.2   Virtual Tagging of Poorly Opacified Feces

The observed radiodensity of tagged material tends to be diluted by the partial-volume effect at the interface between lumen air and tagged materials [8]. In non-cathartic CTC, such regions can imitate the appearance of colorectal lesions. To enhance the tagging effect within these regions, we model the colon surface based upon the Bayes' theorem as

$$P(C|V,G) = \frac{P(C)P(V,G|C)}{P(V,G)} \sim P(C)P(V,G|C), \tag{2}$$

where C is a binary category variable with two outcomes, "S" (surface) or "N" (non-surface), and V and G denote statistical feature variables of the observed CT number and its gradient magnitude at a voxel. The category $L \in \{S, N\}$ that best explains the observed CT number v and the gradient magnitude g can be derived from the maximum a posteriori estimate,

$$\hat{C} = \text{argmax}_L P(C = L)P(V = v, G = g|C = L). \tag{3}$$

Voxels that are not indicated as colonic surface by the model are assigned a high CT number: this complements physical tagging by enhancing poorly tagged residual materials (Fig. 3).

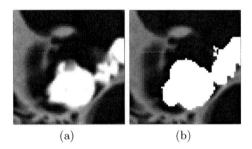

(a)   (b)

Fig. 3. (a) Poorly tagged region with untagged stool. (b) Virtual tagging complements physical tagging by enhancing poorly tagged regions in the CTC data.

2.3   Pseudo-subtraction of Tagged Materials

Because positive-contrast tagging can have unpredictable effects on shape calculations [6], we perform pseudo-subtraction of tagged materials from CTC data according to

$$\dot{v}_p = -1000 + \frac{1000 + t_T}{1 + \exp(v_p - \frac{1}{2}(t_T + t_U))}, \tag{4}$$

where v_p is the observed CT number with $t_U < v_p < t_T$, and $t_U \approx 100$ HU and $t_T \approx 200$ HU are predefined CT-number thresholds of the highest clearly untagged and lowest clearly tagged materials in the HU scale, respectively. If $v_p \leq t_U$, $\dot{v}_p = v_p$, whereas if $v_p \geq t_T$, $\dot{v}_p = -1000$. This application of soft thresholding compensates for measurement errors in the observed CT numbers.

2.4   Detection of Colorectal Lesions

The region of the colon is extracted automatically from CTC data by use of a fully automated scheme that tracks the colonic lumen based upon automatically identified, anatomy-based landmarks in the colon [6]. The region of the colon is tracked completely even if there are several collapsed lumen regions.

For detection of lesions, a thick volumetric region encompassing the colonic mucosa is extracted. Local volumetric shape features are calculated within the extracted region [6,9]. The regions of detected lesions are extracted by use of a dedicated segmentation algorithm [6].

False-positive (FP) detections are minimized by use of a neural network based on shape and texture features of candidate detections [6]. The neural network calculates the likelihood that a detection represents a true lesion. The final detected lesions are the detections with the highest lesion-likelihood values [9].

2.5   Evaluation Methods

Before evaluation, the CAD scheme was trained to detect colorectal lesions from an independent training database of 82 reduced-preparation CTC cases. These patients were prepared for CTC with a reduced volume of laxatives and with fecal tagging by 50 mL of barium [10].

The detection performance of the pre-trained CAD scheme was evaluated by use of *free-response receiver operating characteristic* (FROC) analysis that yields lesion-specific detection sensitivity as a function of the number of FP detections. The FROC curves were generated by thresholding of the lesion-likelihood values calculated by the CAD scheme. A computer-detected lesion candidate was considered as a true-positive detection if the distance between the center of the lesion candidate and that of a colonoscopy-confirmed lesion was within the diameter of the lesion in CTC data. All other detections, including multiple FP detections of the same region, were counted as different FP detections.

The performance of the proposed scheme was compared with that of a conventional CAD scheme that had been developed previously for cathartic CTC [9]. Statistical significance was assessed by use of the paired Student's t-test.

Sources of FP detections were analyzed by visual review of the detections reported by the CAD scheme. Standard 2D and 3D views of a CTC reading workstation were used.

3   Materials

The independent testing set included 46 patients. No bowel cleansing was performed in preparation for CTC. Instead, 30 patients were advised to drink an apple-flavored barium suspension with meals for one or two days prior to CTC, and the other 16 patients were advised to drink 10 mL of non-ionic iodine diluted in beverages with meals for two days prior to CTC. The CT acquisition was performed in the supine and prone positions by use of a total of four CT scanners (LightSpeed Plus, LightSpeed Ultra, or LightSpeed 16, GE Medical Systems, Milwaukee, WI, USA; Sensation 64, Siemens Medical Solutions, Malvern, PA, USA) with $1.0 - 2.5$ mm collimations, $0.7 - 2.5$ mm reconstruction intervals, $28 - 110$ mA currents, and $120 - 140$ kVp voltages.

To establish the ground truth, we performed conventional colonoscopy on the patients within one week after the CTC. Expert radiologists correlated the colonoscopy findings with the CTC image data.

4   Results

There were 10 colonoscopy-confirmed, biopsy-proved adenomas or carcinomas. There were 4 adenomas or carcinomas ≥ 10 mm in three patients, and 6 adenomas $6 - 9$ mm in three other patients.

Figure 4 shows the FROC curve for the detection of lesions ≥ 6 mm, where the proposed scheme (solid line) yielded a per-lesion detection sensitivity of 90% (9/10) with 5.0 FP detections per patient (i.e., per two volumetric CT scans). The dotted line indicates the performance of the CAD scheme that did not use the pseudo-enhancement correction, virtual tagging, and pseudo-subtraction methods. The improvement in detection sensitivity by the proposed scheme was statistically significant ($p < 0.05$). For lesions ≥ 10 mm, the detection sensitivity was 100% (4/4), with 3.7 FP detections per patient.

The largest sources of FP CAD detections included untagged solid feces adhering to the colonic wall (55%), prominent folds (10%), and inhomogeneously tagged feces (8%).

5   Discussion

The results of this pilot study indicate that CAD can yield high accuracy in the detection of clinically significant lesions in non-cathartic CTC. The detection performance is comparable to that reported previously for CAD in cathartic CTC [11].

Analysis of the sources of FP detections indicates that untagged feces adhering to the colonic wall are the single largest source of false positives in automated detection for non-cathartic CTC. This indicates that CAD may not be able to compensate fully for all shortcomings of bowel preparation. It is desirable to improve and optimize the physical non-cathartic preparation to minimize the presence of completely untagged feces.

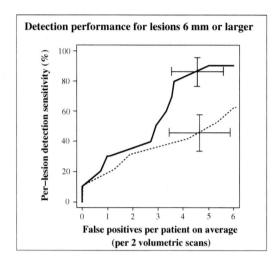

Fig. 4. FROC curves of the per-lesion accuracy of automated detection of lesions ≥6 mm: solid line indicates the detection performance with and dotted line without the pseudo-enhancement correction, virtual tagging, and pseudo-subtraction methods

6   Conclusions

Cathartic cleansing is a major barrier to implementing clinically acceptable large-scale screening programs for colorectal cancer, which is currently the second leading cause of cancer deaths in the Western countries. We developed a fully automated CAD scheme for the detection of colorectal lesions in non-cathartic CTC. Pilot evaluation with an independent testing database of 46 clinical non-cathartic CTC cases demonstrated that the CAD scheme can yield a clinically acceptable accuracy in the detection of clinically significant lesions in non-cathartic CTC.

Acknowledgments. The project described was partly supported by a grant from the Prevent Cancer Foundation and Grant Numbers R21CA140934, R03CA139600, R01CA095279, and R01CA131718 from National Cancer Institute (NCI). We thank Partners Research Computing for providing high-performance computing services.

References

1. Levin, B., Lieberman, D.A., McFarland, B., Andrews, K.S., et al.: Screening and Surveillance for the Early Detection of Colorectal Cancer and Adenomatous Polyps, 2008: a Joint Guideline from the American Cancer Society, the US Multi-Society Task Force on Colorectal Cancer, and the American College of Radiology. Gastroenterology 134, 1570–1595 (2008)

 2. Beebe, T., Johnson, C.D., Stoner, S.M., Anderson, K.J., Limburg, P.J.: Assessing Attitudes Toward Laxative Preparation in Colorectal Cancer Screening and Effects on Future Testing: Potential Receptivity to Computed Tomographic Colonography. Mayo Clinic. Proc. 82, 666–671 (2007)
 3. Meissner, H.I., Breen, N., Klabunde, C.N., Vernon, S.W.: Patterns of Colorectal Cancer Screening Uptake among Men and Women in the United States. Cancer Epidemiol Biomarkers Prev. 15, 389–394 (2006)
 4. Johnson, C.D., Manduca, A., Fletcher, J.G., MacCarty, R.L., Carston, M.J., Harmsen, W.S., Mandrekar, J.N.: Noncathartic CT Colonography with Stool Tagging: Performance with and without Electronic Stool Subtraction. Am. J. Roentgenol. 190, 361–366 (2008)
 5. Näppi, J., Yoshida, H.: Automated Scheme for Preparation-Independent Detection of Colorectal Lesions with Comparison to Conventional CAD in CT colonography. In: H. Yoshida (ed.) Proc MICCAI 2008 Workshop on Computational and Visualization Challenges in the New Era of Virtual Colonoscopy, pp. 127–134 (2008)
 6. Näppi, J., Yoshida, H.: Fully Automated Three-Dimensional Detection of Polyps in Fecal-Tagging CT Colonography. Acad. Radiol. 25, 287–300 (2007)
 7. Näppi, J., Yoshida, H.: Adaptive Correction of the Pseudo-Enhancement of CT Attenuation for Fecal-Tagging CT Colonography. Med. Image Anal. 12, 413–426 (2008)
 8. Näppi, J., Lefere, P., Gryspeerdt, S., Yoshida, H.: Two Automated Methods for Excluding Polyp-Imitating Residual Feces in Laxative-Free CT Colonography. Int. J. Comp. Assisted Radiol. Surg. 3(S1), 192–193 (2008)
 9. Yoshida, H., Näppi, J.: Three-Dimensional Computer-Aided Diagnosis Scheme for Detection of Colonic Polyps. IEEE Trans. Med. Imaging 20, 1261–1274 (2001)
10. Lefere, P., Gryspeerdt, S., Marrannes, J., Baekelandt, M., Van Holsbeeck, B.: CT Colonography after Fecal Tagging with Reduced Cathartic Cleansing and a Reduced Volume of Barium. Am. J. Roentgenol. 184, 1836–1842 (2005)
11. Yoshida, H., Näppi, J.: CAD in CT Colonography without and with Oral Contrast Agents: Progress and Challenges. Comput. Med. Imaging Graphics 31, 267–284 (2007)

Integration of Valley Orientation Distribution for Polyp Region Identification in Colonoscopy

Jorge Bernal, Javier Sánchez, and Fernando Vilariño

Computer Vision Center and Computer Science Department, Campus Universitat
Autònoma de Barcelona, 08193 Bellaterra, Barcelona, Spain
jbernal@cvc.uab.es

Abstract. This work presents a region descriptor based on the integration of the information that the depth of valleys image provides. The depth of valleys image is based on the presence of intensity valleys around polyps due to the image acquisition. Our proposed description method consists of defining, for each point, a series of radial sectors around it and then accumulate the maxima of the depth of valleys image only if the orientation of the intensity valley coincides with the orientation of the sector above. We apply our descriptor to a prior segmentation of the images and we present promising results on polyp detection, outperforming another approach that also integrates depth of valleys information.

Keywords: Colonoscopy, Polyp Detection, VO-DOVA descriptor.

1 Introduction

Colon cancer's survival rate depends on the stage in which it is detected, decreasing from rates higher than 95% in the first stages to rates lower than 35% in stages IV and V [9]; hence the importance of detecting it early by using screening techniques, such as colonoscopy [4].

Intensity valleys appear to surround polyps as the light of the colonoscope and the camera are in the same direction, and for this reason, they are proposed as a cue to detect polyps by means of computer vision techniques [2]. In this paper we present a novel region descriptor built on the concept of the depth of valleys image (DoV image), which combines valley localization given by a valleys detector with the intensity information provided by morphological gradient.

We present in this paper the Valley Orientation-Depth of Valleys Accumulation descriptor (VO-DOVA) which consists of accumulating, by using a series of radial sectors, the maxima of the DoV image. This descriptor will be incorporated into a polyp detection scheme in order to classify previously segmented regions into polyp containing or not. In this case, if a point is surrounded by a boundary constituted by points with high value in the DoV image, the accumulation value for this point will be high. We also consider the orientation of the valleys that were used to build the DoV image in a way such if the orientation of a maxima of the depth of valleys image is not similar to the orientation of the sector that would accumulate it, this value would not be considered.

H. Yoshida et al. (Eds.): Abdominal Imaging 2011, LNCS 7029, pp. 76–83, 2012.
© Springer-Verlag Berlin Heidelberg 2012

The structure of the paper is as it follows: in Section 2 we introduce previous approaches on polyp detection in colonoscopy videos. In Section 3 we present our polyp detection method. In Section 4 we show our experimental setup along with polyp detection results. Finally we finish this paper in Section 5 with the main conclusions extracted from our work and our proposals for future work.

2 Related Work

Polyp detection in colonoscopy videos has been an active field of research during the last 20 years and it has gained the interest of several research groups, although the lack of a public database makes it difficult to make a proper comparison between different approaches. If we had to divide the different approaches, we would do it into shape-based (which normally approximate polyps as elliptical shapes) and texture-based approaches.

Shape-based approaches aim to fit the shapes which polyps commonly have on the test images. Many of them start with a basic segmentation such as watershed and try to fit polyp shapes in the segmented regions. Belonging to this group we have the work of [5], which consists of fitting ellipses into the frontiers obtained after a first segmentation, and then classifying candidate regions by considering curvature, distance to edges and intensity value. The work presented in [6], relies on a first watershed segmentation and then performs an edge detection in each of the R, G and B channels after applying a contrast enhancement algorithm. In order to classify the several regions (connected by closed edges) this method uses area, color and elliptical shape.

Texture-based approaches aim at selecting an adequate texture descriptor and apply it to the image. In the work shown in [7], polyps are detected by combining wavelets coefficients extraction and co-ocurrence matrices and then learning via neural networks. A method which combines the use of local binary patterns and grey-level co-ocurrence matrices is presented in [1].

3 Valley Orientation-Depth of Valleys Accumulation Descriptor

Before explaining the VO-DOVA descriptor, we will introduce the DoV image. This DoV image [2] combines the information obtained from the ridges and valleys detector [8] with the one that the morphological gradient provides (see equation 1), to define valleys in both localization and intensity:

$$\forall i, j \in \mathbf{I} \quad DoV(i,j) = V(i,j) \cdot MG(i,j) \tag{1}$$

where DoV stands for the DoV image, V for the output of the ridges and valleys detector and MG for the morphological gradient image, being their corresponding values normalized to unit (although this does not mean they are binarized) and their corresponding scale parameters equal. Under the assumption that polyps generally present elliptical shapes with soft boundaries (that

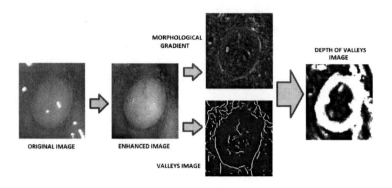

Fig. 1. Definition of the depth of valleys image

show extremal values in the valleys image), our aim is to define a descriptor that is able to to accurately find those image regions that are inside either completely or even partially closed boundaries in the DoV image (see Figure 1).

One first approach could be to fit elliptical shapes inside the boundaries that appear on the DoV image, following the basis of some of the methods depicted in Section 2. The Ellipse Fitting-Depth of Valleys Accumulation algorithm (EF-DOVA) presented in [3] is also built on this idea, although in this case the method does not fit ellipses to boundaries but aims at approximating ellipses using accumulative information from the entire region.

In our case, we will integrate the information from the DoV image by using a series of radial sectors to accumulate the maxima of the DoV image. The VO-DOVA algorithm has the following steps:

- *Obtaining the enhanced DoV image:* The first step will consist of calculating the DoV image. As specular highlights have an impact in the valleys detection [2] we mitigate their effect by approximating what should really should be under them, by substituting the affected pixels by a linear combination of the values around them. The valley detector used to obtain the DV image needs of two parameters, differentiation and integration sigma [8]. The latter should be equal to the size of the structural element used in the calculation of the morphological gradient in order to work in the same scale.
- *Depth of Valleys accumulation:* We denote a point as interior to a structure if it is surrounded by boundaries constituted by pixels with high value in the DoV image (up to a threshold value). We define a series of radial sectors centred in each point and we accumulate, for each sector, the maxima of the portion of the DoV image that falls under it. We use the orientation of the valleys provided by the valleys detector in order to filter which maxima points should be accumulated. As each sector will comprise a series of angles, we will only accumulate maxima of the DoV image whose orientation is within a range of angles defined from those that the sector covers. The accumulation algorithm needs three parameters: 1) Minimum radius of the sector; 2) Maximum radius of the sector, and 3) number of sectors.

We can see how VO-DOVA works by observing Figure 2. For each point we define a series of sectors, shown in red, and we only accumulate those maxima points with similar orientation to the particular sector. In this case we will only accumulate those maxima whose orientation coincides with the range of angles covered by the sector (depicted as green arrows surrounded by yellow boxes) and not those whose orientation is very different (depicted as blue arrows).

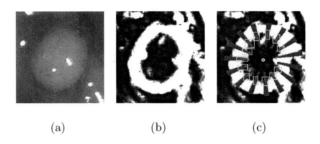

(a)   (b)   (c)

Fig. 2. VO-DOVA descriptor: (a) Original image; (b) Depth of valleys image. (c) VO-DOVA descriptor, where points with suitable orientation are marked with green arrows and surrounded by a yellow box, points with wrong orientation are marked with blue arrows and sectors are shown in red.

We show in Figure 3 how VO-DOVA algorithm would perform in the whole frame. We can see in Figure 3 (c) VO-DOVA accumulation results. Brighter areas in the image correspond to pixels whose accumulation value is high, conversely to dark areas which correspond to pixels with low accumulation value. In order to make the results more understandable, we shown in Figure 3 (d) how VO-DOVA descriptor places points with high accumulation value inside the polyp region, placing also the maxima of the accumulation inside the polyp region.

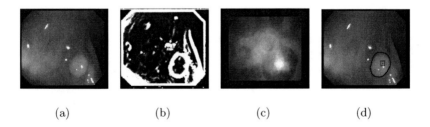

(a)   (b)   (c)   (d)

Fig. 3. Example of VO-DOVA (a) Original image; (b) Depth of Valleys image, and (c) Accumulation image. (d) Result image, where the polyp is surrounded by a blue line, the points with high accumulation value are shown in green and the maxima of the VO-DOVA descriptor is marked as an orange square surrounded by a red frame.

4   Experimental Results

To test the performance of our novel VO-DOVA descriptor, we have created a database with different studies of polyp appearance. We were provided 15 random cases, in which the experts (physicians) annotated all the sequences showing polyps, and a random sample of 20 frames per sequence was obtained. The experts guaranteed that all these 20 frames showed a significantly different point of view (as it can be seen in Figure 4 (c) and (d)) which resulted in the rejection of similar frames. This allows us to maximize the variability of the images used, while not jeopardizing any bias at all. As we are interested in the performance of our descriptor when detecting polyps, our database will contain only frames with polyps, up to 300 different images.

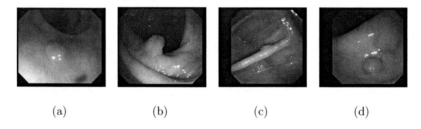

(a)   (b)   (c)   (d)

Fig. 4. Polyp examples (a) flat (b) peduncular (c) lateral view (d) overhead view

Our whole polyp detection scheme consists of 3 stages, namely: region segmentation, region description and region classification. As we mentioned in Section 1, we will use as the region segmentation stage the results provided in [2], which provides, for each image, a reduced number of regions one of them containing a polyp. In the case of region description, we will use both EF-DOVA [3] and the novel VO-DOVA. In the case of EF-DOVA we will use the combination of parameters values that gave better detection results whereas for VO-DOVA we have used the following set of parameters values: 1) Minimum radius ([30, 40, 50]); 2) Maximum radius ([80, 100, 120]), and 3) Number of sectors ([60, 120, 180]).

We will classify the final segmented regions according to their maxima of the DOVA descriptor. In this case we have considered two possible classification scenarios, namely region-based and frame based. In the former we will classify for each frame each one of the final segmented regions according to their descriptor value whereas in the latter we will only consider two regions in each frame: the one that we predict the polyp is inside (according to the value of the DOVA descriptor) and the one where we predict there is no polyp inside. In order to evaluate the performance of both descriptors we calculate, for each image, the number of True Positives (TP), False Positives (FP), True Negatives (TN) and False Negatives (FN). We will also present precision, recall, accuracy, and specificity results for the best combination of parameters in terms of highest additive value for the cited measures, along with providing ROC and PR curves.

As it can be seen in Table 1, there is a difference between the performance of both descriptors for both mentioned criteria (frame-based criteria only affects the number of FP and TN, which improves EF-DOVA results, damaged by the high number of FP). EF-DOVA outperforms VO-DOVA in terms of TP and FN, that is, it detects polyps better but we can also observe that it performs worse in terms of FP and TN. Therefore, the difference between EF-DOVA and VO-DOVA is that the former places more maxima of accumulation in the image whereas the latter, where it places a maxima, it is more likely to be a polyp. We can observe this in the precision, accuracy or specificity results, where VO-DOVA outperforms EF-DOVA, which is only better in terms of recall.

Table 1. EF-DOVA and VO-DOVA performance results

	EF-DOVA		VO-DOVA	
	Region-based	Frame-based	Region-based	Frame-based
TP	291	293	267	265
FP	655	147	31	31
TN	1638	153	2262	269
FN	9	7	33	35
Precision	30.76%	66.59%	89.59%	89.52%
Recall	97%	97.66%	89%	88.33%
Accuracy	74.61%	74.33%	97.53%	89%
Specificity	71.43%	51%	98.64%	89.66%
AUC ROC	0.85	0.63	0.96	0.77
AUC PR	0.3	0.38	0.67	0.46

We show in Figure 5 a graphical comparison in polyp detection between EF-DOVA and VO-DOVA. We can observe how EF-DOVA places more maxima inside the polyp region (shown in yellow) but also places maxima outside the polyp region (shown in red). We can also see how EF-DOVA places the maxima of accumulation (marked as an orange square) outside the polyp for the two examples, whereas VO-DOVA places them inside the polyp region.

We can also observe the superior performance that VO-DOVA provides by observing the ROC and PR curves in Figure 6. In terms of area under curve values, we outperform EF-DOVA, for our best combination of parameter values, for ROC and PR curves, as it can be seen in Table 1. The curves for EF-DOVA present more abrupt changes because we only consider 33 possible accumulation values from 0 to 8, therefore we can only have 33 threshold values. In the case of VO-DOVA the accumulation value and threshold values can go from 0 to 255.

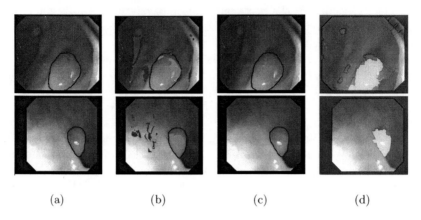

(a)   (b)   (c)   (d)

Fig. 5. Comparative results (a) Original images (b) Polyp detection via EF-DOVA (c) Polyp detection via VO-DOVA. (d) Classified image (yellowish part denote polyp regions, reddish part non-polyp regions.

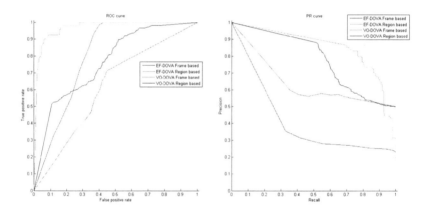

Fig. 6. ROC and PR curves for both EF-DOVA and VO-DOVA

5   Conclusions

In this paper a novel approach to polyp detection in colonoscopy images has been presented by using valley information of the image. The combination of the output of a ridges and valleys detector and the morphological gradient image give us information about valleys' location and intensity. We introduce our novel VO-DOVA descriptor that defines when a pixel is interior to a depth of valleys boundary (complete or incomplete) and when it is not. The direct application of VO-DOVA descriptor into a detection scheme provides promising results on polyp detection, specially when detecting what is not a polyp in the image, letting discard most of the image with no risk of losing polyp information.

The future work may consist of introducing VO-DOVA results earlier in the detection process to help segmentation by, for instance, developing marker-based segmentation using the maxima of the VO-DOVA descriptor. Another possible research line could be to study which description cues (such as color or texture) can be added to improve results. Finally, VO-DOVA's could probably benefit from a multi-scale approach that may also lead to have less parameters.

Acknowledgements. This work was supported in part by a research grant from Universitat Autònoma de Barcelona 471-01-3/08, by the Spanish Government through the founded project "COLON-QA" (TIN2009-10435) and by research programme Consolider Ingenio 2010: MIPRCV (CSD2007-00018).

References

1. Ameling, S., Wirth, S., Paulus, D., Lacey, G., Vilarino, F.: Texture-based polyp detection in colonoscopy. In: Bildverarbeitung für die Medizin 2009, pp. 346–350 (2009)
2. Bernal, J., Sánchez, J., Vilariño, F.: A Region Segmentation Method for Colonoscopy Images Using a Model of Polyp Appearance. In: Vitrià, J., Sanches, J.M., Hernández, M. (eds.) IbPRIA 2011. LNCS, vol. 6669, pp. 134–142. Springer, Heidelberg (2011)
3. Bernal, J., Sánchez, J., Vilariño, F.: Depth of Valleys Accumulation Algorithm for Object Detection. In: Pattern Recognition and Image Analysis. Proceedings of the 14th International Conference of the Catalan Association of Artificial Intelligence, CCIA 2011 (2011)
4. Hassinger, J.P., Holubar, S.D., et al.: Effectiveness of a Multimedia-Based Educational Intervention for Improving Colon Cancer Literacy in Screening Colonoscopy Patients. Diseases of the Colon & Rectum 53(9), 1301 (2010)
5. Hwang, S., Oh, J.H., Tavanapong, W., et al.: Polyp detection in colonoscopy video using elliptical shape feature. In: IEEE International Conference on Image Processing, ICIP 2007, vol. 2. IEEE (2007)
6. Kang, J., Doraiswami, R.: Real-time image processing system for endoscopic applications. In: IEEE Canadian Conference on Electrical and Computer Engineering, vol. 3, pp. 1469–1472 (May 2003)
7. Karkanis, S.A., Iakovidis, D.K., Maroulis, D.E., et al.: Computer-aided tumor detection in endoscopic video using color wavelet features. IEEE Transactions on Information Technology in Biomedicine 7(3), 141–152 (2003)
8. López, A.M., Lumbreras, F., et al.: Evaluation of methods for ridge and valley detection. IEEE Transactions on Pattern Analysis and Machine Intelligence 21(4), 327–335 (1999)
9. Tresca, A.: The Stages of Colon and Rectal Cancer. New York Times (About.com) p. 1 (2010), http://tinyurl.com/3y4acut

Automated Detection and Diagnosis
of Crohn's Disease in CT Enterography

Janne J. Näppi[1], Dushyant V. Sahani[1], Joel G. Fletcher[2], and Hiroyuki Yoshida[1]

[1] Department of Radiology, Massachusetts General Hospital and Harvard Medical School,
25 New Chardon Street, Suite 400C, Boston, MA 02114, USA
jnappi@partners.org, yoshida.hiro@mgh.harvard.edu
[2] Department of Radiology, Mayo Clinic, 200 First Street SW, Rochester, MN 55905, USA

Abstract. Crohn's disease is an inflammatory bowel disease that has a variety of symptoms and that is increasing in prevalence. There is a need for diagnostic tools that would provide objective and reproducible measurements for guiding therapy. We developed a computer-assisted diagnosis (CAD) scheme for diagnosing mural enhancement and for detecting small-bowel obstructions of Crohn's disease in computed tomographic enterography (CTE). The scheme was evaluated on 69 patients. The values of quantitative features calculated by CAD were significantly different in the case of Crohn's disease than in normal patients. The per-patient detection sensitivity for obstructions was 93%. The results indicate that CAD can be used to provide radiologists with reliable automated quantitative interpretation of CTE data.

Keywords: Crohn's disease, enterography, computer-assisted diagnosis, computer-aided detection, small bowel, small intestine, mural enhancement.

1   Introduction

Crohn's disease (CDS) is a chronic inflammatory bowel disease that is increasing in prevalence and that affects more than half a million individuals in the United States and Canada [1]. It can cause a variety of symptoms, including abdominal pain, diarrhea, vomiting, arthritis, skin rash, inflammation of the eyes, weight loss, tiredness, and lack of concentration. Bowel obstructions are another common complication of CDS.

Currently adopted measures for characterizing inflammatory activity are largely subjective. There is an urgent need for diagnostic tools that would provide objective and reproducible measurements of inflammatory activity for stratifying Crohn's patients with global objective markers for guiding therapy [2].

CT enterography (CTE) is being used increasingly for evaluation of the small bowel [3]. However, there are several critical barriers to the usage of CTE, such as large inter-observer variability, time-consuming interpretation, and irreproducible measurements. Furthermore, the diagnostic interpretation of CTE images can be challenging (Fig. 1).

H. Yoshida et al. (Eds.): Abdominal Imaging 2011, LNCS 7029, pp. 84–90, 2012.

Our purpose in this study was to develop a *computer-assisted diagnosis* (CAD) scheme for image-based detection and characterization of CDS. We performed a pilot evaluation to characterize the performance of the scheme in identifying Crohn's patients by CTE.

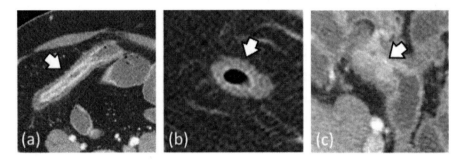

Fig. 1. Examples of active CDS (arrows) in CTE. (a) Application of neutral lumen contrast enables visualization of mural thickening. (b) Even if a contrast agent is used, the lumen may be filled partially with air. (c) In the case of an obstruction, the bowel lumen may be invisible, and the image contrast is often low.

2   Methods

2.1   Extraction of Small Bowel

Normal abdominal anatomy surrounding the small intestine was subtracted automatically by cascade application of thresholding, region growing, mathematical morphology, connected component analysis, and anatomy-based geometric contraints [4]. Surrounding air was extracted by use of region growing, and the skin line and subcutaneous fat were excluded by iterative application of intensity-based morphologic dilation, followed by 5-mm dilation to exclude the external oblique muscle layer. Next, osseous components were extracted by intensity thresholding to exclude the region outside the rib cage. Because the small bowel is located mostly below the liver, the vertical region of the liver was identified and excluded as the largest connected component with elevated intensity at the top region of the abdomen. Also, the regions of vessels with HU values >150 HU originating from the liver were excluded by application of region growing, because large vessels can imitate thread-like types of bowel obstruction.

After subtraction of the surrounding normal anatomy, an adaptive region-growing method was used for extraction of the bowel lumen. Seed points were identified as voxels that satisfy either of the primary seed tests of (1) $\mu_C - \sigma_C < x_s < \mu_C + \sigma_C$ or (2) $x_s < \mu_A$ with $\|\nabla x_s\| < t_A$, where μ_C and σ_C are the mean and standard deviation of the CT intensity values of the lumen contrast agent, and μ_A and t_A are the mean intensity of air and the largest gradient magnitude of the bowel lumen, respectively.

Because of the wide variation of the appearance of small-bowel images (Fig. 1), the primary-seed-point test may fail to establish a satisfactory number of seeds. In this case, the seeds were recomputed by use of secondary tests of (1) $\mu_C - \sigma_C < x_s < \mu_C + \sigma_C$ or (2) $x_s < \mu_A$ without the constraint of the gradient magnitude, or by use of the tertiary tests of (1) $x_0 < x_s < \max\{\mu_C + \sigma_C, x_0 + \sigma_C\}$ or (2) $x_s < \mu_A$, where x_0 is the average CT intensity value at the center of a local region. The secondary and tertiary tests tend to be effective for the types of cases illustrated in Fig. 1c, where CT intensity values are elevated and the gradient magnitude is low.

After a satisfactory number of seeds were established, region-growing was performed for definition of the outer surface of the bowel wall and mural region.

2.2   Detection of Mural Enhancement

To extract features for characterizing mural enhancement by CDS, the bowel wall region was sampled three-dimensionally by application of sample lines in the direction of the surface normal at each point of the extracted bowel surface (Fig. 2). The samples were enhanced by use of polynomial fitting [5].

Three mural features were calculated from the line samples. The *peak enhancement feature* is the highest intensity along the line sample:

$$f_{max} = \max\{f_i\}, \tag{1}$$

where f_i are the CT intensity values of the line sample. The *wall-thickness feature* characterizes the perceived horizontal magnitude, or relative thickness, of the enhanced wall region. It is calculated as

$$F_W = f_e - f_b = \tag{2}$$

$$\min\{\xi \mid f(\xi) < \mu_C, \xi > \xi_{max}\} - \max\{\xi \mid f(\xi) < \mu_C, \xi < \xi_{max}\},$$

where ξ_{max} is the location of f_{max} within the sample. The *hyper-enhancement feature* characterizes the perceived vertical magnitude, or relative intensity, of the enhancement within the wall region. It is calculated as

$$F_H = 100\% \times \frac{f_{max} - max\{f_e, f_b\}}{f_{max}}. \tag{3}$$

If the maximum intensity within the sample is higher than that at both ends of the sample, the wall will be perceived as hyper-enhanced and the value of F_H is close to 100%. On the other hand, if the maximum intensity within the sample does not differ significantly from the intensity at either end of the sample, there is no perceived hyper-enhancement, and the value of F_H will be close to 0%.

To characterize the distribution of these mural 3 features in each region of interest, we calculated the mean, standard deviation, skewness, kurtosis, and maximum values of the 3 features within each sample. Therefore, a total of 15 aggregate features were calculated to characterize mural enhancement.

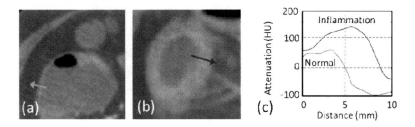

Fig. 2. (a) Blue arrow illustrates a line sample of normal bowel wall. The line samples are three-dimensional normals of the bowel surface. (b) Red arrow illustrates a line sample of inflammated wall. (c) Profile plots of the normal wall (blue line) and inflammated wall (red line) in the direction of the arrow. Normal wall (blue line) is thin and has low enhancement, whereas the inflammated wall (red line) is thick and has significant enhancement.

A *support vector machine* (SVM) classifier [6] was used to predict the presence of CDS based upon the 15 aggregate features. To avoid overfitting, the number of input features was reduced by calculation of the *Pearson correlation* between the feature statistics as $\sigma_{X,Y} = \frac{cov(X,Y)}{\sigma_x \sigma_y}$, where $cov(X,Y)$, σ_x and σ_y are the covariance and standard deviations of two features, respectively. The four least correlated features were chosen for training of the SVM. The internal SVM parameters were optimized by use of leave-one-out evaluation.

2.3   Detection of Bowel Obstructions

Thread-like strictures are bowel obstructions that appear as linear image patterns with higher intensity than that of their surrounding region.

To detect thread-like strictures, we developed a *multi-scale template matching method*. A template with orientation d_i and thickness t_j is placed at each point of the CTE image data (Fig. 3a). The accuracy of the template match is calculated as $S(d_i, t_j) = F(d_i, t_j) - R(d_i, t_j)$, where $F(d_i, t_j)$ is the average intensity of voxels under the template and $R(d_i, t_j)$ is the average intensity of voxels in the surrounding background region. The accuracy is highest when the orientation of the template matches that of the underlying linear image pattern, and the average intensity under the template is higher than that of the surrounding background.

For identifying the template parameters that yield an optimal match at a point, the calculations are performed at different thicknesses and orientations of the template (Fig. 3b and c). The most accurate match (Fig. 3d) is provided by the orientation d_{max} and thickness t_{max} for which

$$S(d_{max}, t_{max}) \geq S(d_i, t_i) \text{ for all } i = 1, .. D; j = 1, .. T. \tag{4}$$

To reduce the number of *false-positive* (FP) CAD detections, the regions detected by the method also need to satisfy a minimum value for the accuracy of the match and a minimum volumetric size [7]. The threshold values are determined from training data.

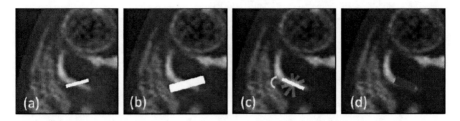

Fig. 3. Detection of obstructions based on thread-like strictures. (a) A stricture template (white rectangle) on a true obstruction (thread-like stricture). (b) A coarser-scale template. (c) The template is tested in multiple orientations. (d) Orientation and scale of the underlying linear pattern is indicated by the best-matching template (red rectangle).

To detect types of obstructions other than strictures, we developed a *blob-filtering method* to detect luminal effacament or air bubbles. These kinds of image patterns appear within partial bowel obstructions. First, the CT image function is thresholded with a value μ_o to determine potential regions of obstruction. Next, the resulting region is convoluted with the Wald kernel

$$f(x; \mu, \lambda) = [\lambda/(2\pi x^3)]^{1/2} \exp\left(-\lambda(x - \mu)^2/(2\mu^2 x)\right), \tag{5}$$

where μ and λ are the mean and scaling parameters, respectively [8]. Three-dimensional connected component analysis is used for identifying the detected lumen regions (Fig. 4). The number of FP detections is reduced based upon the clinically expected size and intensity of luminal effacement within bowel obstructions.

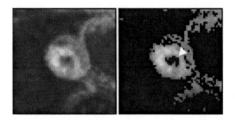

Fig. 4. Detection of obstructions based on luminal effacament. Left: obstruction with blob-like luminal effacament. (b) The red region indicated by arrowhead shows the region of detected effacement. Black regions were not considered as obstruction candidates because of their low CT value.

2.4   Clinical Materials

Sixty-nine patients with known or suspected CDS were included in the study. Prior to the CTE, the patients ingested a large volume of neutral enteric contrast to distinguish the bowel wall from water-signal luminal contents and perienteric fat. Intravenous contrast was administered to provide direct images of the entire small bowel wall and perienteric mesentery. The patients were imaged by use of high-resolution CT scanners.

To provide the ground truth regarding CDS, an unblinded gastroenterologist established the presence or absence of active CDS by use of ileocolonoscopy, the CDS activity index, serum C-reactive protein, and CTE results. An unblinded radiologist correlated the gastroenterologist's assessment with radiographically visible CTE image findings.

To provide the ground truth regarding bowel obstructions, an independent unblinded reader reviewed the operative details of surgical records of the patients from electronic hospital database. Based on the records, the locations of surgically confirmed bowel obstructions were identified visually in CTE images. There were 22 surgically confirmed strictures in 15 patients.

3   Results

3.1   Detection of Mural Enhancement

The average value of the wall-thickness feature calculated by the CAD scheme was significantly higher in the case of CDS (4.0±0.9 mm) than for normal patients (2.9±0.9 mm).   Also, the values of the hyper-enhancement feature were higher in patients with CDS (3.9±0.9%) than in normal patients (3.3±0.8%). The values of the peak enhancement feature did not differ significantly between CDS and normal patients. The result suggests that CAD can be used to provide diagnostically meaningful quantitative information for characterizing CDS.

To evaluate the potential of CAD in resolving challenging CTE cases, first the CAD scheme was trained to diagnose CDS in 46 CTE cases in which two experienced abdominal radiologists blinded to the ground truth agreed on the presence of active CDS. Next, the CAD scheme was tested with 8 CTE cases in which the radiologists disagreed on their diagnosis regarding the presence of CDS. For these 8 challenging CTE cases, the area under the receiver operating characteristic curve (A_z) of the per-patient detection accuracy of CAD for predicting the presence of CDS correctly was 0.92 [0.87,0.97]. The high detection accuracy indicates that CAD has the potential to assist radiologists in resolving challenging CTE cases.

3.2   Detection of Bowel Obstructions

Two 6-mm and 12-mm thick templates with a 15-degree angular resolution were used for detection of bowel obstructions. The CAD scheme detected 5 obstruction-like image patterns per patient, on average. The per-patient detection sensitivity for obstructions was 93%. Most of the FP CAD detections could be dismissed easily by radiologists.

The FP analysis of CAD detections indicates that image patterns of muscle and vessels generate a large number of image patterns imitating bowel obstructions (Fig. 5). This indicates that the detection accuracy of CAD could be improved significantly by improvement in the accuracy of extracting the region of the small bowel from abdominal CTE data.

Sources of FP CAD detections

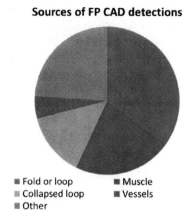

■ Fold or loop   ■ Muscle
▨ Collapsed loop   ■ Vessels
▨ Other

Fig. 5. Major sources of FP obstruction candidates (n=67) detected by the CAD scheme

4   Conclusions

The preliminary results indicate that CAD may be used for identifying active Crohn's patients and image-based sites of bowel obstruction in CTE at high sensitivity. The image-based features calculated by the CAD scheme can provide clinically meaningful quantitative information about the small bowel. Therefore, CAD can provide a useful tool for objective and reproducible diagnosis of Crohn's patients in CTE.

References

1. Loftus, E.J.: Clinical Epidemiology of Inflammatory Bowel Disease: Incidence, Prevalence, and Environmental Influences. Gastroenterology 126, 1504–1517 (2004)
2. Haens, G.R., Fedorak, R., Lemann, M., et al.: Endpoints for Clinical Trials Evaluating Disease Modification and Structural Damage in Adults with Crohn's Disease. Inflamm. Bowel Dis. 15, 1599–1604 (2009)
3. Bodily, K.D., Fletcher, J.G., Solem, C.A., et al.: Crohn Disease: Mural Attenuation and Thickness at Contrast-Enhanced CT Enterography – Correlation with Endoscopic and Histologic Findings of Inflammation. Radiology 238, 505–516 (2006)
4. Sainani, N.I., Näppi, J.J., Sahani, D.V., Yoshida, H.: Computer-Aided Detection of Small Bowel Strictures in CT Enterography (CTE) in an Emergency Setting: a Pilot Study. In: 93rd Scientific Assembly and Annual Meeting of Radiological Society of North America, p. 256 (2007)
5. Dyer, S.A., He, X.: Least-Squares Fitting of Data by Polynomials. IEEE Instrumentation & Measurement Magazine 4, 46–51 (2001)
6. Cortes, C., Vapnik, V.: Support-Vector Networks. Machine Learning 20, 273–297 (1995)
7. Sainani, N.I., Näppi, J., Sahani, D.V., Yoshida, H.: Computer-Aided Detection of Small Bowel Strictures for Emergency Radiology in CT Enterography. In: Proc. MICCAI 2010 Workshop on Computational Challenges and Clinical Opportunities in Virtual Colonoscopy and Abdominal Imaging, pp. 129—134 (2010)
8. Wald, A.: Sequential Analysis. Wiley, New York (1947)

Quantitative Evaluation of Lumbar Disc Herniation Based on MRI Image

Hongtao Jiang[4], Wei Qi[2], Qimei Liao[1], Haitao Zhao[3], Wei Lei[3], Li Guo[4],
and Hongbing Lu[1]

[1] Department of Computer Application, Fourth Military Medical University, Xi'an, China
[2] Department of Orthopaedics, Xijing Hospital, Xi'an, China
[3] Department of Radiology, Xijing Hospital, Xi'an, China
[4] Department of Medical Engineering, People's Liberation Army Hospital 89, Wei Fang, China
luhb@fmmu.edu.cn

Abstract. Lumbar disk herniation (LDH) is a common cause of low back pain in the world. Clinical studies have indicated that morphological characteristics of lumbar discs and signal intensity of patient's MRI image have close relationship with clinical outcome. In this paper, a visualization and quantitative analysis framework for LDH was developed. Based on the framework, six indexes, such as the distribution of the protruded disc, the ratio between the protruded part and the dural sac, relative signal intensity and etc, were extracted from patient MRI images and evaluated. Preliminary results indicate that there is a close relationship between these indexes and the grading of LDH.

Keywords: Lumbar disc herniation, VTK, MRI, 3D reconstruction, classification.

1   Introduction

Lumbar disk herniation (LDH) is a common cause of low back pain in the world. In China, LDH occurs in approximately 18% on average [1] and worldwide reported incidence varies from 15.2% to 30% [1]. Early diagnosis and treatment of LDH is extremely important because the earlier a slipped disc is detected, the simpler and more effective is the treatment. With the fast development of imaging technology, pre-operative studies of disc herniation morphology based on radiograph, CT and MRI images have been increased greatly for more accurate diagnosis. Among them, studies based on MRI imaging has shown great potential due to its capability on better imaging of lumbar disc and surrounding non-bone structures [2],[3].

Due to complete description and direct view of the anatomical information around disc, three-dimensional imaging has been employed as an alternative technique aiming to accurately classify and treat LDH recently. However, which quantitative index or criterion would be better to evaluate the grading of lumbar disc herniation, is still unclear. In this study, based on qualitative indexes and criteria that are used in clinics or

H. Yoshida et al. (Eds.): Abdominal Imaging 2011, LNCS 7029, pp. 91–98, 2012.

have been reported useful for disc herniation [4],[5],[6], we extract six quantitative indexes, such as the distribution of the protruded disc (DPD), the ratio between the protruded part and the dural sac (RPPDS) and relative signal intensity (RSI), and evaluate their potential for the grading of lumbar disc herniation preliminarily.

2   Methods

2.1   MRI Image Acquisitions

The patient MRI datasets of spine used for 3D reconstruction and analysis were acquired from a 3.0 Tesla scanner (SIEMENS). The scanning sequence included T2WI with parameters of matrix size: 320*320, TR/TE =4500/104ms, field of view (FOV): 240*240mm, and slice thickness: 1.489mm.

2.2   The Index Analysis System

To make quantitative analysis more accurate, the system first extracts regions of interest (ROIs) such as the whole lumbar disc between lumbar vertebra L4-L5 or L5-S1. Then fast-marching based segmentation was used to extract dural sac around. Finally contours of disc and other ROIs in each slice were further refined manually by the experienced radiologists.

2.3   Index Analysis

Based on qualitative or semi-qualitative indexes and criteria that are used in clinics or have been reported useful for disc herniation, six indexes were extracted and analyzed in this study, as described below.

The Distribution of the Protruded Disc (DPD): Previous study has indicated that the distribution of herniation along axial, sagittal and coronal direction correlates greatly with the severity degree of LDH [1]. To reflect the 3D distribution of disc herniation, a 3D coordinate was proposed in this study and several indexes was calculated based on the new coordinate. In 3D space, three orthogonal planes (plane A, plane B and plane C) were first defined, where each plane crossed the midpoint of the longest line along coronal, sagittal and axial direction respectively, as shown in Fig. 1(a). The width and height of the lumbar disc were calculated by the function of getwidth() and getheight() from VTK automatically. Then two perpendicular planes (PA and PC) were identified from the middle point while plane PB crossed the middle point of line PA. The point that three planes intersects was defined as the origin and the disc was separated into eight regions in space. Based on the build-up coordinates, the apex of the protrusion was traced and its coordinate was obtained as (x, y, z).

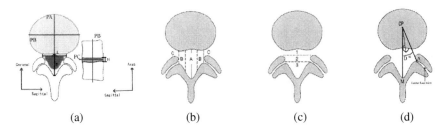

(a) (b) (c) (d)

Fig. 1. (a) The definition of the new coordinate   (b) Distribution of disc protrusion in transverse (c) Distribution of disc protrusion in coronal   (d) Horizontal deviation angle

In Fig.1, L represents the width of spinal canal, W represents the length of spinal canal and H represents the height of the posterior edge of disc. Considering irregular shape of individual canal, L and W were calculated manually with the tool of widget from VTK, and the procedure was repeated for three times to get their average values. The height of lumbar disc H was calculated by the function of getheight (). In order to eliminate value variations caused by difference patient, x/L, y/W, z/H were calculated. x/L and y/W denotes the relative degree of the disc protrusion along transverse and coronal direction respectively, as shown in Fig.1(b) and Fig.1(c). z/H represents the relative degree of the disc along axis. As shown in Fig.1 (d), horizontal deviation angle indicates the degree of deviation along the horizontal position of the disc. To make the index more robust, the three lines of CPM, CPD and CPA can easily be find by the program automatically. Then the ratio of $\angle A1/\angle A2$ is adopted in order to eliminate patient differences.

The Ratio Between the Protruded Part and the Dural Sac (RPPDS): In order to characterize the protruded degree of the nucleus pulposus, a new 3D index was designed. As shown in Fig. 2(b), two red lines represent the lower edge of the upper vertebral and the upper edge of the lower vertebral, respectively, it can be calculated as:

$$R P P D S = V_1 /(V_1 + V_2)$$

(1)

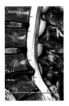

Fig.2. (a) The original MRI image   (b) Definition of RPPDS

where V_1 indicates the volume of the protruded part and V_2 indicates the corresponding volume of the spinal canal.

Relative Signal Intensity (RSI): Previous studies have indicates that signal intensity of the nucleus pulposus is closely related to disc degeneration, where disc degeneration has great relationship with lumbar disc herniation. Lumoa [7] has investigated the usefulness of RSI as an indicator of disc degeneration. In this study, RSI was also included to evaluate LDH.

To calculate RSI, regions of interest above and below the central intranuclear cleft in each nucleus pulposus and in cerebrospinal fluid (CSF) in the anterior part of the adjacent dural sac behind each vertebra were extracted, and RSI can be calculated from:

$$RSI = \frac{(SI_A \times n_A + SI_B \times n_B)/(n_A + n_B)}{SI_{CSF}} \tag{2}$$

where n_A and n_B stand for the number of pixels of ROI above and below the central intranuclear cleft in each nucleus pulposus, respectively, and SI_{CSF} for the median value of the signal intensity measurements of the CSF in the subject.

3   Results

MRI image datasets acquired from 20 patients with scanning parameters described above were used for preliminary evaluate of the proposed method. The improved low back pain evaluation table recommended by the Orthopetic Association of Japan is employed to rank patients' (nine males and eleven females) conditions. The total score is 30 points. Points no higher than 10 indicate a mild condition and points between 10 and 20 indicate a mediate condition. A severe condition is characterized by points higher than 20. The 20 patients are named from A to T, with increased severity of condition. The first seven patients (A-G) were diagnosed as bulge, patients H-S were diagnosed as protrusion, and patient T was extrusion.

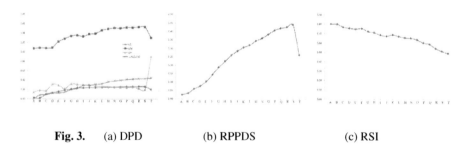

Fig. 3.   (a) DPD   (b) RPPDS   (c) RSI

The scatter diagrams between each index and patients are shown in Fig.3(a)-(c). From Fig.3, we could see that except for patient T, indexes x/L, y/W, $\angle A1/\angle A2$ and RPPDS increase with the severity of LDH, and RSI decreases with the severity. The RSI value of patient T is below 0.5, the rest are over 0.5. There is no regular trend for the change of z/H.

The number of patients with extrusion is only one. Therefore statistical test has been performed only to patients with bulge and protrusion.

According to the result of rank sum test shown in table 1, we can conclude that indexes x/L, y/W, $\angle A1/\angle A2$, RPPDS, and RSI are statistically significant (p<0.05). Index z/H has no statistically significant difference between different groups (p=0.499).

The result of Spearman rank correlation test is shown in table 2. RIS is negatively correlated to the severity of LDH and the correlation is relatively high (r=-0.837, p<0.05), which is statistically significant.

Table 1. Result of Rank Sum Test

Indexes	Group	Num	Mean Rank	Sum of Ranks	Z	P value
	Bulge	7	4.57	32.00		
x/L*	Protrusion	12	13.17	158.00	-3.212	<0.001
	Total	19				
	Bulge	7	4.00	28.00		
y/W*	Protrusion	12	13.50	162.00	-3.550	<0.001
	Total	19				
	Bulge	7	8.86	62.00		
z/H	Protrusion	12	10.67	128.00	-0.676	0.499
	Total	19				
	Bulge	7	4.00	28.00		
RPPDS*	Protrusion	12	13.50	162.00	-3.550	<0.001
	Total	19				
	Bulge	7	4.00	28.00		
$\angle A1/\angle A2$*	Protrusion	12	13.50	162.00	-3.550	<0.001
	Total	19				
	Bulge	7	16.00	112.00		
RSI*	Protrusion	12	6.50	78.00	-3.550	<0.001
	Total	19				

Note: *, p<0.05, has statistically significant difference

Table 2. Spearman's Rank Correlation Analysis

Indexes	Group	Num	r	P value
x/L*	Bulge	7	0.757	<0.001
	Protrusion	12		
y/W*	Bulge	7	0.837	<0.001
	Protrusion	12		

Table 2. (*continued*)

z/H	Bulge	7	0.159	0.515
	Protrusion	12		
RPPDS*	Bulge	7	0.837	<0.001
	Protrusion	12		
∠A1/∠A2*	Bulge	7	0.837	<0.001
	Protrusion	12		
RSI*	Bulge	7	-0.837	<0.001
	Protrusion	12		

Note: *, p<0.05, has statistically significant difference

x/L, y/W, ∠A1/∠A2 and RPPDS are all positively correlated to the severity of LDH and the correlation is also high (r=0.837, p<0.05), which is statistically significant. For z/H, r=0.159, p=0.515, low correlation is shown without statistically significance.

According to the statistical test results, Fisher distinction formula was derived using the Fisher discriminant approach which does not require the sample to be normally distributed. The prior probability is calculated according to the sample size when the distinction is carried out, which means the prior probability of each type is proportional to its sample size. The discriminant function of LDH classification is obtained after preliminary calculation and its coefficients. The discriminant formula is as follow:

$$C_1 = (-1557.038, -640.287, 572.612, 237.853, 2999.606)$$

$$C_2 = (-1680.725, -626.4, 556.753, 1778.672, 344.475, 3140.734)$$

$$X = (1, X_1, X_2, \cdots X_5) \qquad \begin{cases} Y_1 = X \cdot C_1 \\ Y_2 = X \cdot C_2 \end{cases} \tag{3}$$

In the Fisher discriminant function, Y_1 and Y_2 represent functions for bulge group and protrusion group respectively, while C_1 and C_2 are corresponding coefficients. Formula (3) is derived using the proposed five indexes of patients. If $Y_1 < Y_2$ the patient is more likely to belong to the type of bulge and otherwise the type of protrusion. Fisher discriminatory analysis was obtained and 94.7% of cross-validated grouped were correctly classified.

4   Discussion and Conclusion

In the present study, a visualization and quantitative analysis framework for the evaluation of lumbar disc herniation were developed. Based on patient MRI datasets, six indexes were extracted to evaluate the relationship between these indexes and the severity of lumbar disc herniation. Preliminary results indicate that five of them have a close relationship with the grading of LDH.

Among the indexes extracted, $\angle A1/\angle A2$ and x/L describe the deviation degree of protruded nucleus pulposus from the central of spinal canal. The nucleus pulposus protruded outside can easily enter the intervertebral foramen, affecting the nerve root and causing pain. Small debris of protruded nucleus broken into the intervertebral foramen can lead to more serious symptoms because of the limited capacity of the foramen. Preliminary results indicate that the two indexes have a good correlation with severity of patients and the conclusion was also verified by statistical tests ($\angle A1/\angle A2$:r=0.757, p<0.05; x/L:r=0.837,p<0.05).

Indexes RPPDS and y/W are used to describe the compression degree of the nucleus pulposus protruded into spinal cord or cauda equine, and RPPDS describes the situation from the perspective of 3D. Since the capacity of the spinal canal varies along with the individual difference, designing the indexes in the form of ratio can eliminate the individual difference of patients. With the increase of the degree of nucleus pulposus protruded into spinal canal, more severe clinical symptoms are usually observed, along with increased RPPDS and y/W. However, for patient T, y/W and RPPDS cannot be calculated because of the nucleus debris in the spinal canal.

Index RSI reflects the water content of the disc and surrounding structure. The smaller the value of RSI is, the lower water content that the disc has. Under normal condition, the signal intensity of nucleus pulposus is slightly lower than that of adjacent cerebrospinal fluid. With increased degree of disc degeneration, a huge loss of water appeared in the disc and annulus, making the difference between intensities of nucleus pulposus and adjacent CSF more significant. Lower water content leads to decreased toughness of disc and annulus, followed by the instability of the lumbar spine, increasing the severity of LDH [7, 8]. The statistical results indicate that there is a close relationship between RSI and the severity of LDH. The statistical analysis on z/H suggests that, it has a weak correlation with the grading of LDH, which means the axial distribution of protruded nucleus pulposus has less impact on the severity of LDH.

Fisher discriminatory analysis based on 5 indexes i.e., x/L, y/W, $\angle A1/\angle A2$, RPPDS and RSI, demonstrates that 94.7% of cross-validated grouped cases were correctly classified. This indicates that these indexes have potential in LDH grading and could be used for quantitative classification of LDH.

In conclusion, preliminary analysis shows the effectiveness of the system and proposed indexes, and explores the feasibility of LDH quantitative classification based on proposed indexes. Further investigation should be performed for computer-aided detection and grading of LDH based on larger clinical database.

Acknowledgments. This work was supported in part by the National Natural Science Foundation of China under Grant No. 81071220 and the National Key Technology Research and Development Program of China under grant No. 2011BAI12B03.

References

1. Halldin, K., Lind, B., Rönnberg, K.: Three-Dimensional Radiological Classification of Lumbar Disc Herniation in Relation to Surgical Outcome. International Orthopaedics (SICOT) 33, 725–730 (2009)
2. Vucetic, N., Astrand, P., Guntner, P.: Diagnosis and Prognosis in Lumbar Disc Herniation. Clin. Orthop. Relat. Res. 361, 116–122 (1999)
3. Barlocher, C.B., Krauss, J.K., Seiler, R.W.: Central Lumbar Disc Herniation. Acta Neurochirurgica 142, 1369–1375 (2000)
4. Carragee, E.J., Kim, D.H.: A Prospective Analysis of Magnetic Resonance Imaging Findings in Patients with Sciatica and Lumbar Disc Herniation: Correlation of Outcomes with Disc Fragment and Canal Morpholohy. Spine 22, 1650–1660 (1997)
5. Guo, J., Liu, D., Zhang, G.: The Influence of Intervertebral Discs or lumbar Spinal Stenosis on the Lumbar Spinal Curvature. Progress of Anatomical Sciences 13, 219–220 (2007)
6. Bernhardt, M., Gurganious, L.R., Bloom, D.L.: Magnetic Resonance Imaging Analysis of Percutaneous Disectomy: A Perliminary Report. Spine 18, 211–217 (1993)
7. Katariina, L., DMedSc, V.T.: Disc Height and Signal Intensity of the Nucleus Pulposus on Magnetic Resonance Imaging as Indicators of Lumbar Disc Degeneration. Spine 26, 680–686 (2001)
8. Hu, Y.: MRI Diagnosis of Disc Degeneration. Acta Academiae Medicinae Qin Dao Universitys 41, 189–191 (2005)

Liver Tumor Segmentation Using Kernel-Based FGCM and PGCM

Rajeswari Mandava[1], Lee Song Yeow[1], Bhavik Anil Chandra[1],
Ong Kok Haur[1], Muhammad Fermi Pasha[1], and Ibrahim Lutfi Shuaib[2]

[1] School of Computer Sciences, Universiti Sains Malaysia, 11800, Penang, Malaysia
mandava@cs.usm.my
[2] Advanced Medical and Dental Institute, Bertam, Penang, Malaysia
ibrahim@amdi.usm.edu.my

Abstract. Low contrast between tumor and healthy liver tissue is one of the significant and challenging features among others in the automated tumor delineation process. In this paper we propose kernel based clustering algorithms that incorporate Tsallis entropy to resolve long range interactions between tumor and healthy tissue intensities. This paper reports the algorithm and its encouraging results of evaluation with MICCAI liver Tumor Segmentation Challenge 08 (LTS08) dataset. Work in progress involves incorporating additional features and expert knowledge into clustering algorithm to improve the accuracy.

Keywords: Tumor Segmentation, Tsallis Entropy, Kernelized Fuzzy C-Mean, Liver Tumor, Multi Feature Fuzzy C-Mean.

1 Introduction

Liver tumor is one of the most frequently occurring and leading cause of cancer related deaths. Accurate localization and volumetric analysis of the tumor are crucial for early diagnosis, further treatment monitoring and surgical planning. The use of computed tomography (CT) imaging to help diagnose liver tumors is proven to be accurate by medical professionals for years. Manual delineation, requiring localizing multiple tumors in hundreds of slices tends to be approximate in quantification [10,7] and is time consuming.

There have been numerous attempts to automate liver tumor segmentation. Broadly, these attempts include (i) machine learning [10,9,16,3] (ii) clustering [7] (iii) region based [1,14] (iv) edge detection [15] and (v) partial differential equation [13,12] based approaches. In these approaches, the image feature employed range from simple intensity features to a battery of texture features. Although there is some success with the existing tumor segmentation approaches, the major issue affecting performance is the high similarity between tumor and healthy tissue, both in terms of intensity as well as texture. Here we quote two works that will later be used to compare our proposed approach:

In the first, Kubota [6] reports a fully automated two step process to detect tumors. In the initial step they localize the candidate tumor regions by detecting

H. Yoshida et al. (Eds.): Abdominal Imaging 2011, LNCS 7029, pp. 99–107, 2012.
© Springer-Verlag Berlin Heidelberg 2012

local minima of the intensity fields. The second step has two parts: The first part is for the initial segmentation of low intensity regions and the second part, named as competition diffusion, is to combine the multiple low intensity regions belonging to a single tumor by region tracing process. In their initial step, they down sample the image and this is followed by smoothing operations. Because of this there may be a danger of missing small tumors and thus the limitation of the algorithm in locating tumors that are larger than $1cm^3$.

The second work by Hame [4] also reports a two step process. The first step is a simple thresholding and morphological operations to generate tumor candidates. In the second step, they apply morphological dilation and generate a mask around the tumor candidates to isolate tumor regions. The candidate tumor regions are clustered with fuzzy clustering approaches and segmented using thresholding. The contours of the tumor segments are traced using Geometric Deformation Models. Even though they report very encouraging results, they emphasize on the need for an improved first step rough segmentation process to improve the overall performance of their system.

In radiologist terms, density which may be translated to intensity is one is of the primary features to localize and delineate tumor. In the case of liver tumor, it may either be lower or higher or same density as the healthy tissue. Additional markers include unusual visual appearance as compared to the healthy tissue and abnormal bumps (convex) or depressions (concave) on the surface of the liver. Where ambiguity persists, the radiologists routinely refer to the neighboring axial slices to confirm tumor/non tumor tissues.

In this work we focus on density difference between the tumor and healthy tissue to localize as well as delineate tumor tissue based on intensity differences. This shall serve as an initial step in the tumor segmentation process. The algorithms may then be extended to incorporate additional features and expert knowledge to emulate the expert with an intention to aid the expert in delineating and quantifying tumor.

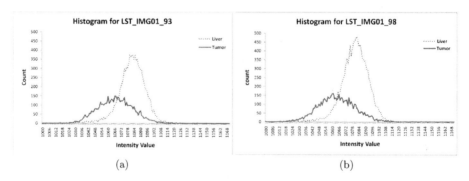

(a)   (b)

Fig. 1. Comparing intensity difference in tumor and healthy tissue in two sample images

The histograms in Figure 1 illustrate the high similarities in the intensities between tumor and healthy tissue. In statistical mechanics terms this phenomena is described as long range interactions between the two classes. In this study, we extend the most popular Fuzzy C-Means (FCM) clustering algorithm to include Tsallis entropy principle to cater for long range interactions and apply it to liver tumor segmentation in order to maximize the separability between classes. We also introduce kernelized distances to further enhance differences between the foreground and background to aid the clustering process.

We are inspired by the work of [11] where fuzzy and possibilistic generalized C-Means algorithms are combined to improve the class separability of adipose tissue from the noisy background. Class interactions between tumor and healthy tissue are much more severe. This prompted us to extend the generalized C-Means algorithms with kernelized distances to further improve the class separability. Our contribution lies in proposing this idea to tumor delineation, extending the Generalized C-Means algorithms to include kernelized distances and experimentally evaluating its efficacy in localizing and delineating tumor regions based on the intensity differences.

The rest of the paper is organized as follows: Section 2 contains the proposed method; Section 3 is devoted to experimental results and discussion and finally section 4 concludes the proposed methodology and provides future directions.

2 Materials and Methods

In FCM the clusters have higher mobility to converge to global minimum, whereas the clusters in PCM have lower mobility. In PCM the data points see one cluster at a time and thus PCM is more focused on optimizing the class association of the data points [10]. Thus concatenating FCM and PCM is particularly attractive in the case of tumor delineation where there is large overlap in the clusters related to tumor and non tumor pixels. FCM helps to define the number of clusters and PCM assists in the fine tuning process of class association to produce optimum results.

This idea, inspired by the work of Roullier et.al [11], is extended to combine the Kernel-based Fuzzy Generalized C-Means (KFGCM) and Kernel-based Possibilistic Generalized C-Means (KPGCM). This section describes formulation of KFGCM and KPGCM and presents the methodology adapted in this work.

2.1 Kernel-Based FGCM and PGCM (KFGCM & KPGCM)

The Generalized Fuzzy C-Means formulation proposed by Menard et. al. [8] and later adapted by Roullier et. al.[11] is based on the minimization of the following objective function :

$$J(U, V; Y) = \sum_{k=1}^{n} \sum_{i=1}^{c} \mu_{ik}^m D_{ik}^2 + \frac{1}{\lambda(m-1)} \sum_{k=1}^{n} \sum_{i=1}^{c} \mu_{ik}^m - \frac{1}{\lambda} \sum_{k=1}^{n} \gamma_k (\sum_{i=1}^{c} \mu_{ik} - 1) \quad (1)$$

where:

x_k is the kth data point, c_i is the ith cluster center, c is the number of clusters, n is the number of data points, D_{ik} is the distance between the data point and the cluster, $m(> 1)$ is the fuzzifier component that controls the extent of membership sharing between clusters, μ_{ik} is the degree of membership of the kth data point to the ith cluster, λ is the Lagrange regularization parameter and $\gamma_k = \frac{\sum_{k=1}^{N} \mu_{ik}^m D_{ik}^2}{\sum_{k=1}^{N} \mu_{ik}^m}$ determines the distance at which the membership value of a point in a cluster becomes 0.5 [5].

Cluster membership update function is

$$\mu_{ik} = \frac{[1 + \lambda(m-1)D_{ik}^2]^{(\frac{-1}{m-1})}}{\sum_{i=1}^{C}[1 + \lambda(m-1)D_{ik}^2]^{(\frac{-1}{m-1})}} \tag{2}$$

Cluster center update function is

$$v_i = \frac{\sum_{k=1}^{N} \mu_{ik}^m x_k}{\sum_{k=1}^{N} \mu_{ik}^m} \tag{3}$$

Kernelizing transforms data points x_k and cluster centers c_i into higher dimensional feature space as $\phi(x_k)$ and $\phi(c_i)$ respectively, using a non-linear transformation $\phi(\ldots)$. Clustering is then performed in the feature space. The distance between k^{th} data point and the ith cluster, in the feature space, using the most common Euclidean distance metric known as the kernel distance is given by

$$\begin{aligned} D_{ik}^2 &= \|x_k - c_i\|^2 \\ &= \|\phi(x_k) - \phi(c_i)\|^2 \\ &= [\phi(x_k) - \phi(c_i)] \cdot [\phi(x_k) - \phi(c_i)] \\ &= \phi(x_k) \cdot \phi(x_k) + \phi(c_i) \cdot \phi(c_i) - 2(\phi(x_k) \cdot \phi(c_i) \\ &= [k(x_k, x_k)] + [k(c_i, c_i)] - 2[k(x_k, c_i)] \end{aligned} \tag{4}$$

Using the popular Gaussian kernel :

$$k(x_k, x_i) = \exp(-\frac{\|x_k - x_i\|^2}{2\sigma^2}) \tag{5}$$

$k(x_k, x_k)$ reduces to 1. With this, Equation (4) reduces to $D^2(x_k, c_i) = 2[1 - k(x_k, c_i)]$.

Substituting the kernel distance into Equations (1), (2) and (3) produces kernel-based Fuzzy Generalized C-Means (KFGCM) formulation. This is given by the following equations.

KFGCM objective function :

$$J(U, V; Y) = 2\sum_{k=1}^{n}\sum_{i=1}^{c} \mu_{ik}^m[1 - k(x_k, c_i)] + \frac{1}{\lambda(m-1)}\sum_{k=1}^{n}\sum_{i=1}^{c} \mu_{ik}^m - \frac{1}{\lambda}\sum_{k=1}^{n} \gamma_k(\sum_{i=1}^{c} \mu_{ik} - 1) \tag{6}$$

The new objective function is minimized by the following function:

$$\mu_{ik} = \frac{[1 + \lambda(m-1)[1 - k(x_k, c_i)]]^{(\frac{-1}{m-1})}}{\sum_{i=1}^{C}[1 + \lambda(m-1)[1 - k(x_k, c_i)]]^{(\frac{-1}{m-1})}} \quad (7)$$

Centroid update function is updated as follows:

$$v_i = \frac{\sum_{k=1}^{N}\mu_{ik}^m[k(x_k, c_i)]x_k}{\sum_{k=1}^{N}\mu_{ik}^m[k(x_k, c_i)]} \quad (8)$$

Similarly, Kernel-based Possibilistic Generalized C-Mean (KPGCM) is formulated extending the PGCM proposed by Menard et.al [8]. This formulation for KPGCM is as given by Equation (9), (10) and (11).

$$J(U,V;Y) = 2\sum_{k=1}^{N}\sum_{i=1}^{C}\mu_{ik}^m[1 - k(x_k, c_i)] + \frac{1}{\lambda(m-1)}\sum_{k=1}^{N}\sum_{i=1}^{C}[\mu_{ik}^m - \mu_{ik}] - \frac{1}{\lambda}\sum_{k=1}^{N}(\sum_{i=1}^{C}\mu_{ik}) \quad (9)$$

$$\mu_{ik} = \frac{1}{[1 + \lambda(m-1)[1 - k(x_k, c_i)]]^{(\frac{-1}{m-1})}} \quad (10)$$

$$v_i = \frac{\sum_{k=1}^{N}\mu_{ik}^m[k(x_k, c_i)]x_k}{\sum_{k=1}^{N}\mu_{ik}^m[k(x_k, c_i)]} \quad (11)$$

2.2 Methodology

Figure 2 illustrates the methodology of the proposed work together with some of the associated intermediate results. It begins with clustering the intensities in the input image with a predetermined number of clusters using KFGCM. The cluster centers produced are then fed into the KPGCM to fine tune the cluster membership. Each of the resulting clusters are then mapped to a pre-specified intensity. The clusters containing tumor pixels are identified using prior knowledge. The clusters associated with tumor are then selected as foreground and the remaining clusters are identified as background and segmented using thresholding operation. From this point onwards, to limit the data for processing to liver region alone, a manually pre-segmented liver mask is applied to isolate the liver region. The clusters in the liver region are further treated with morphological opening, closing and small region deletion to remove noise.

3   Experimental Results and Discussions

The proposed algorithm is evaluated with MICCAI Liver Tumor Segmentation Challenge 2008 (LTS 2008) training dataset which consists of 4 patient datasets

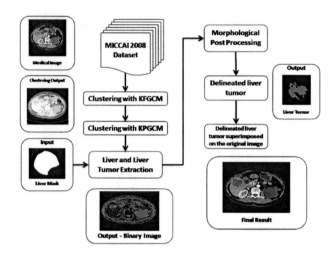

Fig. 2. Methodology of the proposed work

with selected tumors manually labeled by experts. Each patient is given different number of labels.The evaluation metrics are the same as those proposed in LTS 2008. These are: Volume overlap ($m1$); Relative absolute volume difference ($m2$); Average symmetric surface distance ($m3$); RMS symmetric surface distance ($m4$) and Maximum symmetric surface distance ($m5$) [2]. For the purpose of discussion, we present 4 out of the 5 evaluation metrics in Table 1.

The parameters of the algorithm are empirically determined. Number of clusters for KFGCM and KPGCM is 8 and $\lambda = 5000$. A 12 connected disc is used for morphological operations. Table 1 presents the quantitative results of the experiments and their comparison with similar works by Kubota [6] and Hame [4]. The proposed method performed better than the other two for datasets IMG01, IMG02 and IMG03. However the performance is very poor for dataset IMG04. The reasons for this poor performance may be analyzed through visual comparisons.

In addition to the quantitative comparison, results are visually compared with the tumor labels available on LTS 2008. For all labeled tumor regions in images IMG01, IMG02 and IMG03 the results are in close agreement with expert labeling. However in some of the images of IMG04_L2 and IMG04_L3 where the selected tumor is in close proximity to another tumor, the two tumor regions merge and appear as a single tumor region. Additionally if the tumor texture or multiple low intensity sites with abnormal appearance the proposed method does not produce acceptable results. Figure 3 illustrates sample images of manual comparison. The merge between two labeled tumors of IMG04_L2 and IMG04_L3 is clearly visible. Abnormal appearance in IMG04_L3 is not delineated accurately. This explains large differences in the quantitative results presented in Table 1.

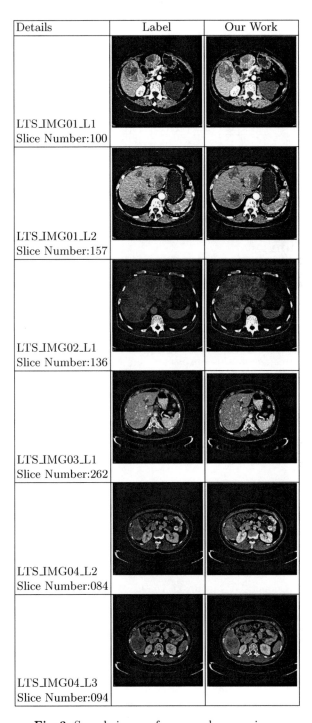

Fig. 3. Sample images for manual comparisons

Table 1. Comparing the proposed work results with similar works

Image	Vol. Overlap Error ($m1$)			Vol. Difference ($m2$)			Avg. Surf. Dist.($m3$)			RMS Surf. Dist. ($m4$)		
	K	H	PW	K	H	PW	K	H	PW	K	H	PW
IMG01_L1	41.75	51.40	40.33	28.10	49.72	40.33	2.73	4.10	3.65	3.65	5.29	4.86
IMG01_L2	60.13	37.96	12.46	59.72	37.77	12.46	2.64	1.36	0.79	3.00	1.65	1.69
IMG02_L1	95.10	41.70	18.57	95.10	39.80	18.57	8.52	1.66	0.72	9.74	2.04	1.10
IMG02_L2	78.12	23.63	42.82	78.12	20.24	42.82	4.85	0.82	1.69	5.49	1.29	2.81
IMG02_L3	72.63	95.16	59.92	72.63	95.16	59.92	3.80	7.06	2.22	4.19	7.44	2.86
IMG03_L1	76.02	42.93	45.41	153.67	36.07	45.41	4.24	1.05	0.71	6.02	1.56	1.14
IMG04_L1	53.66	18.26	9.44	40.93	12.95	9.44	4.59	1.37	1.12	5.85	1.84	2.26
IMG04_L2	70.41	9.79	51.12	70.41	2.59	51.12	4.57	0.35	1.71	4.89	0.60	2.81
IMG04_L3	40.15	12.44	58.97	32.42	7.88	27.56	3.28	0.86	2.81	4.29	1.37	4.81
IMG04_L4	50.49	15.52	4.76	50.42	11.54	4.76	3.58	0.80	0.70	4.03	1.47	2.08

(PW - Proposed work, K - Kubota [6], H - Hame [4])

4   Conclusion

Even though the proposed method is solely based on intensities, the preliminary experiments are encouraging. It is able to produce results that are comparable or better than some of the other methods and it shows promise in delineating the tumor successfully. In cases where the tumor consists of abnormal appearance, the proposed approach may fail. Thus this algorithm is currently being extended to include texture features. Future work shall include extensive validation and testing of the algorithm with more datasets.

Acknowledgement. This work was supported in part by Universiti Sains Malaysia APEX Delivering Excellent grant no. 1002/PKOMP/910304.

References

1. Ben-Dan, I., Shenhav, E.: Liver Tumor segmentation in CT images using probabilistic methods. Image (Rochester, N.Y.) pp. 1–11 (2008)
2. Deng, X., Du, G.: Editorial: 3D segmentation in the clinic: a grand challenge IILiver Tumor Segmentation. In: International Conference on Medical Image Computing and Computer Assisted Intervention (2008)
3. Freiman, M., Cooper, O., Lischinski, D., Joskowicz, L.: Liver tumors segmentation from CTA images using voxels classification and affinity constraint propagation. International Journal of Computer Assisted Radiology and Surgery (June 2010)
4. Hame, Y.: Liver tumor segmentation using implicit surface evolution. The Midas Journal, 1–10 (2008)
5. Krishnapuram, R., Keller, J.: A possibilistic approach to clustering. IEEE Transactions on Fuzzy Systems 1(2), 98–110 (1993)
6. Kubota, T.: Efficient Automated Detection and Segmentation of Medium and Large Liver Tumors: CAD Approach. In: Workshop Proceedings of the 11th International Conference on Medical Image Computing and Computer Assisted Intervention-MICCAI (2008)

7. Massoptier, L., Casciaro, S.: A new fully automatic and robust algorithm for fast segmentation of liver tissue and tumors from CT scans. European Radiology 18(8), 1658–1665 (2008)
8. Ménard, M., Eboueya, M.: Extreme physical information and objective function in fuzzy clustering. Fuzzy Sets and Systems 128(3), 285–303 (2002)
9. Militzer, A., Hager, T., Jager, F., Tietjen, C., Hornegger, J.: Automatic Detection and Segmentation of Focal Liver Lesions in Contrast Enhanced CT Images. In: 20th International Conference on Pattern Recognition, pp. 2524–2527 (August 2010)
10. Pescia, D., Paragios, N., Chemouny, S.: Automatic detection of liver tumors. In: 5th IEEE International Symposium on Biomedical Imaging: From Nano to Macro, ISBI 2008, pp. 672–675. IEEE (2008)
11. Roullier, V., Cavaromenard, C., Calmon, G., Aube, C.: Fuzzy algorithms: Application to adipose tissue quantification on MR images. Biomedical Signal Processing and Control 2(3), 239–247 (2007)
12. Smeets, D., Loeckx, D., Stijnen, B., De Dobbelaer, B., Vandermeulen, D., Suetens, P.: Semi-automatic level set segmentation of liver tumors combining a spiral-scanning technique with supervised fuzzy pixel classification. Medical Image Analysis 14(1), 13–20 (2010)
13. Smeets, D., Stijnen, B., Loeckx, D., De Dobbelaer, B., Suetens, P.: Segmentation of liver metastases using a level set method with spiral-scanning technique and supervised fuzzy pixel classification. 3D Segmentation in the Clinic: A Grand Challenge IILiver Tumor Segmentation (2008)
14. Wong, D., Liu, J., Fengshou, Y., Tian, Q., Xiong, W., Zhou, J., Qi, Y., Han, T., Venkatesh, S., Wang, S.: A semi-automated method for liver tumor segmentation based on 2D region growing with knowledge-based constraints. The Midas Journal (2008)
15. Zhang, X., Lee, G., Tajima, T., Kitagawa, T., Kanematsu, M., Zhou, X., Hara, T., Fujita, H., Yokoyama, R., Kondo, H., Hoshi, H., Nawano, S., Shinozaki, K.: Segmentation of liver region with tumorous tissues. In: Proceedings of SPIE 6512, pp. 651235–651235-9 (2007)
16. Zhou, J., Xiong, W., Tian, Q., Qi, Y., Liu, J., Leow, W., Han, T., Venkatesh, S., Wang, S.: Semi-automatic segmentation of 3D liver tumors from CT scans using voxel classification and propagational learning. In: Proceedings of MICCAI Workshop on 3D Segmentation in the Clinic: A Grand Challenge II, New York, NY, USA., vol. 25 (2009)

Improving Diagnosis and Intervention: A Complete Approach for Registration of Liver CT Data

Marius Erdt[1], Cristina Oyarzun Laura[1], Klaus Drechsler[1], Stefano De Beni[2], and Luigi Solbiati[3]

[1] Fraunhofer IGD, Cognitive Computing & Medical Imaging,
Fraunhoferstrasse 5, 64283 Darmstadt, Germany
[2] Esaote, Ultrasound Division,
Via Siffredi 58, 16153 Genoa, Italy
[3] Hospital of Busto Arsizio, Department of Radiology,
Piazzale Solaro 3, 21052 Busto Arsizio, Italy
marius.erdt@igd.fraunhofer.de

Abstract. Registration of liver CT scans from different points in time or different phases of contrast agent saturation is a highly demanded tool for computer aided diagnosis, operation planning and intervention. This work presents a complete registration workflow to precisely overlap scans from 4 different application scenarios including registration of pre-treatment and post-treatment data as well as registration of multi-phase CT. Various state of the art techniques in shape modeling and matching, visualization as well as augmented interaction are applied to cover all of the described scenarios in a clinically usable system. Our system has been in use for clinical evaluation under real life conditions and has been tested on more than 30 patients.

Keywords: liver, registration, computed tomography, intervention.

1 Introduction

Multiphase liver registration has great potential improving diagnosis and operation planning since it allows the fusion of complementary information from *routinely* gathered CT scans. Usually physicians have to compare the different phases slice-by-slice and map them mentally. This is especially problematic if precise knowledge about the location of structures is needed, e.g. the distance of a vessel to a tumor which are not visible in the same phase. Furthermore, the comparison of pre- and post-treatment CT scans is of great importance. It allows, for example, to determine if all tumor areas have been burned correctly in the application of radio frequency ablation. Fig. 1 gives an overview of the 4 different scenarios that have to be taken into account for a computer guided liver registration system. The green arrows indicate the registration of scans from different phases of contrast agent saturation from either pre- or post-treatment. Registration is problematic, because the internal structures cannot be used to guide

H. Yoshida et al. (Eds.): Abdominal Imaging 2011, LNCS 7029, pp. 108–115, 2012.

arterial-phase   portal-phase

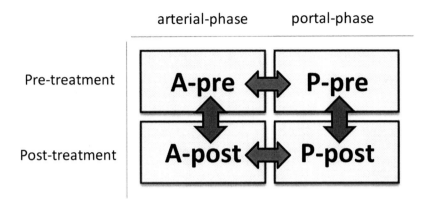

Pre-treatment   A-pre ⇔ P-pre

Post-treatment   A-post ⇔ P-post

Fig. 1. Registration variants of liver CT scans useful for clinical practice: pre-post CT of the same phase (red arrows) and inter-phase registration between arterial and portal venous CT scans (green arrows)

the deformation, since usually complementary information is visible in different phases. The red arrows depict the registration between pre- and post-treatment scans of the same phase. Here, usually the same internal structures, i.e. vessel trees, are visible. However, the appearance of those structures can differ due to resections, tissue burning or tumor growth.

In this work, we make use of several state of the art modeling, visualization and interaction techniques to cover all of the described scenarios in a clinically usable system. At first, 3D single- and multiple-surface organ models are created to segment the liver in all phases. For the pre-post registration scenario, the vasculature is segmented and converted into a graph representation. An augmented interactive tree-matching method is then used by the clinician to match branching points between the trees of each scan. The resulting point correspondences are used to guide an elastic registration in order to overlap pre and post data. In case of registering different phases, the 3D shape information of the liver is used as input to a landmark and voxel-based registration scheme.

2   Modeling Liver Shapes

Model based methods are commonly used for segmentation of organs in CT data [7], since they incorporate prior knowledge about the expected shape of the structure to segment. For segmentation of the portal phase we use a locally constrained statistical shape model that is based on automatically adapting a polygonal mesh to the image data [4]. The advantage of this method is that it is robust to model initialization errors and segmentation leakage, because it incorporates the expected local elasticity of the organ and makes use of a multi-tiered adaptation where the degrees of freedom of the model are stepwise increased. Fig. 2 shows the model and an exemplary segmentation result. Average mean surface distance error of this method is between 1.3 mm and 1.85 mm compared

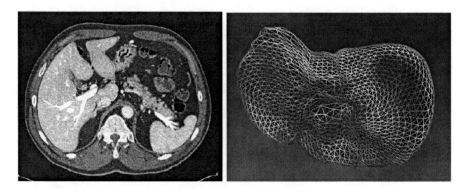

Fig. 2. Liver model with non-uniform local elasticity (blue areas denote regions of high stiffness while red areas denote regions of high elasticity

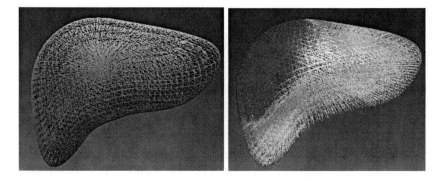

Fig. 3. Multi-layer model without (left) and with local adaptation constraints mapped to all layers of the model

to ground truth depending on the image resolution and tested on 86 scans. In order to also robustly segment the arterial phase, a volumetric point based multi-layer deformable model that consists of many interconnected polygonal surfaces (cf. Fig. 3) [5] is used. It extends common parametric deformable models to incorporate regional information in order to improve the robustness of segmentation in case of the low contrast arterial phase. In contrast to other volumetric approaches, the optimization of the model can be performed very efficiently. The accuracy of the method is 1.96 mm average mean surface distance error tested on 20 scans.

3   Registration of Arterial and Portal Phase CT

Fig. 4 shows the workflow of the registration of arterial and portal phase scans. The volumes are coarsely registered using a landmark based registration. Subsequently, deformations caused by the patient's breathing are compensated by an elastic Demons algorithm with a boundary distance based speed function. This allows for a high accuracy natural deformation without having to rely on the liver's internal structure in complementary phases. Furthermore, since shape information is given, surrounding structures can be omitted which significantly speeds up registration.

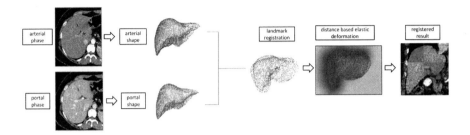

Fig. 4. Workflow of the automatic registration framework. The liver is extracted in the portal phase. The resulting mesh position is used as initialization for the extraction of the arterial phase. Afterwards shapes are registered based on their corresponding landmarks. The final registration is computed by a distance based deformable registration.

4   Registration of Pre- and Post-treatment CT

For registering pre- and post-treatment data, we use the branching points of the vessel trees of the liver as guiding landmarks for an elastic registration based on volume splines. This allows an accurate deformation of the liver's interior. We use a vessel enhancement technique to segment the vessels in the extracted livers [2]. The vasculature is then transformed into a graph representation [1]. Tree matching algorithms have being designed to match branching points of such vasculature. They have been used on the human airway [6,10] or on the liver vessels [8]. In addition to this it is necessary to get the most accurate possible results. Every tree matching algorithm however gives some incorrect matches as result. Motivated by that we decided to enhance a tree matching algorithm to be able to interactively fix those incorrect matches provided by the algorithm [3,9]. It is necessary that it is easy to use so that the doctor does not need to put effort on it and can concentrate on the clinical use of it. With this goal in mind we developed a series of interaction features that will be described in the following section.

4.1   Interactive Augmented Tree Matching

The tree matching algorithm used [9] is an enhancement of that presented by Graham et al. [6]. We enhanced the algorithm by making it able to get some preselected matches as input. In this way the automatic tree matching algorithm is then guided by the clinical user, who can decide the correspondences that are of importance for him to be taken into account by the algorithm.

This process in addition to give more freedom to the doctor makes the algorithm more efficient.

4.2   Interactive Features

The goal of the interaction features is mainly to help the clinical user to easily identify those matches that are incorrectly provided by the tree matching algorithm. Since the rate of correct matches provided is high, it is not necessary to visualize all the matches when trying to find incorrect matches. This would make the task of finding them much harder (Figure 5, 1st row). To avoid this we visualize the different matched node-pairs with different colors depending on their probability to be correct: green when the probability is high, yellow when it is not so high and red for the rest. Our measure to decide which nodes are in each group is based on the similarity between the attributes of the nodes and edges of both trees. This way the doctor can focus on the red or yellow nodes which makes his task easier and faster (Figure 5, 2nd row). In addition to this we let the doctor visualize only the matches corresponding to a determined group (Figure 5, 3rd row) or to visualize the nodes one by one (Figure 5, 4th row). Some additional features were developed. For better identification of node-pairs two visualization features were used, on the one hand lines joining node-pairs, on the other hand showing the same number near both nodes belonging to a node-pair. It is usual that trees from different modalities do not show the same number of branches. A feature was developed that can reduce the number of branches of a tree that are shown with the goal of making it more similar to the other tree.

7 persons participated in the experiments to evaluate the developed interactive features. The goal of the experiments was to find those features which make the interaction with the application easier. On the other hand we also where interested on measuring which one of the features allowed the clinical user to find faster those correspondences that were incorrectly matched by the tree matching algorithm. The mean time required by the participants to find the incorrect matches was of 107 seconds (71.28% of the incorrect matches found) for the feature showing the node-pair in groups of colors and 122 seconds (78.43% found) for the feature that showed the nodes with different colors and one by one. In addition to the measured results the participants were asked to give an opinion about the evaluated features. They all coincided saying that the feature showing the node-pairs differenced by colors and one-by-one was the easier to use one.

5   Evaluation and Results

Currently, our system has been used in clinical evaluation on the data of more than 30 patients. Fig. 6(a) shows exemplary results of the multiphase registration. For evaluation of the phase registration quality, in 22 scans from 11 patients the liver was divided into 3 parts. The overlap errors were 4.4 mm, 2.2 mm and 2.1 mm on average for the different parts judged by experienced radiologists.

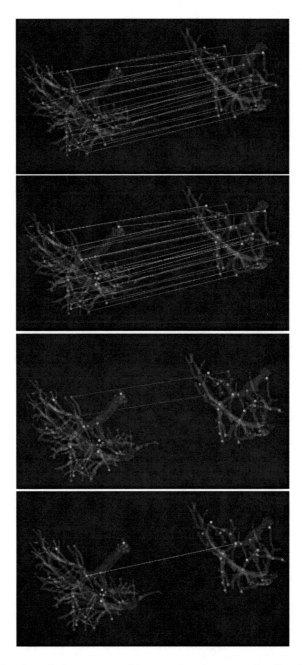

Fig. 5. Visualization of the tree matching results. 1st row: visualization that shows in green the matched nodes and in blue the unmatched ones. 2nd row: visualization using different colors to represent how likely a node-pair is correctly matched. 3rd row: visualization showing only the group of nodes of a specific color. 4th row: visualization showing the nodes with different colors and one by one.

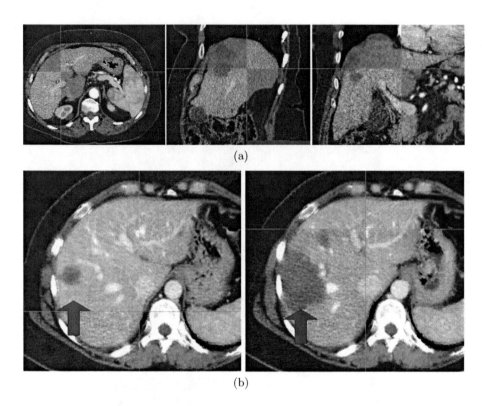

(a)

(b)

Fig. 6. Split views of registration results: (a) Multiphase-registration of arterial and portal contrast enhancement phase. (b) Pre-treatment (left) and post-treatment (right) registration. Arrows indicate initial lesion in pre-treatment scan (left) and ablated area in post-treatment scan (right).

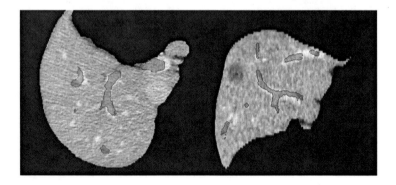

Fig. 7. Deformed post-treatment vessel tree overlayed with pre-treatment liver volume

Fig. 6(b) shows the registration of a pre-treatment and a post-treatment scan. By overlaying the registered images, it can be assessed whether enough tissue around the lesion has been ablated in the operation. Fig. 7 shows the deformed vessel system of the post-treatment scan overlayed with the pre-treatment scan using the results of the tree matching algorithm.

6   Discussion and Conclusion

This work presents a complete registration workflow to precisely overlap scans from 4 different application scenarios including registration of pre-treatment and post-treatment data as well as registration of multi-phase CT. The system has been tested on more than 30 patients. Using the registered pre-treatment and post-treatment CT images, the result of an operation such as a radiofrequency ablation can be assessed more precisely in contrast to a slice-by-slice comparison. Registration of multiphase CT data can be used to enhance operation planning. In future work we plan to improve intervention and navigation procedures in an application scenario where the fused phases can be registered with ultrasound data.

References

1. Drechsler, K., Oyarzun Laura, C.: Hierachical decomposition of vessel skeletons for graph creation and feature extraction. In: Proc. BIBM (2010)
2. Drechsler, K., Oyarzun Laura, C.: A novel multiscale integration approach for vessel enhancement. In: IEEE CBMS, pp. 92–97 (2010)
3. Drechsler, K., Oyarzun Laura, C., Chen, Y., Erdt, M.: Semi automatic anatomical tree matching for landmark-based elastic registration of liver volumes. Journal of Healthcare Engineering 1(1), 101–123 (2010)
4. Erdt, M., Kirschner, M., Steger, S., Wesarg, S.: Fast automatic liver segmentation combining learned shape priors with observed shape deviation. In: IEEE CBMS, pp. 249–254 (2010)
5. Erdt, M., Schlegel, P., Wesarg, S.: Multi-layer deformable models for medical image segmentation. In: IEEE ITAB, p. 4 (2010)
6. Graham, M.W., Higgins, W.E.: Globally optimal model-based matching of anatomical trees. In: Medical Imaging: Image Processing, vol. 6144 (2006)
7. Heimann, T., van Ginneken, B., Styner, M., et al.: Comparison and Evaluation of Methods for Liver Segmentation from CT datasets. IEEE Trans. Med. Imaging 28(8), 1251–1265 (2009)
8. Metzen, J.H., Kröger, T., Schenk, A., Zidowitz, S., Peitgen, H.-O., Jiang, X.: Matching of Tree Structures for Registration of Medical Images. In: Escolano, F., Vento, M. (eds.) GbRPR. LNCS, vol. 4538, pp. 13–24. Springer, Heidelberg (2007)
9. Oyarzun Laura, C., Drechsler, K.: Computer assisted matching of anatomical vessel trees. Computers & Graphics 35(2), 299–311 (2011)
10. Tschirren, J., McLennan, G., Palágyi, K., Hoffman, E.A., Sonka, M.: Matching and anatomical labeling of human airway tree. IEEE Trans. Med. Imaging 24(12), 1540–1547 (2005)

Abdominal Images Non-rigid Registration Using Local-Affine Diffeomorphic Demons

Moti Freiman[1], Stephan D. Voss[2], and Simon Keith Warfield[1]

[1] Computational Radiology Laboratory, Children's Hospital,
Harvard Medical School, Boston, USA
[2] Department of Radiology, Children's Hospital,
Harvard Medical School, Boston, USA
moti.freiman@childrens.harvard.edu

Abstract. Abdominal image non-rigid registration is a particularly challenging task due to the presence of multiple organs, many of which move independently, contributing to independent deformations. Local-affine registration methods can handle multiple independent movements by assigning prior definition of each affine component and its spatial extent which is less suitable for multiple soft-tissue structures as in the abdomen. Instead, we propose to use the local-affine assumption as a prior constraint within the dense deformation field computation. Our method use the dense correspondences field computed using the optical-flow equations to estimate the local-affine transformations that best represent the deformation associated with each voxel with Gaussian regularization to ensure the smoothness of the deformation field. Experimental results from both synthetic and 400 controlled experiments on abdominal CT images and Diffusion Weighted MRI images demonstrate that our method yields a smoother deformation field with superior registration accuracy compared to the demons and diffeomorphic demons algorithms.

Keywords: abdominal registration, computed tomography, magnetic resonance imaging.

1 Introduction

Longitudinal intra-patient non-rigid image registration is a widely required pre-processing step in many abdomen related clinical applications. Examples include: 1) Quantitative evaluation of tumor response to therapy using imaging-based biomarkers [4]. 2) Motion-compensation for Diffusion-Weighted imaging acquisition protocols [10], and; 3) pre/intra/post operative comparison of patient images to quantitatively evaluate the surgical procedure's success.

The non-rigid registration task is an ill-posed problem which may produce accurate but non realistic solutions. Usually, a regularization scheme is used to constrain the solutions domain to only the realistic ones. Existing regularization approaches can be classified roughly into two categories: 1) Spatial smoothing of the non-parametric dense deformation field, and 2) Using a parameterized transformation model.

H. Yoshida et al. (Eds.): Abdominal Imaging 2011, LNCS 7029, pp. 116–124, 2012.

Spatial smoothing of the non-parametric dense deformation field methods apply a smoothing kernel onto the pre-computed dense deformation field to ensure its spatial coherence. For instance, the demons algorithm [16] applies a Gaussian kernel on the deformation field to ensure its spatial coherence. The kernel can be applied uniformly to the entire field as in the original implementation, or by using adaptive weighting schemes to represent different prior assumptions on tissue properties or lesion progression/regression [7,12,15]. Since the kernel is applied to the motion vectors themselves, it assumes only a local translational motion and cannot preserve more complex models such as local-affine motion. In addition, there is a well-known trade-off between the registration accuracy and the smoothness of the deformation field [19]. However, both properties are of interest. In [9], an adaptive smoothing scheme which account for the locally affine structure of the deformation field was proposed. However, this method highly depends on the anisotropic smoothing parameters.

Parameterized transformation model methods use a constrained optimization scheme in which a global similarity measure is optimized with respect to a limited pre-defined number of transformation parameters. For instance, a B-spline transformation model with mutual information as a similarity measure is used in [13]. These methods are sensitive to the pre-defined grid points that are used to parameterize the transformation, and cannot represent different tissue properties naturally.

Recently, a new transformation model that is constrained to a local-affine motion for pre-defined structures was proposed by several researchers. In [8,2,18], a set of local-affine transformations associated with a set of pre-defined structures is computed by optimizing each component's transformation separately, and then combining all components into a smooth diffeomorphic dense deformation field. The main advantage of this approach is that it yields smoother deformation fields compared to the dense deformation field registration approaches [16,17]. However, current local-affine methods are using a fixed, pre-defined set of structures. Thus, they are less useful for longitudinal intra-patient registration where prior segmentation is not available. In addition, they use "ad-hoc" solutions to define the set of components and their associated spatial extent, which may not represent the actual affine components, especially in soft tissue structures such as abdominal structures, and therefore may affect the registration accuracy.

Subdivisions schemes such as [5] apply an iterative subdivision of the image grid into multiple affine components and then merge all of them together. The main drawback of this approach is that it is limited to axis-aligned affine components, which is less suitable for medical images.

In this paper we present a new approach for local-affine registration. In our approach, the local-affine assumption is introduced as a hidden variable that moderates between a dense correspondences field and the desired deformation field. Our approach does not rely on a pre-defined set of structures and is not limited to axis-aligned structures. Thus, it is more flexible than previously published local-affine methods, and can be useful in cases where prior segmentation is not available.

Evaluation of our method using both quantitative evaluation of the registration of both synthetic images and intra-patient abdominal CT images with 400 controlled deformations and qualitative evaluation of the registration of intra-patient longitudinal Diffusion Weighted MRI (DWI) images shows that our method produces much smoother deformation fields compared to those produced by the demons [16] and diffeomorphic demons [17] methods, with comparable and even superior accuracy.

2   Method

2.1   Registration Framework

Given a floating image $I_f(i) : i \to \mathbb{R}$, the goal of the non-parametric registration is to find a dense deformation field $D_f^r(i) : i \to i + D_f^r(i)$ that minimizes its dissimilarity to the reference image $I_r(i) : i \to \mathbb{R}$. The registration can be formulated as a regularized optimization problem:

$$\widehat{D_f^r} = \operatorname*{argmin}_{D_f^r} E(I_f, I_r, D_f^r) + \lambda S(D_f^r) \tag{1}$$

where $E(I_f, I_r, D_f^r)$ is the dissimilarity measure between the reference and deformed images, $S(D_f^r)$ is usually the harmonic regularization criteria: $\|\nabla D_f^r\|^2$ and λ is a weighting parameter that controls the balance between the smoothness and the accuracy of the solution. The regularization ensures the smoothness and spatial coherence of the resulting deformation field.

The demons algorithm [16] computes the deformation field that minimizes the energy in Eq. 1 by minimizing each of the energy terms separately instead of the complex global optimization. Thus, it is often considered an "ad-hoc" solution. In order to cast the demons algorithm into a well-posed energy minimization problem, Cachier et al [6] introduced an auxiliary variable which serves as a moderator between the correspondences C_f^r as computed by minimizing the dissimilarity measure and the actual dense transformation D_f^r. Their energy minimization is formulated as:

$$\widehat{D_f^r} = \operatorname*{argmin}_{D_f^r} E(I_f, I_r, C_f^r) + \sigma\|C_f^r - D_f^r\|^2 + \lambda S(D_f^r) \tag{2}$$

where $\|C_f^r - D_f^r\|^2$ is the vectorial norm between the correspondences and the deformation field and σ is a weighting parameter.

By replacing the vectorial norm between the displacement and deformation fields with a generalized minimization formulation:

$$D_f^r \leftarrow \operatorname*{argmin}_{D_f^r \in \Omega_{D_f^r}} \|D_f^r - C_f^r\|^2 \tag{3}$$

where $\Omega_{D_f^r}$ is the domain of the transformations of interest, we may integrate prior information on the deformation field into the registration framework. The assignment: $D_f^r \leftarrow C_f^r$ is a private case of the generalized minimization in Eq. 3, where $\Omega_{D_f^r}$ is the entire domain of the dense deformation fields.

The local-affine motion model assumes that the motion of each voxel i is associated with some local affine motion of its similar nearby voxels. Thus, the minimization of Eq. 3 can be replaced by a sum of voxel-associated minimization problems:

$$\underset{D_f^r \in \Omega_{D_f^r}}{\operatorname{argmin}} \| D_f^r - C_f^r \|^2 \sim \sum_i \underset{A}{\operatorname{argmin}} \| A(i) - C_f^r(i) \|^2 \qquad (4)$$

where A is an affine transformation and $A(i)$ is the deformation of voxel i resulting from applying A_i on i. The minimization of Eq. 4 can be formulated as a fitting problem in which we seek an affine transformation that best represents the correspondence of voxel i based on its nearby voxels.

2.2   Robust Local Affine Transformation Fitting

The fitting of local affine transformation for each voxel is done using the hybrid expectation-maximization iterative closest point approach proposed in [1]. We describe the method in detail next.

For each voxel i, our goal is to find an affine transform A_i that best approximates the deformation of the structure in this region with respect to its neighboring voxels $j \in \Omega_i$ and their correspondences $C_f^r(j)$. Considering all voxels $j \in \Omega_i$ equally may introduce motions of different organs. Therefore, we use a hybrid weighting function that prefers voxels with intensity values similar to that of voxel i and have affine motion similar to the motion of their nearby voxels. Consequently, the local affine fitting is formulated as a weighted least-squares problem:

$$\widehat{A_i} = \underset{A}{\operatorname{argmin}} \sum_{j \in \Omega_i} w_j \cdot \| A(j) - C_f^r(j) \|^2 \qquad (5)$$

The weights w_j are defined as:

$$w_j = \alpha \cdot e^{\left(-\frac{(I(i) - I(j))^2}{2\sigma_{sig}^2} \right)} + (1 - \alpha) \cdot e^{\left(-\frac{(A_i(j) - C_f^r(j))^2}{2\sigma_{dist}^2} \right)} \qquad (6)$$

where σ_{sig} is a predefined scaling parameter representing the expected variability in the local structure intensity, σ_{dist} is a predefined scaling parameter representing the expected deviation of the current voxel motion from the local structure affine motion, and α is a weighting parameter that balances between these two weighting terms.

The transformation $\widehat{A_i}$ that minimizes Eq. 5 is computed by applying the following two successive steps iteratively:

1. Update the weights w_j based on the difference between the observed correspondence $C_f^r(j)$ and the current estimated affine transform A_i
2. Solve Eq. 5 using [3] with updated weights.

Where at the first iteration: $A_i = id$.

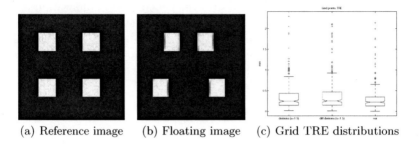

(a) Reference image   (b) Floating image   (c) Grid TRE distributions

Fig. 1. Synthetic example: (a) Reference image, (b) Deformed image, (c) Box-plots of the TRE distributions measured on the grid points for the demons algorithm (left), the diffeomorphic demons algorithm (center) and our algorithm (right)

2.3   Diffeomorphic Update Rule

The demons algorithm iterative scheme [16] uses additive or compositive up-date rules, where the deformation that computed at current iteration is added or composed into the overall deformation. However, these update steps do not ensure the diffeomorphic property of the resulting transformation. Therefore, we use an exponential update rule as proposed in [17].

3   Experimental Results

3.1   Synthetic Example

A synthetic image (Fig. 1a) consisting of 4 squares with 10% additive noise was deformed by a synthetically generated deformation field, and produced the de-formed image (Fig. 1b). The synthetic transformation was generated by defining a different translational component to each square, and constructing a global Thin-Plate Spline (TPS) transformation from these local translations. Next, the images were registered using our approach, the demons registration [16] with compositive update rule, and with the diffeomorphic demons algorithm [17]. For all of the algorithms, we used a multi-resolution scheme with 3 resolutions and 15,10,5 iterations at each resolution, respectively, and an elastic smoothing kernel where $\sigma = 1.5$. The additional specific parameters for our local affine fitting were: $\sigma_{dist} = 2mm$, $\sigma_{sig} = 15$, $\alpha = 0.2$. The neighborhood size that was used for the local affine computation was 5x5, and 7 iterations were used in Eq. 5.

Targets were distributed equally on a uniform grid over the image domain. The Target Registration Error (TRE) was measured for each of the algorithms. Fig. 1c presents the TRE distribution for each of the algorithms in box-plot presentation. Our algorithm produced the most accurate deformation field. The harmonic energy values of the fields were as follows: Our method: 0.0825, dif-feomorphic demons: 0.095, and for the demons algorithm: 0.1. This synthetic example shows that our method produces smoother deformation fields compared to the other approaches, while improving the registration accuracy.

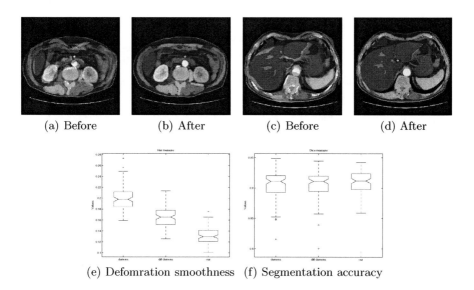

(a) Before   (b) After   (c) Before   (d) After

(e) Defomration smoothness   (f) Segmentation accuracy

Fig. 2. Controlled clinical registration example: (a)-(d) Representative axial slices from abdominal CT scan with the deformed manual annotation overlaid before (a,c) and after registration (b,d). (e) Box-plot representation of the harmonic energy values of the deformation fields produced by the demons algorithm (left), by the diff. demons algorithm (middle), and by our method (right), for 400 experiments. (f) Box-plot representations of the accuracy of multiple organ segmentation produced by the registration using the demons algorithm (left), by the diffeomorphic demons algorithm (middle), and by our method (right), measured by Dice measure, for 400 experiments.

3.2   Controlled Experiment

To evaluate our method on real images, we used a publicly available abdominal CT atlas [14]. The data size was 256x256x113 voxels with physical spacing of 0.94x0.94x1.5mm³.

We randomly selected 4 axial slices from different parts of the abdomen. A total of 400 random TPS transformations were generated by defining a uniform grid over the image domain, defining a random translation of each grid vertex in the range of $[-10, 10]$mm on each axis, and building a global TPS transformation from these vertices. Then, the 100 TPS transformations were applied to each slice. Next, we applied our non-rigid registration method and compared its results to that of the original demons [16] and the diffeomorphic demons [17] algorithms. For all of the algorithms we used a multi-resolution scheme with 5 resolutions and 60,30,15,10,5 iterations at each resolution, respectively. We used only a elastic smoothing kernel with $\sigma = 1.5$. The additional specific parameters for our local affine fitting were: $\sigma_{dist} = 2mm$, $\sigma_{sig} = 40$, $\alpha = 0.2$. The neighborhood size that was used for the local affine computation was 3x3, and 7 iterations were used in Eq. 5. The registration quality was evaluated by measuring the accuracy

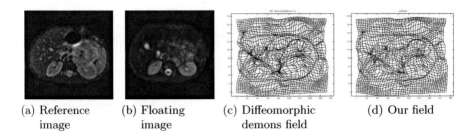

(a) Reference   (b) Floating   (c) Diffeomorphic   (d) Our field
    image   image   demons field

Fig. 3. DWI registration: (a) Abdominal Diffusion MR image with bvalue=0 from pre-treatment stage, used as a reference image, (b) Abdominal Diffusion MR image with bvalue=0 from post-treatment stage, used as a floating image, (c) The deformation field computed using the diffeomorphic demons algorithm. (d) The deformation field computed using our algorithm. Our method produced smoother deformation field.

of the projected segmentation of multiple organs as compared to the manual annotation using the Dice similarity measure, and by the smoothness of the deformation fields.

Fig. 2(a-d) presents representative slices with the deformed segmentation overlaid before and after registration. Fig. 2(e-f) presents the distributions of the Harmonic energy and the computed deformation fields as well as the multiple organs segmentation accuracy using our method, the demons [16], and the diffeomorphic demons [17] algorithms from 400 experiments. Our method produced smoother deformation fields with slightly superior accuracy. This is in contrast to previous methods that suffer from a trade-off between the smoothness of the deformation field and the projected segmentation accuracy [19].

3.3   Longitudinal DWI Experiment

In order to demonstrate the application of our method to intra-patient longitudinal abdominal Diffusion MR image registration, we randomly selected a patient with a kidney Wilms tumor who underwent chemotherapy. Quantitative assessment of the tumor response to therapy using the method in [11] requires registration of the pre and post therapy images. The images were 176x176x50 voxels in size with physical spacing of $1.36 \times 1.36 \times 8 mm^3$. The images first globally aligned. Next, a representative slice was extracted from each volume and registered using our method, and with the demons and the diffeomorphic demons algorithms. Fig. 3(a)-(b) presents the images that were used in this experiment, and Fig. 3(c)-(d) presents the deformation fields as computed by the diffeomorphic demons algorithm (c) and by our algorithm (d). The harmonic energy of the field computed by our algorithm was lower than the energy of the field computed by the diffeomorphic demons algorithm.

4   Conclusions

We have presented a method to integrate a local-affine prior model into a non-parametric non-rigid registration framework. Our approach uses the auxiliary variable of correspondences to introduce prior models into the dense-deformation computation. The local-affine model is used to moderate between the observed correspondences and the desired dense-deformation field. Both quantitative and qualitative evaluation shows that the integration of our approach into the diffeo-morphic demons framework produced smoother deformation fields with superior accuracy as compared to the original diffeomorphic demons method.

Acknowledgements. This investigation was supported in part by NIH grants R01 RR021885, R01 EB008015, R03 EB008680 and R01 LM010033.

References

1. Akselrod-Ballin, A., Bock, D., Reid, R., Warfield, S.: Improved registration for large electron microscopy images. In: IEEE Int. Sym. Biomedical Imaging: From Nano to Macro, ISBI 2009, pp. 434–437 (2009)
2. Arsigny, V., Commowick, O., Ayache, N., Pennec, X.: A fast and log-euclidean polyaffine framework for locally linear registration. Journal of Mathematical Imaging and Vision 33(2), 222–238 (2009)
3. Arun, K., Huang, T., Blostein, S.: Least-Squares Fitting of Two 3-D Point Sets. IEEE Trans. Patt. Anal. Mach. Intell. 9(5), 698–700 (1987)
4. Ma, B., Meyer, C.R., Pickles, M.D., Chenevert, T.L., Bland, P.H., Galbán, C.J., Rehemtulla, A., Turnbull, L.W., Ross, B.D.: Voxel-by-Voxel Functional Diffusion Mapping for Early Evaluation of Breast Cancer Treatment. In: Prince, J.L., Pham, D.L., Myers, K.J. (eds.) IPMI 2009. LNCS, vol. 5636, pp. 276–287. Springer, Heidelberg (2009)
5. Buerger, C., Schaeffter, T., King, A.: Hierarchical adaptive local affine registration for respiratory motion estimation from 3-D MRI. In: IEEE Int. Sym. Biomedical Imaging: From Nano to Macro, ISBI 2010, pp. 1237–1240 (2010)
6. Cachier, P., Bardinet, E., Dormont, D., Pennec, X., Ayache, N.: Iconic feature based nonrigid registration: the PASHA algorithm. Comp. Vis. Image Und. 89(2–3), 272–298 (2003); nonrigid Image Registration
7. Cahill, N., Noble, J., Hawkes, D.: A Demons Algorithm for Image Registration with Locally Adaptive Regularization. In: Yang, G.-Z., Hawkes, D., Rueckert, D., Noble, A., Taylor, C. (eds.) MICCAI 2009, Part I. LNCS, vol. 5761, pp. 574–581. Springer, Heidelberg (2009)
8. Commowick, O., Arsigny, V., Isambert, A., Costa, J., Dhermain, F., Bidault, F., Bondiau, P.Y., Ayache, N., Malandain, G.: An efficient locally affine framework for the smooth registration of anatomical structures. Medical Image Analysis 12(4), 427–441 (2008)
9. Freiman, M., Voss, S., Warfield, S.: Demons registration with local affine adaptive regularization: application to registration of abdominal structures. In: Proceedings of the 8th IEEE International Symposium on Biomedical Imaging: From Nano to Macro, ISBI 2011, pp. 1219–1222 (2011)

10. Koh, D., Thoeny, H. (eds.): Diffusion-Weighted MR imaging: applications in the body. Springer, Heidelberg (2010)
11. Moffat, B., Chenevert, T., Meyer, C., McKeever, P., Hall, D., Hoff, B., Johnson, T., Rehemtulla, A., Ross, B.: The functional diffusion map: an imaging biomarker for the early prediction of cancer treatment outcome. Neoplasia 8(4), 259–267 (2006)
12. Risholm, P., Samset, E., Talos, I., Wells, W.: A Non-Rigid Registration Framework that Accommodates Resection and Retraction. In: Prince, J.L., Pham, D.L., Myers, K.J. (eds.) IPMI 2009. LNCS, vol. 5636, pp. 447–458. Springer, Heidelberg (2009)
13. Rueckert, D., Sonoda, L., Hayes, C., Hill, D., Leach, M., Hawkes, D.: Nonrigid registration using free-form deformations: application to breast MR images. IEEE Trans. Med. Imaging 18(8), 712–721 (1999)
14. Talos, I., Jakab, M., Kikinis, R.: Spl abdominal atlas (2008),
http://www.spl.harvard.edu/publications/item/view/1266
15. Tang, L., Hamarneh, G., Abugharbieh, R.: Reliability-Driven, Spatially-Adaptive Regularization for Deformable Registration. In: Fischer, B., Dawant, B.M., Lorenz, C. (eds.) WBIR 2010. LNCS, vol. 6204, pp. 173–185. Springer, Heidelberg (2010)
16. Thirion, J.: Image matching as a diffusion process: an analogy with maxwell's demons. Med. Image Anal. 2(3), 243–260 (1998)
17. Vercauteren, T., Pennec, X., Perchant, A., Ayache, N.: Diffeomorphic demons: Efficient non-parametric image registration. NeuroImage 45(1, supplement 1), S61–S72 (2009)
18. Xiahai, Z., Rhode, K., Razavi, R., Hawkes, D., Ourselin, S.: A Registration-Based Propagation Framework for Automatic Whole Heart Segmentation of Cardiac MRI. IEEE Trans. Med Imaging 29(9), 1612–1625 (2010)
19. Yeo, B., Sabuncu, M., Desikan, R., Fischl, B., Golland, P.: Effects of registration regularization and atlas sharpness on segmentation accuracy. Med. Image Anal. 12(5), 603–615 (2008)

FIST: Fast Interactive Segmentation of Tumors

Sebastian Steger and Georgios Sakas

Fraunhofer IGD,
Department of Cognitive Computing & Medical Imaging,
Fraunhoferstrasse 5, 64283 Darmstadt, Germany
Sebastian.Steger@igd.fraunhofer.de

Abstract. Automatic segmentation methods for tumors are typically only suitable for a specific type of tumor in a specific imaging modality and sometimes lack in accuracy whereas manual tumor segmentation achieves the desired results but is very time consuming. Interactive segmentation however speeds up the process while still being able to maintain the accuracy of manual segmentation.

This paper presents a novel method for fast interactive segmentation of tumors (called FIST) from medical images, which is suitable for all somewhat spherical tumors in any 3d medical imaging modality. The user clicks in the center of the tumor and a belief propagation based iterative adaption process is initiated, thereby considering image gradients as well as local smoothness priors of the surface. During that process, instant visual feedback is given, enabling to intervene in the adaption process by sketching parts of the contour in any cross section.

The approach has successfully been applied to the segmentation of liver tumors in CT datasets. Satisfactory results could be achieved in 15.21 seconds on the average. Further trials on oropharynx tumors, liver tumors and the prostate from MR images as well as lymph nodes and the bladder from CT volumes demonstrate the generality of the presented approach.

Keywords: tumor segmentation, interactive segmentation, belief propagation.

1 Introduction

The accurate 3d segmentation of tumors in medical images is required for analysis, therapy planning and visualization. An example application scenario is the preoperative target definition for radio frequency ablation of tumors in the abdomen, e.g. liver tumors.

The size and shape of tumors can vary tremendously. However for many types of tumors – including liver tumors – the shape is typically somewhat spherical. The appearance in prevalent imaging modalities also varies from type to type and from instance to instance. Whereas some tumors show a strong image gradient at the boundary and therefore can easily be segmented with high accuracy, the boundaries of other tumors are hardly visible or even not at all in any common

H. Yoshida et al. (Eds.): Abdominal Imaging 2011, LNCS 7029, pp. 125–132, 2012.

imaging modality. In those cases the boundary of a tumor can only be guessed by an experienced observer based on indirect signs like irregularities in anatomy due to tumor growth. Even for some tumors with seemingly visible boundaries, the actual tumor may be larger and can only be guessed based on the experience of the observer.

Whereas manual contouring is very time consuming and therefore prone to errors due to fatigue of the operator, automatic or semi-automatic segmentation techniques may in some cases not yield in the required accuracy. Furthermore automatic and semi-automatic segmentation methods are typically tailored and fine-tuned to a very specific segmentation problem (e.g. [5]). A generalization to different imaging modalities or different types of structures is in many cases not possible.

Interactive segmentation does usually not suffer from these problems. For a successful fast interactive segmentation the following key requirements must be met:

- The algorithm shall adapt to user interaction in the sense that a manual delineation always overrules any automatization. This guarantees that accuracy identical to manual segmentation can be achieved.
- The smaller the amount of interaction is, the faster a segmentation can be achieved.
- All interactions shall be performed using a user friendly GUI. The user shall receive instant visual feedback from the GUI during the segmentation process.
- The method shall be as general as possible, meaning that it should perform well across different types of tumors in different imaging modalities.

Many interactive segmentation techniques exist. Popular methods are based on *seeded region growing* [1], *interactive graph cuts* [4], *simple interactive object extraction* [7] or *binary partition trees* [11]. A comparative evaluation of those interactive segmentation algorithms can be found in [9]. Furthermore interactive methods based on the adaption of contours have been presented [8].

In this work a novel interactive 3d segmentation method for more or less spheric structures such as tumors is presented. It has successfully been applied to the segmentation of liver tumors from CT and MR images as well as to other structures.

2   Segmentation Process

The workflow of the segmentation process from the user's perspective is as follows: In a cross section view of a 3d medical volume the user initially sets a seed point in the approximate center of the target structure (Fig. 1(a)). An initial surface around that point purely based on image features is shown (Fig. 1(b)). In many cases this initial contour is rather discontinuous. Within very few seconds this contour iteratively adapts in order to meet a compromise between smoothness and image criteria (Fig. 1(c)). During this adaption process the user

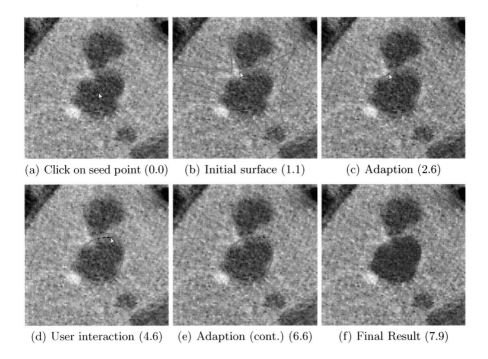

(a) Click on seed point (0.0)   (b) Initial surface (1.1)   (c) Adaption (2.6)

(d) User interaction (4.6)   (e) Adaption (cont.) (6.6)   (f) Final Result (7.9)

Fig. 1. Interactive segmentation workflow (duration in seconds)

may navigate through the volume and observe the adaption process. In case he or she is not satisfied with the adaption, the user can intervene by manually sketching parts of the boundary in any cross section (Fig. 1(d)). The adaption process then incorporates this input as a constraint in the subsequent iterations (Fig. 1(e)). The user must stop the process as soon as he or she is satisfied with the segmentation result (Fig. 1(f)).

3   Adaption Algorithm

3.1   Data Structure

The target structures are assumed to be somewhat spherical. For such objects at least one central point – the seed point – exists, which can be directly connected to each point on the object's surface without intersecting the surface elsewhere. Thus the surface can uniquely be described by assigning a single radius to each member of a set of m angles uniformly covering all possible angles in the 3d space (see Fig. 2): $[0, .., m-1] \mapsto \mathbb{R}^+$, or $[0, .., m-1] \mapsto \mathbb{N}$ in the discrete version. Very similar data structures are used for the segmentation of gliomas from MRI [6] and lymph nodes from CT images [2].

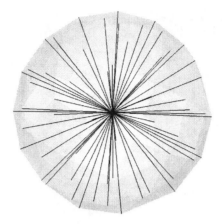

Fig. 2. Rays are sent out from a given seed point. Segmentation is given by an assignment of a radius to each ray. It is obtained jointly by globally minimizing an energy function using belief propagation.

An energy is assigned to each possible configuration $r \in \mathbb{N}^m$, a low energy for likely surfaces and high energy for unlikely surfaces. It depends on the image, the user input and local shape priors. The actual segmentation process then comes down to an energy optimization problem.

3.2 Energy Functional

The energy to be minimized is given by

$$E(r) = \sum_{i=0}^{i<m} \left(c(r_i \cdot a_i) + \lambda \cdot \sum_{j \in N(i)} c(r_i, r_j) \right) , \tag{1}$$

where λ is a balancing weight, a_i denotes a unit vector in the direction of ray i, the unary term $c(x)$ represents a cost for a single point and the pairwise term $c(r_i, r_j)$ represents a cost for the transition between the assignment of two neighboring rays. The neighborhood is denoted by $N(i)$ and includes all neighboring rays.

Image Based. The image based contribution to the unary cost term $c(x)$ may depend on many different image properties. The more is known about the target structure, the more specific this term can be. For example if a typical gray value range was known, the term could penalize configurations in which parts of interior are not within that range, as seen in [12]. Furthermore the term could incorporate gray value homogeneity in the interior and/or exterior or even learnt gray value profiles.

All of these examples have in common that something about the structure has to be known in advance and thus generality is lost. Instead we only deploy an image gradient based cost which is given by

$$c(\boldsymbol{x}) = \max(0, g_{\max} - |\nabla(G_\sigma * I(\boldsymbol{x}))|), \tag{2}$$

where $g_{\max}$ is the maximal gradient strength, ∇ is the gradient operator, $*$ is the convolution operator and G_σ is a gaussian kernel. Please note that the costs are bound to $[0, g_{\max}]$ in order to not favor very large gradients potentially not belonging to the object's boundaries. The gaussian kernel is used to suppress noise. A non local minimum suppression technique can additionally be used in order to favor the exact object boundary in areas that all have a larger image gradient than $g_{\max}$.

Shape Preserving Cost. To ensure a smooth contour, similar radii of neighboring rays shall be preferred. This is reflected by the shape preserving cost:

$$c_{\text{shape}}(i, j) = \frac{r_{\max}}{n} \cdot |r_i, r_j|^\alpha , \tag{3}$$

where r_i and r_j represent the radii of two neighboring rays, $\frac{r_{\max}}{n}$ is the distance between two neighboring radii and α allows to over proportionally penalize large differences of neighboring radii.

User Input. As soon as the user draws a contour the unary costs are adapted in the following way: For all drawn points, the closest ray with the direction $\hat{a}$ and the euclidean distance $\hat{d}$ to the seed point is computed. Then the costs are set to

$$c(d \cdot \hat{a}) = \begin{cases} 0 & d = \hat{d} \\ \infty & \text{otherwise} \end{cases} . \tag{4}$$

This ensures that the optimal solution – the segmentation surface – will go through the manually drawn points. Due to the shape preserving cost, similar radii will be assigned to the surrounding rays.

Optimization. In [2], a gradient descent like approach was successfully used in a similar optimization problem. However, due to the interactive change of the energy functional, the optimal solution may "jump" from one to another local optimum and thus local optimization approaches are not suitable.

Since the energy given by equation (1) depends on a unary term and pairwise connections between direct neighbors only, the energy minimization problem is suited to be minimized by the belief propagation algorithm [10] or the graph cut algorithm [3]. Even though the latter showed slightly superior optimization performance in some cases [13], we decided to use the former as the interactive adaption of the energy functional can easily be incorporated.

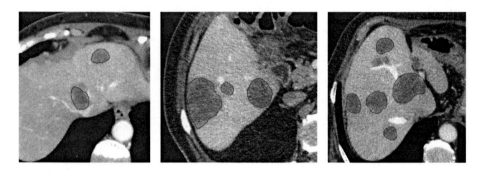

Fig. 3. Segmentation of liver tumors from CT images

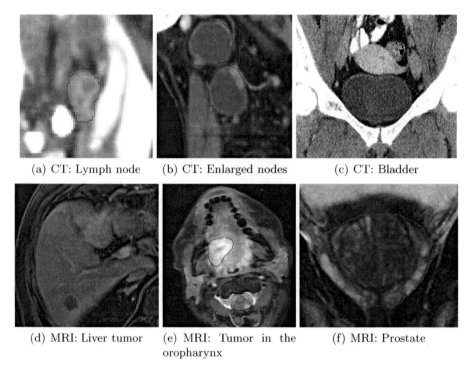

(a) CT: Lymph node   (b) CT: Enlarged nodes   (c) CT: Bladder

(d) MRI: Liver tumor   (e) MRI: Tumor in the   (f) MRI: Prostate
                         oropharynx

Fig. 4. Application to different somewhat spherical structures from different imaging modalities

The general idea of the algorithm is that messages are iteratively passed from nodes to neighboring nodes thereby inferring the most likely assignment. In our case we use the algorithm to jointly infer the most likely radius for each ray. Messages are passed between neighboring rays. After each iteration the most likely assignment is computed and the corresponding surface is shown in the graphical user interface, giving the operator instant feedback and the chance to intervene.

4   Experiments

The presented approach has been applied to the segmentation of 24 liver tumors from 3 CT images. The operator clicked in the center of the lesion and then interacted with the system until the expected contour was shown. In all cases this was possible because the boundaries of all tumors could be directly connected from the seed point without intersecting the contour elsewhere. For spherical tumors almost no interaction was required, whereas for others with corners required heavy interaction. The interactive segmentation of a single tumor took 15.21 seconds on the average. The standard deviation was 16.64 seconds. Figure 3 shows some sample results.

In order to test the generality of the presented interactive segmentation technique, it was applied to various somewhat spherical structures from different imaging modalities: Lymph nodes and the urinal bladder from CT as well as the prostate, liver tumors and tumors in the oropharynx from MR images. All of these structures could be satisfactorily segmented. Results can be seen in Figure 4.

5   Conclusion

This paper presented a novel method for fast interactive segmentation of tumors (FIST). From all possible surfaces around a user defined seed point, the most likely surface is computed by minimizing an energy functional using belief propagation. The energy of a surface depends on the image gradient and the local smoothness. During the adaption process the user gets instant visual feedback and is able to interactively set specific points of the surface in all three orthogonal cross sections. The approach has successfully been tested on liver tumors in CT images as well as on other kind of structures in CT and MR images.

While achieving similar accuracy than manual segmentation, it is a lot faster (on the average only 15.21 seconds for each entity) and therefore feasible to use it in clinical routine, for example for target definition in abdominal intervention. In contrast to automated segmentation techniques, FIST is not limited to a specific type of structure in a single imaging modality, but can be used on any somewhat spherical in any 3d imaging modality. Furthermore the user has a major impact on the segmentation result, so that even tumors with only little contrast can still be segmented based on the operator's experience.

Future work includes research on further image based and shape preserving costs in order to require less user interaction to obtain segmentation results even faster. This may however sacrifice generality.

Acknowledgements. This work is partially funded within the NeoMark project (FP7-ICT-2007-2-224483) by the European Commission.

References

1. Adams, R., Bischof, L.: Seeded region growing. IEEE Transactions on Pattern Analysis and Machine Intelligence 16(6), 641–647 (1994)
2. Barbu, A., Suehling, M., Xu, X., Liu, D., Zhou, S., Comaniciu, D.: Automatic Detection and Segmentation of Axillary Lymph Nodes. In: Jiang, T., Navab, N., Pluim, J.P.W., Viergever, M.A. (eds.) MICCAI 2010, Part I. LNCS, vol. 6361, pp. 28–36. Springer, Heidelberg (2010)
3. Boykov, Y., Veksler, O., Zabih, R.: Fast approximate energy minimization via graph cuts. IEEE Transactions on Pattern Analysis and Machine Intelligence 23(11), 1222–1239 (2001)
4. Boykov, Y.Y., Jolly, M.P.: Interactive graph cuts for optimal boundary & region segmentation of objects in n-d images. In: Proc. Eighth IEEE Int. Conf. Computer Vision, ICCV 2001, vol. 1, pp. 105–112 (2001)
5. Dornheim, L., Dornheim, J., Rossling, I., Monch, T.: Model-based segmentation of pathological lymph nodes in ct data, vol. 7623, p. 76234V. SPIE (2010)
6. Egger, J., Bauer, M., Kuhnt, D., Carl, B., Kappus, C., Freisleben, B., Nimsky, C.: Nugget-Cut: A Segmentation Scheme for Spherically- and Elliptically-Shaped 3d Objects. In: Goesele, M., Roth, S., Kuijper, A., Schiele, B., Schindler, K. (eds.) DAGM 2010. LNCS, vol. 6376, pp. 373–382. Springer, Heidelberg (2010)
7. Friedland, G., Jantz, K., Rojas, R.: Siox: simple interactive object extraction in still images. In: Proc. Seventh IEEE Int. Multimedia Symp. (2005)
8. Kass, M., Witkin, A., Terzopoulos, D.: Snakes: Active contour models. International Journal of Computer Vision 1(4), 321–331 (1988)
9. McGuinness, K., O'Connor, N.E.: A comparative evaluation of interactive segmentation algorithms. Pattern Recognition 43(2), 434–444 (2010)
10. Pearl, J.: Probabilistic Reasoning in Intelligent Systems: Networks of Plausible Inference. Morgan Kaufmann Publishers Inc., San Francisco (1988)
11. Salembier, P., Garrido, L.: Binary partition tree as an efficient representation for image processing, segmentation, and information retrieval 9(4), 561–576 (2000)
12. Steger, S., Erdt, M.: Lymph node segmentation in ct images using a size invariant mass spring model. In: 10th IEEE International Conference on Information Technology and Applications in Biomedicine (ITAB) pp. 1–4 (2010)
13. Tappen, M.F., Freeman, W.T.: Comparison of graph cuts with belief propagation for stereo, using identical mrf parameters. In: Proc. Ninth IEEE Int. Computer Vision Conf., pp. 900–906 (2003)

Intraoperative Registration
for Liver Tumor Ablation

Cristina Oyarzun Laura[1], Klaus Drechsler[1], Marius Erdt[1], Matthias Keil[1],
Matthias Noll[1], Stefano De Beni[2], Georgios Sakas[1,3], and Luigi Solbiati[4]

[1] Fraunhofer Institute for Computer Graphics Research IGD
[2] Esaote Spa
[3] Technische Universitaet Darmstadt
[4] General Hospital of Busto Arsizio
cristina.oyarzun@igd.fraunhofer.de

Abstract. Computer aided navigation augments intraoperatively gathered U/S with planning information that the doctor carries out before
the intervention on a CT volume. A crucial step for the navigation is the
registration between CT and U/S. Our approach consists on a landmark
based registration. The correspondences between both modalities are
found automatically using a graph to graph matching algorithm. Therefore, liver and vessels are previously segmented. The whole process has
being tested on 15 pairs of real clinical data. The results are promising.

Keywords: Intervention, liver, tumor ablation, registration, segmentation, graph matching, navigation.

1 Introduction

Tumor ablation interventions require of a previous planning in which the doctor
checks where the tumor is and how should he proceed during the intervention.
Unfortunately planning information remains on the preoperatively gathered CT,
while the modality used during the intervention is U/S. With the U/S information alone the doctor needs to guess where the target is and proceed accordingly.
Computer aided navigation tries to overcome those problems. The CT containing the planning information is registered to the intraoperative U/S showing
the doctor where the target is on the resulting registered image. Each time the
doctor acquires a new U/S volume it is registered to the CT augmenting the
U/S with the planning information.

Lange et al. [1] faced the challenge with a combined landmark and intensity
based registration method. The results show qualitatively good results, however
they assume that in the time available during the intervention it is possible
to identify 5-6 corresponding landmarks. In our first approach we were also
preselecting corresponding landmarks manually. The preselection task was easy
in those pairs of data containing very small deformations, however in most of
the data, the preselection showed to be difficult and time consuming. That is
why in this work we present a different approach in which the correspondences
are found automatically using a graph to graph matching algorithm.

H. Yoshida et al. (Eds.): Abdominal Imaging 2011, LNCS 7029, pp. 133–140, 2012.

2   Methods

Fig. 1 shows the workflow of our approach. The first step before a surgery is to plan the intervention. This is carried out on a preoperatively gathered CT. To augment the intraoperative U/S with the planning information a registration between CT and U/S is necessary. Our approach consists on a landmark based registration. The liver and its vessels are segmented out of the CT volume before the surgery. During the intervention the doctor acquires a series of U/S images to guide himself. After a U/S is taken its vessels are segmented and the corresponding bifurcation points between the CT and U/S vessel trees are automatically identified. Once all the landmarks are known a rigid registration is carried out.

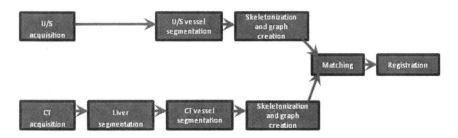

Fig. 1. Workflow of the whole process. First the liver and the vessels are segmented, after that a graph is generated out of the segmented vessels and corresponding landmarks are automatically identified using a graph matching algorithm. Finally CT and U/S are rigidly registered.

2.1   Liver Segmentation

The shape of the liver strongly varies between subjects and may also be influenced by diseases or treatment procedures. In order to segment the liver robustly for a large set of individual liver shapes, a statistical shape model based approach is used [2]. In a recent comparison of liver segmentation methods [3], the majority of the best scoring automatic approaches were using statistical shape information. The chosen method has the advantage of being very robust to initialization errors. This is important, since a correct model placement can often not be guaranteed due to different patient positioning, low contrast images etc. Fig. 2 shows an exemplary segmentation result.

2.2   Vessel Segmentation and Graph Creation

We use a multi-scale analysis approach to segment the vessels. We detect the tubular structures at each scale by using the vesselness function introduced by Sato et al. [4], which has shown to keep the connection at the vessel junctions better [5] that other popular functions. We use a weighted additive response

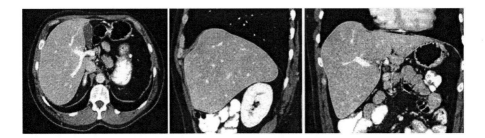

Fig. 2. The yellow line shows the surface of the segmented liver

(WAR) for the combination of the results at each scale. With this approach introduced in [6] the separation between nearby vessels is better compared to the results obtained by using maximum response approach. To create a formal graph out of the segmented vessels we first need to calculate their centerline. Therefore we use the thinning-based algorithm proposed by Lee et al. in [7]. The approach proposed by Drechsler et al. [8] makes use of the generated skeleton to get the graph representation that will be used as input for the graph matching algorithm.

2.3   U/S Acquisition

Naturally ultrasound imaging is a low resolution image modality especially if compared to other image modalities like high resolution CT or MRI. To generate a 3D ultrasound volume of equal quality to the ultrasound input data, the tracked image acquisition and the 3D reconstruction have to be very sophisticated [9,10]. Furthermore depending on the patients liver condition (e.g. normal, fat or cirrhotic liver) the acquisition quality may be negatively influenced. Thus the extraction of vessel information from B-mode 3D ultrasound data is a challenging task and the quality that can be achieved depends highly on the available 3D ultrasound data. Since we are mainly interested in the liver vessel information we can utilize the ultrasound transducer capability to acquire color flow images that show blood flow information and therefore vessels. But even here good balances of power and persistency options of the ultrasound have to be found to acquire usable data. A 3D intraoperative ultrasound can generally be performed percutaneous or subcutaneous with mechanical probes or by utilizing freehand methods. We believe that, while each acquisition method has its advantages and disadvantages, a freehand based acquisition with small transducers is the best approach in open liver surgery scenarios due to space constrictions between mobilized organ and the body cavity. Here the employed ultrasound probe should have a good field of view to minimize moving artifacts in the 3D reconstruction compared to the prolonged acquisition time of small field of view transducers. To enable a good freehand reconstruction an accurate freehand ultrasound calibration is required [11]. How to obtain such a calibration is thoroughly described in the literature. The acquisition itself should be performed with homogeneous speed, equal direction and angle to minimize reconstruction artifacts.

2.4   Interactive Graph Matching

Doctors are very experienced on working on CT and U/S 2D slices. However, when it comes to work with the segmented vessels in 3D the interaction becomes difficult. We have implemented a series of interaction features to make this interaction easier (Fig. 3). On the one hand we show on the 3D view (top part of the figure) not only the vessels in 3D but also two perpendicular slices of the corresponding CT and U/S volumes. On the other hand we show two 2D views (bottom part of the figure) showing the CT and U/S slices respectively. The doctor can change the slice that is shown as well as the view (sagittal, coronal or transversal). When the doctor needs to interact with the matching algorithm to refine the results or to preselect matches that will be used by the manual algorithm, he can do it either in the 3D or in the 2D views. In any case the selected or removed node will appear or disappear automatically in the opposite window (3D or 2D). The selectable vessels are highlighted in white in the 2D view. When the doctor clicks near a selectable bifurcation in 2D, the corresponding bifurcation in 3D is highlighted and vice versa.

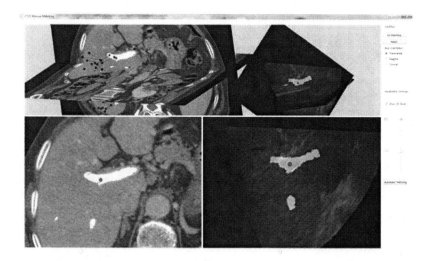

Fig. 3. Interactive application window. The upper renderer shows the 3D surface of the segmented vessels of the CT on the left and the U/S on the right side. They are augmented with the addition of two perpendicular slices of CT and U/S respectively. In the lower rendered one of the slices shown in the 3D view are shown. The segmented vessels appear highlighted in white. The doctor can interact either in the 2D or the 3D view and the results are automatically shown in both of them. The preselected correspondence is shown as a pink sphere.

2.5   Automatic Graph Matching

In a first step we developed a point cloud based matching algorithm which required the preselection of two pairs of corresponding nodes in CT and U/S. However, after clinical evaluation the preselection showed to be difficult and time consuming. It is desirable to save that time avoiding also the wrong preselection of points due to stress during the intervention. That is why we decided to apply an automatic graph to graph matching algorithm as proposed in [12]. This algorithm is independent of a known root. Additionally being a graph matching algorithm it does not need tree separation between hepatic and portal vein which also saves time intraoperatively. In this way the algorithm solves two problems that state of the art matching algorithms used in medical imaging have when they are used during interventions.

2.6   Registration

Using grey value information for multimodal registration of ultrasound B-Mode and CT images is insufficient. Even similarity metrics from information theory as Mutual Information are highly error prone, which has been shown in [13]. The main reason for failure is the difference in tissue properties represented by the two modalities. Therefore our goal was to build a common representation of the structures of interest. In our case we chose the vessel structures as internal landmarks for calculating the registration. By adapting the vessel segmentation techniques mentioned above to the ultrasound volume data, it is possible to derive three dimensional vessel structures from clinical ultrasound volumes. Our current application target for ultrasound and CT matching is needle navigation for percutaneous ablation of liver tumors. These interventions are performed under breath hold and therefore only little deformation of the liver parenchyma occurs. For that reason we are currently calculating rigid registrations of the two modalities based on the bifurcation points of the vessel structures. The transformation is calculated by minimizing the root mean squared distance between all matched bifurcation points.

3   Evaluation on Clinical Data

The presented workflow was applied to 15 patients. In 12 of them the results were satisfactory. Fig. 7 show the results of registering the CT and US on one of those 12 patients. The transversal view shows how the vessels and the border of the liver are correctly registered in CT and U/S. The coronal view shows how the gallbladder is also registered. The remaining 11 patient data show similar qualitative results. The process failed in three patients. Those patients had highly cyrrotic livers and the acquired U/S had very low quality and did not show vessel information.

Fig. 4 shows the matching results between the vessels segmented from a CT and U/S. The yellow circle shows an area in which the US segmentation leaked into the parenchyma, in addition to this there was a branch in the U/S that was missing in CT. The reason for this is that a refinement was applied to the CT segmented vessels to reduce the number of branches to be considered and consequently speed up the matching algorithm. Fig. 5 shows a case in which the U/S vessel segmentation leaked into a tumor, the CT segmentation however did not. The nodes inside the circles do not exist in the other graph and are therefore impossible to be matched. Even under these conditions automatic matching seems to work properly. Fig. 6 show some quantitative results of the automatic algorithm. The mean value of wrong matches found is 0.75.

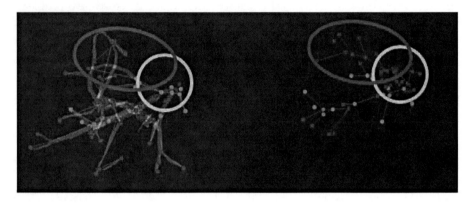

Fig. 4. Results of the matching. The U/S image (right) has a leakage in the parenchyma (yellow circle). An additional branch appears in U/S (red circle). This branch is missing in the CT because of the applied refinement to speed up the matching algorithm.

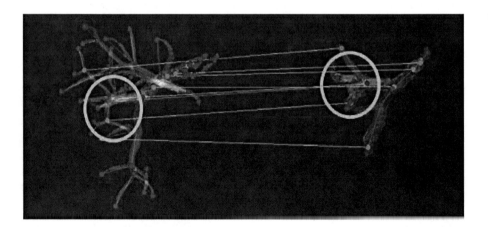

Fig. 5. Results of the matching. The U/S leaked into a tumor (yellow circle) showing false branches.

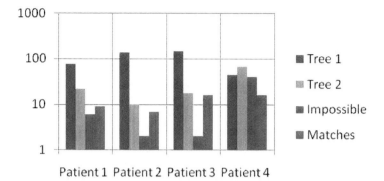

Fig. 6. Quantitative results of the graph matching algorithm on four patients. The red and green columns show the number of nodes that CT and U/S contained. The violet columns show the number of nodes impossible to be matched. The blue column show the number of correspondences found.

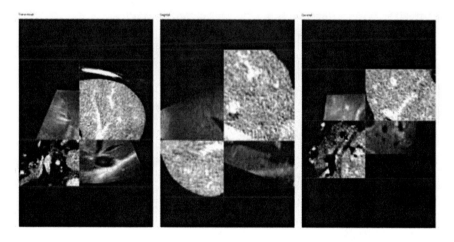

Fig. 7. Results of the rigid registration. Transversal (left), sagittal (middle) and coronal (right) are shown. The results show that vessels liver surface and gallbladder are correctly registered.

4   Conclusion

We present a registration method for computer aided navigation with application on liver tumor ablation. The presented approach is fast and overcomes the need of preselection of corresponding landmarks. It has being tested on 15 pairs of real clinical data presenting good qualitative results in cases where the liver is not highly cyrrotic. The introduction of deformation within the registration is part of our future work.

References

1. Lange, T., Papenberg, N., Heldmann, S., Modersitzki, J., Fischer, B., Lamecker, H., Schlag, P.: 3D ultrasound-CT registration of the liver using combined landmark-intensity information. International Journal of Computer Assisted Radiology and Surgery 79–88 (2009)
2. Erdt, M., Kirschner, M., Steger, S., Wesarg, S.: Fast Automatic Liver Segmentation Combining Learned Shape Priors with Observed Shape Deviation. In: IEEE International Symposium on Computer-Based Medical Systems, pp. 249–254 (2010)
3. Heimann, T., van Ginneken, B., Styner, M., et al.: Comparison and Evaluation of Methods for Liver Segmentation from CT datasets. IEEE Transactions on Medical Imaging 1251–1265 (2009)
4. Sato, Y., Nakajima, S., Atsumi, H., Koller, T., Gerig, G., Yoshida, S., Kikinis, R.: 3D multi-scale line filter for segmentation and visualization of curvilinear structures in medical images. In: Joint Conference Computer Vision, Virtual Reality and Robotics in Medicine and Medical Robotics and Computer-Assisted Surgery, pp. 213–222 (1997)
5. Drechsler, K., Oyarzun Laura, C.: Comparison of vesselness functions for multi-scale analysis of the liver vasculature. In: International Conference on Information Technology and Applications in Biomedicine, pp. 1–5 (2010)
6. Drechsler, K., Oyarzun Laura, C.: A Novel Multiscale Integration Approach for Vessel Enhancement. In: IEEE International Symposium on Computer-Based Medical Systems, pp. 92–97 (2010)
7. Lee, T., Kashyap, R., Chu, C.: Building skeleton models via 3-D medial surface/axis thinning algorithms. CVGIP: Graphical Models and Image Processing 462–478 (1994)
8. Drechsler, K., Oyarzun Laura, C.: Hierarchical Decomposition of Vessel Skeletons for Graph Creation and Feature Extraction. In: IEEE International Conference on Bioinformatics and Biomedicine, pp. 456–461 (2010)
9. Karamalis, A., Wein, W., Kutter, O., et al.: Fast Hybrid Freehand Ultrasound Volume Reconstruction. In: SPIE Medical Imaging (2009)
10. Dai, Y., Tian, J., Dong, D., Yan, G., Zheng, H.: Real-time visualized freehand 3D ultrasound reconstruction based on GPU. IEEE Transactions on Information Technology in Biomedicine, 1338–1345 (2010)
11. Wein, W., Khamene, A.: Image-Based Method for In-Vivo Freehand Ultrasound Calibration. In: SPIE Medical Imaging (2008)
12. Oyarzun Laura, C., Drechsler, K.: Graph to Graph Matching: Facing Clinical Challenges. In: IEEE International Symposium on Computer-Based Medical Systems (2011)
13. Keil, M., Stolka, P., Wiebel, M., Sakas, G., McVeigh, E., Taylor, R., Boctor, E.: Ultrasound and CT registration Quality: Elastography vs. Classical B-Mode. In: IEEE International Symposium on Biomedical Imaging: From Nano to Macro, pp. 967–970 (2009)

Sliding Geometries
in Deformable Image Registration

Danielle F. Pace[1], Marc Niethammer[2], and Stephen R. Aylward[1]

[1] Kitware Inc., Clifton Park NY and Carrboro NC, USA
{danielle.pace,stephen.aylward}@kitware.com
[2] The University of North Carolina at Chapel Hill, Chapel Hill NC, USA
mn@cs.unc.edu

Abstract. Regularization is used in deformable image registration to encourage plausible displacement fields, and significantly impacts the derived correspondences. Sliding motion, such as that between the lungs and chest wall and between the abdominal organs, complicates registration because many regularizations are global smoothness constraints that produce errors at object boundaries. We present locally adaptive regularizations that handle sliding objects with locally planar and tubular geometries. These regularizations allow discontinuities to develop in the displacement field at sliding interfaces and increase the independence with which regions surrounding distinct geometric structures can behave. Validation is performed by registering inhale and exhale abdominal computed tomography (CT) images and artificial images of a sliding tube. The sliding registration methods produce more realistic correspondences that may better reflect the underlying physical motion, while performing as well as the diffusive regularization with respect to image match.

1 Introduction

Within many clinical workflows, the goal of deformable image registration is to (1) quantify treatment effectiveness by measuring change within longitudinal datasets or across subjects, (2) map surgical plans from preoperative images onto intraoperative images for guidance, or (3) align atlases with patient images to map auxilliary information from the atlas, such as expected functional site localizations, into the patient. To successfully accomplish thse tasks, it is critical to establish accurate correspondence between the images. However, establishing correspondence using a deformable image registration method that optimizes image match alone is ill-posed, i.e. there exist many displacement fields that produce the same transformed moving image [5].

To obtain sensible correspondences using deformable image registration, a regularization term is typically introduced to encourage a smooth displacement field. The registration result is therefore a compromise between image similarity and spatial regularity, and the regularization forms a strong prior on the final transformation. This is true for any non-corner or point structure due to spatial ambiguity (the so-called aperture effect). Registration results are dependent on

H. Yoshida et al. (Eds.): Abdominal Imaging 2011, LNCS 7029, pp. 141–148, 2012.

relatively sparse features and regularization drives the estimation of otherwise unobservable deformations within homogeneous regions.

The focus of this paper is on accurately registering images that depict sliding motion between multiple structures. This includes the sliding of the abdominal organs and lungs due to respiration. Here, the assumption of a globally smooth displacement field is inappropriate, as globally smoothing regularizations, such as the diffusive regularization, cannot recover the motion discontinuities that arise at the interfaces between sliding structures. Locally adaptive regularizations [2,9] vary spatially and can more accurately capture complex deformations.

Several regularizations aiming to handle sliding motion have been presented, but have typically been applied to the alignment of lung images. These include investigations of non-quadratic regularizers [4], a volume-preserving regularization that allows shear discontinuities at sliding interfaces [7], and regularizations based on anisotropic diffusion that use supplied organ segmentations [6,8,10]. We take this last approach here. Yin *et al.* [10] tailor their regularization towards the biomechanics of lung lobar fissures using spatially-varying isotropic smoothing. Schmidt *et al.* [8] implement sliding motion by smoothing the displacement components tangential to the sliding interface separately for a sliding object and within its background, using Neumann boundary conditions. We present a regularization that instead applies separate diffusion tensors to the normal and tangential displacements of the entire displacement field. This regularization natively handles multiple sliding organs and has been evaluated preliminarily using synthetic and phantom lung images [6].

The sliding regularizations based on anisotropic diffusion described above, including our own work [6], solely handle displacement field discontinuities at roughly planar interfaces between two sliding organs. By also adding notions of tubular and point-like structures, we present a regularization that handles sliding motion of planes and tubes and that smooths displacement fields according to local structure classifications. We refer to registration methods including this regularization as "geometry conditional registration methods".

We begin by outlining our sliding organ formulation, followed by a description of its extension to a geometry conditional deformable registration method that also considers tubular and point-like structures. Validation is conducted by performing intra-subject registrations between inhale and exhale computed tomography (CT) images and between artificial images depicting a sliding tube. These assessments demonstrate the increased plausibility of the resulting displacement field, which encapsulates the correspondence necessary to use registration in clinical tasks. Additionally, these results demonstrate the advantages of considering sliding motion throughout the abdomen.

2   Methods

2.1   Deformable Non-parametric Image Registration

Given a target image T and a moving image M on the domain Ω, deformable non-parametric image registration aims to find a displacement field u that maps the moving image onto the target such that $T(\mathbf{x}) \approx M(\mathbf{x}-u(\mathbf{x}))$ [5]. This is often performed by minimizing a cost function of the form $C(u) = D[T, M; u]+\alpha S(u)$. $D[T, M; u]$ is an image match distance measure between T and M under the current estimate of the displacement field u, and $S(u)$ is the regularization that penalizes unrealistic displacement fields.

2.2 Principles of Sliding Motion

Writing a regularization for use in registering images depicting sliding organs can be guided by decomposing the displacement field u into normal $(u^{\perp})$ and tangential $(u^{\parallel})$ displacements with respect to the organ boundary along which sliding is expected to occur. One can then consider the following principles [6,8] close to sliding organ boundaries:

1. **Sliding motion:** Sliding causes the tangential displacements to be discontinuous along the normal direction(s).
2. **Intra-organ smoothness:** The displacements must be smooth along the tangential direction(s) to encourage smooth movement within individual structures.
3. **Inter-organ coupling:** Discontinuities in the normal displacements in the surface normal direction(s) are penalized to ensure organs do not pull apart (a valid assumption for many medical images).

2.3 Sliding Organ Registration

For sliding organ registration, we encapsulate these rules in a regularizer based on anisotropic diffusion [6]. Here, diffusion tensors specify the direction and strength of the intra-organ smoothness (IOS) and inter-organ coupling (IOC) constraints:

$$S_{sliding}(u) = \frac{1}{2} \sum_{l=x,y,z} \sum_{\mathbf{x} \in \Omega} \|D_{IOS}(\mathbf{x})\nabla u_l(\mathbf{x}) + D_{IOC}(\mathbf{x})\nabla u_l^{\perp}(\mathbf{x})\|^2 \qquad (1)$$

where ∇ is the gradient operator, $u_l(\mathbf{x})$ is the lth scalar component of the displacement field, and $u_l^{\perp}(\mathbf{x})$ is the lth scalar component of the normal component of the displacement field. If $n(\mathbf{x})$ is the normal to the organ boundary derived from a surface model of the organ and $n_l(\mathbf{x})$ is its lth scalar component, then $u_l^{\perp}(\mathbf{x}) = \left(u(\mathbf{x})^T n(\mathbf{x})\right) n_l(\mathbf{x})$.

The diffusion tensor

$$P(\mathbf{x}) = n(\mathbf{x})n(\mathbf{x})^T \qquad (2)$$

smooths in the normal direction alone, while the diffusion tensor $I - P(\mathbf{x})$ smooths in the tangential plane. We therefore define the intra-organ smoothness and inter-organ coupling diffusion tensors as:

$$\begin{aligned} D_{IOS}(\mathbf{x}) &= I - w(\mathbf{x})P(\mathbf{x}) \\ D_{IOC}(\mathbf{x}) &= w(\mathbf{x})P(\mathbf{x}) \end{aligned} \qquad (3)$$

The weighting term $w(\mathbf{x})$ equals one at organ borders and decreases as a function of the distance $d(\mathbf{x})$ to the organ boundary. $w(\mathbf{x})$ can be formulated as $w(\mathbf{x}) = e^{-\lambda d(\mathbf{x})}$ (exponential decay) or $w(\mathbf{x}) = \frac{1}{1+\lambda\gamma e^{-\lambda d(\mathbf{x})^2}}$ (Dirac function [8,10]). Within organ interiors, $w(\mathbf{x}) \approx 0$ and the sliding organ regularization tends to the diffusive regularization $S_{diffusive}(u) = \frac{1}{2}\sum_{l=x,y,z}\sum_{\mathbf{x}\in\Omega}\|\nabla u_l(\mathbf{x})\|^2$, which enforces smooth motion in all directions and serves as a point of comparison in this study.

2.4   Geometry Conditional Deformable Image Registration

Regions within medical images can be classified into four types: homogeneous regions, and those representing planes, tubes, and small point-like (spherical) structures. We would like to recover sliding motion for both planar and tubular structures. Examples of registrations involving the later include registration of images showing contrast agent flowing through vessels or needles moving through tissue.

In the geometry conditional regularization, we include explicit planar, tubular and point-like structure classifications and aim to recover large and discontinuous deformations. The intra-organ smoothness constraint ensures displacement field smoothness within individual structures and the inter-organ coupling constraint propagates locally detectable displacements to their neighborhood. Discontinuities are allowed to develop where there is tangential movement of planes or tubes. Tube segmentations are stored as centerline+radius+normals measurements and can be extracted using methods such as that described in [1]. Since correspondence for a point-like structure is unambiguous, its displacement vectors should be propagated to its surroundings and the diffusive regularization is appropriate. Forsberg $et\ al.$ [3] also integrate concepts of local structure but do not model sliding motion.

The sliding geometries regularizer is formed by substituting new definitions for $u_l^{\perp}(\mathbf{x})$ and $P(\mathbf{x})$ used in equations (1) and (3). Note that planar, tubular and point-like structures have one, two and three normals, respectively. Based on the local geometry, we include up to three normals at each coordinate, $n_0(\mathbf{x})$, $n_1(\mathbf{x})$, $n_2(\mathbf{x})$, and we add the structure-dependent variables $a_1(\mathbf{x})$ and $a_2(\mathbf{x})$ (planes: $a_1 = a_2 = 0$; tubes $a_1 = 1, a_2 = 0$; points $a_1 = a_2 = 1$). Define $N(\mathbf{x})$ as the $3{\times}3$ matrix $[n_0(\mathbf{x}), n_1(\mathbf{x}), n_2(\mathbf{x})]$, A as a $3{\times}3$ diagonal matrix whose diagonal elements are $(1, a_1(\mathbf{x}), a_2(\mathbf{x}))$, and $N_l(\mathbf{x})$ as the column vector of the lth components of the (up to) three normals. The scalar components of the normal displacements $u^{\perp}(\mathbf{x})$ can now be written as:

$$u_l^{\perp}(\mathbf{x}) = (N(\mathbf{x})A(\mathbf{x})N_l(\mathbf{x}))^T u(\mathbf{x}) \tag{4}$$

Similarly, equation (2) is extended to write the diffusion tensor $P(\mathbf{x})$ that smooths in the normal direction alone as:

$$\begin{aligned}P(\mathbf{x}) &= N(\mathbf{x})A(\mathbf{x})N(\mathbf{x})^T \\ &= n_0(\mathbf{x})n_0(\mathbf{x})^T + a_1(\mathbf{x})n_1(\mathbf{x})n_1(\mathbf{x})^T + a_2(\mathbf{x})n_2(\mathbf{x})n_2(\mathbf{x})^T\end{aligned} \tag{5}$$

This formulation approximates the diffusive regularization at point-like structures, where $a_1(\mathbf{x}) = a_2(\mathbf{x}) = 1$, and within organ interiors, where $w(\mathbf{x})$ approximates zero. Near planar objects, the regularization equals the sliding organ regularization presented earlier.

2.5   Optimization

We use a gradient descent scheme to minimize the cost function $C(u)$ using the regularization defined in equation (1). Without loss of generality, and since we focus on monomodal registration of CT images, we use the sum of squared differences image similarity metric for $D[T, M; u]$. On each registration iteration, the sliding geometries regularization induces an update to the displacement field equal to $-\nabla_u S(u) \triangle t$ at each coordinate $\mathbf{x}$, where $\nabla_u S(u)$ is the gradient of equation (1) with respect to a small perturbation and $\triangle t$ is the time step. Dropping the $(\mathbf{x})$ notation,

$$\nabla_u S(u) = - \sum_{l=x,y,z} \text{div}((I - wP)^T((I - wP)\nabla u_l + wP\nabla u_l^{\perp}))e_l$$
$$+ \text{div}(wP^T((I - wP)\nabla u_l + wP\nabla u_l^{\perp}))NAN_l$$

(6)

where e_l is the lth canonical unit vector (ex. $e_x = [1, 0, 0]^T$). At convergence, this gradient must be balanced with the gradient from the image similarity measure.

3   Validation

3.1   Inhale/Exhale Abdominal CT Registration

Respiration induces significant and complex deformations to the abdominal organs, including sliding motions between several semi-independent organs. An arterial abdominal CT image acquired at inhale (target) was registered with a hepatic-venous abdominal CT image (moving) from the same patient acquired at exhale (size $240 \times 170 \times 150$; spatial resolution 1.5mm^3). Segmentations of the liver, left and right kidneys, and bones were created semi-automatically in the target image and used to generate surface models defining organ boundaries and normals. Following initial rigid alignment between the two images, the sliding organ deformable registration algorithm described in Section 2.3 was applied in a multi-resolution framework using two resolution levels, the first downsampling by a factor of two and the second operating at native resolution. The registrations took 1000 and 3000 iterations, respectively, with time step 0.046875 s, empirically-determined parameters $\lambda = 0.2$ (for exponential decay) and $\alpha = 24/8$, and were repeated using the diffusive regularization for comparison.

Figure 1 shows the alignment between the target and deformed moving images following sliding organ registration. The alignment was validated quantitatively by segmenting the liver, kidneys and bones in the moving image, warping the resulting label map by the registration displacement field, and calculating

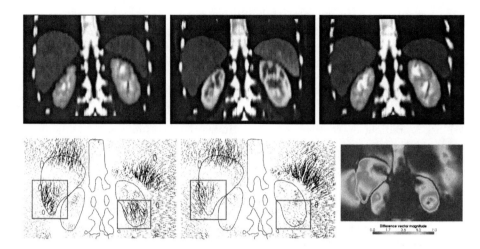

Fig. 1. *Top:* Coronal slice through the (left) moving, (center) target, and (right) transformed moving abdominal CT images using the sliding organ registration. *Bottom:* Coronal slice through the displacement fields from the (left) sliding organ and (center) diffusive registrations, with overlaid anatomical outlines for context, plus (right) the difference vector magnitudes between the displacement fields from the two registrations (best viewed in colour online)

the Dice coefficients between them and segmentations within the target image (Table 1). The results show good overlap between anatomical structures following image registration using the sliding regularization and comparable accuracy to the diffusive regularization.

The improvements of the sliding organ registration lie in the derived correspondences. Figure 1 shows representative coronal slices through the displacement fields from registration with the sliding organ and diffusive regularizations, and the magnitudes of their voxel-wise difference vectors. Unlike the diffusive regularization, the sliding organ regularization preserves the independent and sliding motion of the liver and kidneys. The difference vector magnitude image shows that allowing sliding motion at organ borders causes significant differences in the motion interpolated deep within organs, leading to greatly altered detected correspondences of up to 7mm.

Table 1. Dice coefficient for organ mask overlap between target images and deformed moving images of registered abdominal images, after registration using the sliding organ and diffusive regularizations.

Organ	Sliding	Diffusive
Liver	0.946	0.945
Right Kidney	0.877	0.870
Left Kidney	0.888	0.896
Bones	0.826	0.840

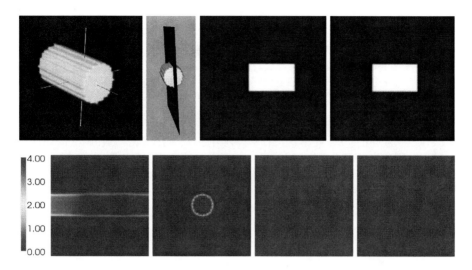

Fig. 2. *Top:* (left) Volume rendering of the sliding tube within the target image, plus slices along the tube's long axis for the (center) target and (right) moving images. *Bottom:* Representative long-axis and cross-sectional slices through the displacement magnitudes resulting from registration with the (left) geometry-conditional and (right) diffusive regularizations (best viewed in colour online).

3.2 Artificial Images of a Sliding Tube

We used the geometry conditional deformable registration algorithm described in Section 2.4 to register artificial images of a tube sliding along its long axis (size $80 \times 80 \times 80$; spatial resolution 1mm^3) (Figure 2). Registration was performed using a single resolution level, and compared to the results from the diffusive regularization (8000 and 190000 iterations required to recover the 4mm motion at the tube's edge, respectively, with time step 0.125, λ=0.25, γ=1000, α=1).

As shown in Figure 2, registration with the geometry conditional regularization nicely recovers and constrains the longitudinal motion within the tube. The background material correctly moves with the tube at its two ends, preventing folding, while motion is not interpolated to the stationary background elsewhere. In contrast, registration with the diffusive regularization incorrectly blends the tube's motion within the entire background.

4 Conclusions

In this paper, we have presented sliding organ and geometry conditional regularizations for deformable image registration, to align image pairs exhibiting large and complex deformations with a focus on handling sliding motion. By taking advantage of local structure information modeled as surfaces and tubular structures, these registration techniques increase the plausibility of the resulting displacement fields while maintaining registration accuracy as measured by image match. In the domain of abdominal imaging, such improved correspondence detection has implications for more accurate image-guided interventions, longitudinal and intersubject analysis, and application of atlas information to individuals. Future work includes additional quantitative validation of correspondence accuracy, application of the geometry conditional regularization to clinical images, and investigations into alternatives to requiring a detailed prior segmentation.

The registration software is available at http://public.kitware.com/Wiki/ TubeTK. This work was sponsored in part by: (1) NIH/NCI 1R01CA138419-01; (2) NIH/NIBIB 2U54EB005149-06; (3) NIH/NCI 1R41CA153488-01; (4) NSF EECS-0925875; (5) NIH/NIMH 1R01MH091645-01A1; (6) NIH/NIBIB 5P41EB002025-27; (7) NIH/NCI 1R41CA153488-01.

References

1. Aylward, S.R., Bullitt, E.: Initialization, noise, singularities, and scale in height ridge traversal for tubular object centerline extraction. IEEE Transactions on Medical Imaging 21(2), 61–75 (2002)
2. Cahill, N.D., Noble, J.A., Hawkes, D.J.: A Demons Algorithm for Image Registration with Locally Adaptive Regularization. In: Yang, G.-Z., Hawkes, D., Rueckert, D., Noble, A., Taylor, C. (eds.) MICCAI 2009, Part I. LNCS, vol. 5761, pp. 574–581. Springer, Heidelberg (2009)
3. Forsberg, D., Andersson, M., Knutsson, H.: Adaptive anisotropic regularization of deformation fields for non-rigid registration using the morphon framework. In: Proc. IEEE ICASSP, pp. 473–476 (2010)
4. Heinrich, M., Jenkinson, M., Brady, M., Schnabel, J.: Discontinuity preserving regularization for variational optical-flow registration using the modified lp norm. In: van Ginneken, B., et al. (ed.) Medical Image Analysis for the Clinic - A Grand Challenge, Workshop MICCAI 2010, pp. 185–194 (2010)
5. Modersitzki, J.: Numerical methods for image registration. Oxford University Press (2004)
6. Pace, D., Enquobahrie, A., Yang, H., Aylward, S., Niethammer, M.: Deformable image registration of sliding organs using anisotropic diffusive regularization. In: Proc. IEEE ISBI, pp. 407–413 (2011)
7. Ruan, D., Esedoglu, S., Fessler, J.A.: Discriminative sliding preserving regularization in medical imaging registration. In: Proc. IEEE ISBI, pp. 430–433 (2009)
8. Schmidt-Richberg, A., Ehrhardt, J., Werner, R., Handels, H.: Slipping Objects in Image Registration: Improved Motion Field Estimation with Direction-Dependent Regularization. In: Yang, G.-Z., Hawkes, D., Rueckert, D., Noble, A., Taylor, C. (eds.) MICCAI 2009, Part I. LNCS, vol. 5761, pp. 755–762. Springer, Heidelberg (2009)
9. Stefanescu, R., Pennec, X., Ayache, N.: Grid powered nonlinear image registration with locally adaptive regularization. Medical Image Analysis 8, 325–342 (2004)
10. Yin, Y., Hoffman, E.A., Lin, C.-L.: Lung Lobar Slippage Assessed with the Aid of Image Registration. In: Jiang, T., Navab, N., Pluim, J.P.W., Viergever, M.A. (eds.) MICCAI 2010, Part II. LNCS, vol. 6362, pp. 578–585. Springer, Heidelberg (2010)

Simulation of Portal Vein Clamping and the Impact of Safety Margins for Liver Resection Planning

Klaus Drechsler and Cristina Oyarzun Laura

Fraunhofer Institute for Computer Graphics Research IGD,
Fraunhoferstr. 5, 64283 Darmstadt, Germany
{klaus.drechsler,cristina.oyarzun}@igd.fraunhofer.de

Abstract. In this work, we present a planning tool for liver interventions. It allows for a simulation of the color change on the liver surface after clamping the portal vein at a user defined position. The result is a patient-specific approximation of the (sub-)segmental borders on the liver surface. Furthermore, the impact of different safety margins around a tumor can be simulated to assess the risk of a resection. In addition, it provides delinated portal- and hepatic vein, which can be overlapped to the 2D CT slices, and 3D visualization of the results.

Keywords: Planning, Liver, Portal Vein Clamping, Risk Analysis, Safety Margin.

1 Introduction

The liver is a vital organ with a wide range of functions, which are necessary for survival. It is currently impossible to compensate for the absence of these functions. In case of tumors, a resection of the liver has to be carefully planned in order to preserve as much of the liver as possible. The liver is located below the diaphragm on the right side of the abdominal cavity and is connected to two large blood vessel systems, namely portal and hepatic vein.

During an intervention, the surgeon can clamp the portal vein at a position that supplies blood to the (sub-)segment where the tumor is located. This leads to a color change on the surface of the liver, which indicates the borders of this (sub-)segment. The surgeon then usually uses a coagulator to 'draw' the borders on the liver surface before releasing the clamped vein. Selle et al. showed that patient-individual liver segments can be calculated by using the portal vein and mathematical methods to approximate the liver segments [11]. They evaluated the accuracy of this method to be between 80-90% overlap compared to the real segments. Jean H.D. Fasel noticed in his work that the concept of eight portal venous segments is challenged by an increasing number of reports. He investigated the branching patterns of the liver and found that the number of second order branches was between 9 and 44 [7]. This indicates that the liver does not consist of eight segments, as proposed by Claude Couinaud, but of many more.

H. Yoshida et al. (Eds.): Abdominal Imaging 2011, LNCS 7029, pp. 149–156, 2012.

It is not unlikely that a tumor is bigger than assumed and often found during a surgery. Thus, it is advantageous to estimate the risk of a resection with respect to different safety margins around a tumor. The bigger the tumor and the bigger the safety margin, the more vessels are affected that supply or drain blood to/from parts of the liver. However, it is crucial that blood supply and drain is not suppressed for parts of the remnant liver, which would result in necrotic liver tissues. Furthermore, a specific amount of remnant liver should remain to ensure a positive outcome for the patient. The analysis of different scenarios based on safety margins is part of our planning tool. This is done by analyzing the vessel structure around a tumor.

In this work, we present a tool that allows for a simulation of the color change on the liver surface after clamping the portal vein at a user defined position. This results in a patient-specific approximation of the (sub-)segmental borders on the liver surface. Furthermore, the impact of different user defined safety margins around a tumor can be assessed. Results are visualized with respect to affected portal- and hepatic venous territories.

2   Methods

The segmentation of the organ is mainly performed for visualization purposes. However, as a side effect the memory footprint of the data to be processed by the following steps is significantly reduced, and algorithms can be executed only on the organ of interest. We use the model-based approach described in [6] which first performs a rigid transformation, followed by an affine transformation and finally a free-form deformation is performed. The organ is automatically placed using anatomical knowledge of the position of the lungs.

Following organ segmentation, the vessels are segmented using a multi-scale analysis approach. The liver is inspected at multiple scales and the eigensystem of corresponding Hessian is analyzed using a vesselness function to detect tubular structures. Afterwards, the analysis results of each scale are integrated to provide the final filter response. We use the vesselness function by Sato et al. [10] to detect tubular structures at each scale. Compared to the popular vesselness funtion proposed by Frangi et al. [8] it has proven to keep vessel better connected at junctions [2]. The final filter response that combines the results from each scale is generated using a weighted additive response (WAR) function as proposed in [5]. Using WAR in comparison to the widely used maximum response approach has the advantage that nearby vessels are much better separated during the segmentation step. The segmentation of the vessels is done using a simple region growing approach with the criteria that starting from a seed point voxels must be connected and within a threshold range.

Next, the centerlines of the vessels are calculated. Therefore, we use the approach proposed by Lee et al. [9]. It belongs to the category of thinning-based skeletonization methods. It repeatedly deletes so called simple voxels until the centerlines remain, keeping topology and shape unchanged.

We now start to create a formal graph using the centerlines of the vessels. Therefore, we use the recently proposed decomposition of vessel skeleton into sub-branches to efficiently create the final graph and calculate several attributes like length, diameter, distance and so on [3]. In order to decompose the skeleton into sub-branches, each skeleton voxel has to be labeled as branch-, regular- and end-voxel. Branch voxel have more than two neighbors, regular voxels have exactly two neighbors and end voxel only have one neighbor. However, voxel constellations exist that makes the classification of branch voxels ambiguous. To resolve for this, we first classify each possible branch voxel as branch candidate and apply a branchness function, which takes the neighborhood relationship into account to decide for which voxel it is more reasonable to be the final branch voxel. Afterwards, the classified skeleton can be decomposed into sub-branches and attributes for each sub-branch can be easily calculated. The formal graph is formally described using the DOT language [1].

Due to partial volume effects, artefacts and imperfect segmentation algorithms, portal- and hepatic vein may seem to be connected and some points. Using the formal graph description of the vessel systems, the semi-automatic separation algorithm proposed in [4] is executed in order to find wrong edges. These edges are then removed from the graph, and the result is transfered back to the imaging data. The algorithm applies model assumptions, like decreasing diameter from the root to leafs, no obtuse angles and so on. Compared to other methods it takes into account that sometimes model assumptions are violated, although nothing is wrong.

To simulate the color change on the surface of the liver after clamping the portal vein at a specific position, we use the Nearest Neighbour Approach originally proposed by Selle et al. [11] to classify each liver tissue voxel. Let L be the set of liver voxels, P_j a portal vein branch with label j, $j = 0, .., n-1$. We define that $g(x, y)$ labels voxel x with label y and $dist(x, y)$ calculates the euclidean distance between voxel x and y. Then $\forall v \in L.g(v, f(v))$, with

$$f(v) = \operatorname*{argmin}_{j=0,\ldots,n-1} \operatorname*{argmin}_{v_i \in B_j} dist(v, v_i) \tag{1}$$

The result is an approximation of the portal venous territory that is supplied starting at the clamping position.

To explore the impact of different safety margins, we have to find all relevant vessel subtrees that supply/drain affected parts of the liver. Directly involved vessels are within the specified safety margin and injured as a result of the resection. As a consequnce, indirectly involved vessels can also not supply/drain blood anymore. Both vessel types must be found to determine the affected liver areas. Therefore, we utilize skeleton and graph representations of both vessel systems. We search for all directly involved vessel branches within a user defined distance around the tumor. Afterwards, we determine all indirectly involved vessel branches that belong to a subtree of these branches. We now have all subtrees that are involved when a tumor is resected with the specified safety margin. All branches are then automatically labeled and portal and hepatic venous territories are calculated and presented independently to the user.

---

[1] http://en.wikipedia.org/wiki/DOT_language

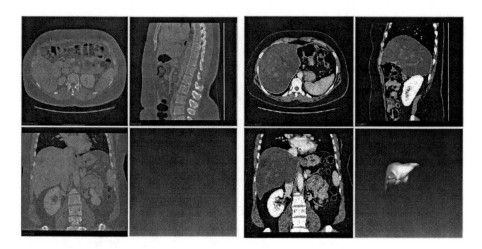

Fig. 1. Left: 2D views of a CT dataset. Right: Fully automatic organ segmentation.

3   Results

In this section, the results of our developed tool at each stage of the application workflow from a user point of view is described. The procedure consists of two stages. In the first stage, the necessary preprocessing of the data is carried out. The second stage deals with simulating the portal vein clamping.

3.1   Stage 1 - Data Processing

First of all, the user has to segment the liver from the CT dataset. This task is carried out fully automatically after pushing a 'Start' button. Figure 1 shows the CT dataset before (left) and after (right) organ segmentation.

Next, the liver vessels are segmented. Therefore, the user has to provide a few seed points in the main branches of the liver veins. After pushing another 'Start' button, an initial segmentation is calculated. Figure 2 shows the segmented organ with three user provided seed points and the initial segmentation (left). The initial segmentation can be refined with a slider until the results are optimal (Figure 2, right).

The segmentation of the vessels contains both, portal and hepatic vein. Because of low resolutions, motion artefacts and imperfect segmentations algorithms both vessel systems appear to be connected at several points in the CT data. Thus, the next step deals with the separation of both vessel systems. The user has to manually mark root nodes of both vessel systems. Our algorithm then automatically suggests edges to be removed. At any time, the user can unmark edges or select additional ones. Figure 3 shows the main steps of separating portal and hepatic vein. From left to right: Graph representation of the segmented vessels, selected root nodes of portal- (red) and hepatic-vein (blue), automatically suggested edges and separation results.

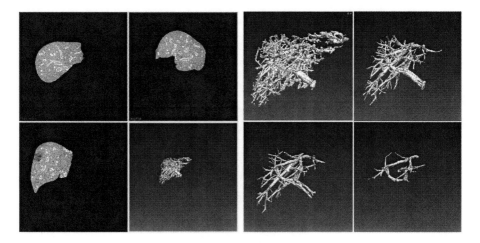

Fig. 2. Left: Vessel segmentation results overlapped on 2D slices of cropped liver and 3D visualization. Right: Possible refinements to the initial segmentation.

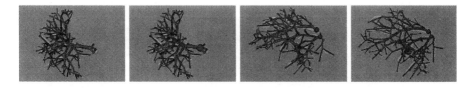

Fig. 3. Separation of portal- and liver vein. From left to right: Interconnected portal- and hepatic vessels, selected root nodes of portal- and hepatic vessel trees, automatically suggested edges to be removed, separation result.

Finally, tumors are marked. Therefore, the user has to click in the center of the tumor to place a sphere around it. With a slider, the size of the sphere can be adjusted. At any time, the user can grab the sphere and move it around to correct the position. Please note that this is not a real tumor segmentation, but just a marker to visualize the position and approximate size of a tumor. Figure 4 shows transversal, sagittal and coronal views in 2D and a 3D view of the organ, vessels and tumor.

3.2   Stage 2 - Simulation and Analysis

At this point, all relevant structures are segmented, namely liver, portal- and hepatic vein and tumors. An abstract version of the portal vein is visualized together with the segmented vessels and tumors as transparent backgrounds. To simulate clamping, the user can select nodes or edges. The corresponding sub-tree is then annotated with a new color to indicate visually which parts of the vessels are affected. Figure 4 shows the initial visualization (right top) and an annotated sub-tree in yellow (right bottom).

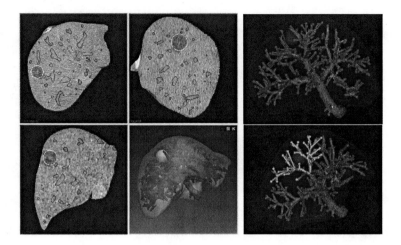

Fig. 4. Left: Marking of tumors and overlapped visualization of portal- and hepatic veins in 2D views and visualization in 3D. Right top: Visualization of the portal vein with an overlapped abstract representation that is used for interaction. Right bottom: After clicking a node, the corresponding sub-tree is automatically annotated.

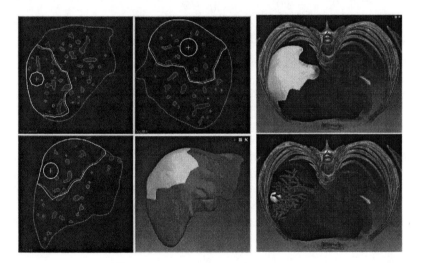

Fig. 5. Left: Results in 2D and 3D. The yellow area visualizes the borders on the liver surface when the portal vein is clamped at the given position. Right: Visualization of 3D structures combined with volume rendering of surrounding structures.

If the annotation is completed, the color change on the liver surface will be calculated. Figure 5 shows the results. On the left side, the results are shown in transversal, sagittal and coronal view. These results can also be overlapped on the original CT data (not shown). On the right side, the results are visualized in the context of surrounding structures using a mix between 3D visualization of surfaces and volume rendering of surrounding structures.

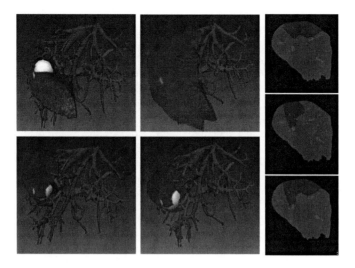

Fig. 6. Top 3D: Portal venous territories with an assumed safety margin of 10mm (left) and 15mm (right). Bottom 3D: Hepatic venous territories with an assumed safety margin of 10mm (left) and 15mm (right). Top 2D: Portal venous territory with an assumed 10mm safety margin. Middle 2D: Hepatic venous territories with an assumed safety margin of 10mm. Bottom 3D: Overlapping territories.

To assess the risk of a planned intervention, the user has to provide a safety margin around the tumor. Our tool then calculates the affected portal and hepatic venous territories. Blood in these parts would not be supplied/drained anymore and should be resected to prevent necrotiv tissues. Figure 6 shows an example for a 10mm and 15mm safety margin. As can be seen, if a slightly bigger safety margin is preferred or the tumor is slightly bigger than assumed, a much bigger portal venous territory is affected. In this example the hepatic venous territories have almost the same size.

4   Conclusion

In this work, we presented a tool to simulate the effects of portal vein clamping and assess the risk of a resection with different safety margins around a tumor. Furthermore, it provides delinated portal- and hepatic vein, which can be overlapped to the 2D CT slices, and 3D visualization of the results.

A priliminary version of the presented tool has been shown to medical experts and tested by a clinical partner. Comments were quite positive. The delineation of portal- and hepatic vein with different colors was very useful and 3D visualization helped to assess better the position of anatomical structures and pathologies. These results are in line with results found by other groups, e.g. [1].

Future work includes clinical evaluation and research in the direction of automatic generation of resection proposals.

References

1. Beermann, J., Tetzlaff, R., Bruckner, T., Schebinger, M., Mller-Stich, B.P., Gutt, C.N., Meinzer, H.P., Kadmon, M., Fischer, L.: Three-dimensional visualisation improves understanding of surgical liver anatomy. Medical Education 44(9), 936–940 (2010), http://dx.doi.org/10.1111/j.1365-2923.2010.03742.x

2. Drechsler, K., Oyarzun Laura, C.: Comparison of vesselness functions for multiscale analysis of the liver vasculature. In: Proceedings of the 10th IEEE International Conference on Information Technology and Applications in Biomedicine (ITAB), pp. 1–5 (November 2010)

3. Drechsler, K., Oyarzun Laura, C.: Hierarchical decomposition of vessel skeletons for graph creation and feature extraction. In: Proceedings of the IEEE International Conference on Bioinformatics and Biomedicine (BIBM), pp. 456–461 (December 2010)

4. Drechsler, K., Oelmann, S., Oyarzun Laura, C.: Separation of interconnected hepatic veins. In: Proceedings of the 24th International Symposium on Computer-Based Medical Systems, CBMS (2011)

5. Drechsler, K., Oyarzun Laura, C.: A novel multiscale integration approach for vessel enhancement. In: Proceedings of the 23rd International Symposium on Computer-Based Medical Systems (CBMS), pp. 92–97 (2010)

6. Erdt, M., Kirschner, M., Steger, S., Wesarg, S.: Fast automatic liver segmentation combining learned shape priors with observed shape deviation. In: Proceedings of the IEEE International Symposium on Computer-Based Medical Systems (CBMS), pp. 249–254 (2010)

7. Fasel, J.H.D.: Portal venous territories within the human liver: an anatomical reappraisal. Anat Rec (Hoboken) 291(6), 636–642 (2008), http://dx.doi.org/10.1002/ar.20658

8. Frangi, A.F., Niessen, W.J., Vincken, K.L., Viergever, M.A.: Multiscale Vessel Enhancement Filtering. In: Wells, W.M., Colchester, A.C.F., Delp, S.L. (eds.) MICCAI 1998. LNCS, vol. 1496, pp. 130–137. Springer, Heidelberg (1998)

9. Lee, T.C., Kashyap, R.L., Chu, C.N.: Building skeleton models via 3-d medial surface/axis thinning algorithms. Graphical Models and Image Process (CVGIP) 56(6), 462–478 (1994)

10. Sato, Y., Nakajima, S., Atsumi, H., Koller, T., Gerig, G., Yoshida, S., Kikinis, R.: 3d multi-scale line filter for segmentation and visualization of curvilinear structures in medical images. In: Proceedings of the First Joint Conference on Computer Vision, Virtual Reality and Robotics in Medicine and Medical Robotics and Computerassisted Surgery (CVRMed-MRCAS), pp. 213–222 (1997)

11. Selle, D., Preim, B., Schenk, A., Peitgen, H.O.: Analysis of vasculature for liver surgical planning. IEEE Transactions on Medical Imaging 21(11), 1344–1357 (2002)

Liver Segmentation in CT Images
for Intervention Using a Graph-Cut Based Model

Yufei Chen[1,2], Weidong Zhao[1,2], Qidi Wu[1,2], Zhicheng Wang[1,2], and Jinyong Hu[1,2]

[1] Research Center of CAD, Tongji University, Shanghai 200092, China
[2] The Engineering Research Center for Enterprise Digital Technology, Ministry of Education,
Tongji University, Shanghai 200092, China
april337@163.com

Abstract. Liver segmentation in computerized tomography (CT) images has been widely studied in recent years, of which the graph cut models demonstrate a great potential with the advantage of global optima and practical efficiency. In this paper, a graph-cut based model for liver CT segmentation is presented. The image is interpreted as a graph, that the segmentation problem is then casted as an optimal cut on the graph. An energy function is then formulated for minimization, which combines both regional properties and boundary smoothness. The prior knowledge on liver is unified into the energy function via fuzzy similarity measure. Finally, the optimal cut can be computed through the max-flow algorithm. Experiments on a variety of CT images show its effectiveness and efficiency.

Keywords: liver CT segmentation, graph-cut model, prior knowledge.

1 Introduction

As a noninvasive and painless medical test, abdominal CT scan has been widely used in hospitals of China for liver cancer diagnosis and treatment [1]. In the field of liver CT image processing, some of the current interests are the automatic diagnosis of liver pathologies and its three-dimensional visualization [2]. The first and fundamental step in all these studies is the liver segmentation. It is of benefit in many aspects for following process [3~5], including basis information provision on focal liver lesions and its spatial relationship with liver vascular system, measurement of tissue volume, computer guided diagnosis and surgery, surgical treatment planning and intervention etc.

However, the topic is still an open and difficult problem because of the following reasons [6]. Firstly, the CT images are often very noisy that inevitably exist ambiguous boundaries between the liver and its adjacent organs, such as abdominal wall, right kidney, heart, stomach and so on. Sometimes, it becomes even worse that the boundaries are disappeared because of the poor image quality. Secondly, there exists large inter-patient and intra-patient variability in liver geometric properties, intensity distributions and so on, which make it difficult to generate a uniform

H. Yoshida et al. (Eds.): Abdominal Imaging 2011, LNCS 7029, pp. 157–164, 2012.

benchmark. Thirdly, there exists diversity problem on intensity of target area, i.e. the bright vessel, the regular liver tissue and the dim tumor. Therefore, the algorithms based on local intensity are often difficult to obtain accurate segmentation results. Finally, the slice-by-slice segmentation approach in two-dimensional space is time consuming, and the results are independent between each other. Therefore, a more efficient and accurate volume segmentation method in three-dimensional space is needed.

There are many segmentation approaches that have been proposed by various researchers, these techniques have varying degrees of success. In recent years, the most popular used models are based on energy minimization [7], among which two kinds of methods are overwhelming adopted: level set based method [8] and graph based method [9]. The widely studied level set based method optimizes a function defined on a continuous contour, which shows its robustness and efficiency in most circumstances. However, it always generates local minima of the energy function, be sensitive to contour initialization and has large computational burden when it comes to liver segmentation [10]. Especially in dealing with tumors located near liver surface, it often tends to eliminate the tumors from target area to obtain an inaccurate liver segmentation result. Furthermore, the vessels need to be additional segmented and then re-merged into the whole final result. The graph based method is not iterative, and can achieve global minimum of the energy functions under a given set of boundary conditions in polynomial time. In this paper, we describe a graph-cut based model to segment liver from abdominal CT data for intervention. Our main contribution is unifying the prior knowledge information from data into a single framework via fuzzy representation, and integrating them into the energy function through semi-supervised strategy.

The paper is organized as follows. In section 2, the basic concept and framework of graph-cut model is introduced. In section 3, the proposed semi-supervised graph-cut based model for liver segmentation in CT images is elaborated. In section 4, the experimental results to evaluate the proposed model are presented and discussed. Section 5 concludes the work.

2   Related Work

The graph-cut theory provides a discrete optimization method for object segmentation through minimize an energy function defined over a finite set of variables to compute the globally optimal partition of an image. In 3D space, such variables are associated with image voxels. An undirected weighted graph $G = (V, E)$ is defined as a set of nodes V and a set of directed edges E connecting neighboring nodes. The nodes represent image voxels. There are also two specially designated special nodes that are called terminals, the source s and the sink t. In the context of segmentation, they correspond to the set of assigned labels that respectively represent object and background. Normally, there are two types of edges in the graph: n-links and t-links. n-links stands for edges between neighboring voxels. t-links is used to connect voxels to terminals.

The goal of the segmentation is to find a labeling L that assigns each voxel a label that is both piecewise smooth and consistent with the observed data. The problem can be naturally formulated in terms of energy minimization. In this framework, one seeks the labeling L that minimizes the following energy [11]

$$E(L) = E_{data}(L) + E_{smooth}(L) = \sum_{p \in P} D_p(L_p) + \sum_{(p,q) \in (V \setminus \{s,t\})} S_{p,q}(L_p, L_q). \quad (1)$$

where $L = \{L_p | p \in P\}$ is a labeling of image P. D_p is a data penalty function indicates individual label references of voxels, which concentrates on regional properties of segmentation L. $S_{p,q}$ is an interaction potential encourages spatial coherence by penalizing discontinuities between neighboring voxels, which represents boundary properties of segmentation L.

Typically, all graph edges are assigned some non-negative weight $c(u, v) \geq 0$ according to the measure of similarity between the two nodes u and v: the higher the edge weight, the more similar they are. Cost of t-links corresponds to data penalty which is normally derived from the term D_p, while the cost of n-links corresponds to $S_{p,q}$. In practice, the graph G can be represented as a flow network, i.e. the nodes of graph G are pairwise interconnected by edges in a regular grid-like fashion with a certain flow on them. A flow in G is a positive real-valued function $f: V \times V \rightarrow R^+$ that satisfies $f(u, v) \leq c(u, v)$.

The s-t cut framework offers a globally optimal method for segmentation. A cut (S, T) of the flow network is a partition of V into S and $T = V$-S such that $s \in S$ and $t \in T$, which respectively corresponds to object and background. The capacity of a cut is defined as the summational costs of the edges that across the cut

$$c(S,T) = \sum_{u \in S, v \in T} c(u,v). \quad (2)$$

The s-t minimum cut method is to find a cut in G that separates s and t with the smallest capacity. As indicated by the following theorem, the cuts in networks have a great relationship with flows [12]. The value of flow is defined as

$$|f| = \sum_{v \in V} f(s,v). \quad (3)$$

Theorem 1. *The maximum flow from source s to sink t, i.e. max ($|f|$), is equal to the value of the capacity $c(s, t)$ of the minimum cut separating s and t.*

With the theorem above, the s-t minimum cut can be computed by using existing max-flow algorithms. In this paper, we adopted the well-known min-cut/max-flow algorithm for combinatorial optimization that was proposed by Boykov and Kolmogorov in 2004 [11]. The practical efficiency of the algorithm was shown that it could solve 3D segmentation problem in close to real-time using regular PCs.

The implementation is straightforward, details can be found in [11], but the difficulty lies on the penalties definition of both regional and boundary terms.

3   Model Description

A graph-cut based model for liver segmentation from abdominal CT images is described in this section. The core of the model is minimizing a fairly general objective function that includes both regional and boundary properties of a segment with certain types of topological constrains that naturally fit into the global minimization framework.

3.1   MAP-MRF

The goal of image segmentation is to find an optimal labeling configuration. In liver CT images, the label assigned to a voxel depends only on the labels assigned to its neighbors. This condition satisfies the Markovian property. Obviously, the Markov random field (MRF) theory provides an elegant mathematical framework for solving the problem [13]. Assuming the labels $L=$ {'object', 'background'} as a field of random variables, wherein each random variable is associated with a voxel. Any possible assignment of labels is essentially a realization of the field. The segmentation problem is formulated as maximum a posterior estimation (MAP) of a MRF that requires minimization of a posterior energy conditioned over the observed data X.

$$
\begin{aligned}
E(L \mid X) &= \sum_{p \in P} D_p(L_p \mid X) + \sum_{(p,q) \in (V \backslash \{s,t\})} S_{p,q}(L_p, L_q \mid X) \\
&= \lambda \cdot \sum_{p \in P} -\log \Pr(L_p \mid x_p) + (1-\lambda) \cdot \sum_{p \in (V \backslash \{s,t\}} \sum_{q \in N_p} K(p,q \mid x_p) \cdot \delta.
\end{aligned}
\tag{4}
$$

where $\lambda > 0$ controls the balance between the two energy terms. $x_p \in \{$'object', 'background'$\}$ is a label that has to be assigned to p. N_p is the set of neighbors of p and $K(p, q)$ is a positive penalty function. δ is a two-valued indicator function with 1 only if $x_p \neq x_q$, otherwise $\delta = 0$.

In most cases, the CT images do not have sufficiently distinct regional properties that more necessary information on topological constraints should be incorporated into the global optimization framework, so as to further restrict the searching space of possible solutions before optimizing. Assume that O and B denote a priori knowledge on subsets of 'object' and 'background'. The hard constraints on both of the subsets should satisfy: $O \cap B = \phi$ & $\forall p \in O : L_p =$'object' & $\forall p \in B : L_p =$'background'. In this paper, the hard constraints are set both automatically and manually.

Automatically set seeds are initialized using the following prior knowledge: the object is almost surrounded by the right kidney, heart, rib and spine, wherein the intensities are much larger than the liver's that can be easily marked as part of the background seeds. Furthermore, based on the prior knowledge that liver cannot exist at the left-down part of abdominal space, all the voxels in the CT image that located in the intersection of right part of spine and down part of abdomen can be directly eliminated from the computing space. On the other hand, manually controlled seeds are obtained by user interactive tool, such as bush and lasso strokes. For a more distinct representation, the object seeds are chosen respectively around the liver tissues, blood vessels and tumors, while the background seeds are marked around the seriously ambiguous boundaries.

Owing to the inherent imprecision or fuzziness that is common in the description of liver CT images [13], we use a fuzzy theoretic framework to unify these prior knowledge for segmentation.

3.2   Construction of Regional Term

The regional term D_p is the individual penalties for assigning voxel p to label 'object' and 'background', which is measured by the probability distribution $\Pr(L_p|x_p)$.

The two distributions are defined on the a priori basis knowledge that is deduced from histograms of object and background. The general method of establishing a statistical model discrimination of the liver from quantities of data sets is time consuming and could not respond sensitively to different liver shapes. In this paper, we use Gaussian distribution to model $\Pr(L_p|x_p)$. The parameters of the Gaussian distributions are derived only from the seed regions. More specifically, as discussed above, the object seeds consist of three intensity-different parts. For a more precise description, a mixture of three Gaussian distributions representing liver tissues, blood vessels and tumors is modeled to describe the object probability distribution. A single Gaussian distribution is established for background.

$$\Pr(L_p \mid x_p = 'object') = \sum_{i=1}^{3} w_i \cdot e^{-\frac{(I_p - \mu_{O(i)})^2}{2\sigma_{O(i)}^2}} \quad (\sum_{i=1}^{3} w_i = 1). \tag{5}$$

$$\Pr(L_p \mid x_p = 'background') = e^{-\frac{(I_p - \mu_B)^2}{2\sigma_B^2}}. \tag{6}$$

where I_p is the intensity of voxel p, w_i is the weight coefficient, μ_O, σ_O are the object Gaussian distribution parameters, while μ_B, σ_B are for background.

3.3   Construction of Boundary Term

The boundary term $S_{p,q}$ is interpreted as a penalty for a discontinuity between neighbor voxel p and q, which is typically used to guarantee that the resulting segmentation has smooth boundaries.

In this paper, q is only searching along the nearest 6-neighborhood of p in 3D space in order to improve efficiency. The more similar p and q are, the larger cost of the penalty is. The penalty will decrease close to zero when the two neighbor voxels are very different. The similarity measure can base on local intensity gradient, Laplacian zero-crossing, gradient direction, geometric and so on [14]. Normally, it is sufficient to adopt local intensity as the criteria which can be expressed as follows:

$$K(p,q) = e^{-\frac{(I_p - I_q)^2}{2\sigma^2}} \quad (q \in N_{p(6)}).$$ (7)

where I_p, I_q are the intensities of voxel p and q, $N_{p(6)}$ stands for the 6-neighborhood of p. σ is a user specified penalty control parameter, which can be empirically set as 10 in our application.

4   Experimental Results and Discussion

The proposed method has been evaluated on numerous of clinical abdominal CT volumes stored as DICOM images, each volume was composed by 512×512 pixel slices. The computer used for runtime measures had a Intel(R) Core(TM)2 Duo CPU (2.6GHz), 2.0GB of RAM and a Windows XP operating system. The parameters are set as follows: λ=0.15, w_1=0.5, w_2=0.3, w_3=0.2, σ=10.

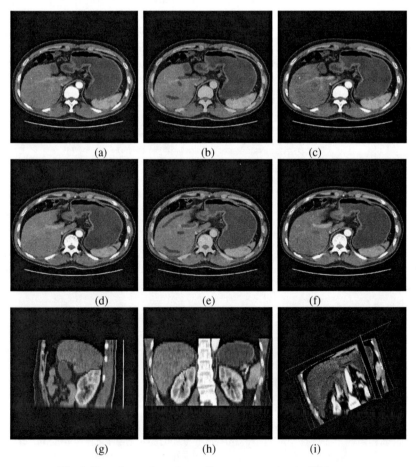

Fig. 1. Experimental results on liver segmentation in CT images

As shown in Fig. 1, the treated abdominal CT images had reliable and satisfied results by our method. (a) and (d) are two slices from an original CT volume. (b) and (e) respectively depict their seed regions for the object and background, in which the red strokes are user-initialized object seeds on tissues, vessels and tumors, while green regions are automatic initialized background seeds. Within the red circle of (c) and (f), there comes the final segmentation result of the two slices in transversal plane. Another two segmentation results of the same volume in sagittal and coronal plane are respectively given in (g) and (h). (i) demonstrates the 3D visualization of the extracted liver.

The proposed method also performed well when it came to efficiency: For each volume, assume N_{slice} stands for the total slice number, N_{liver} means the number of slices that contains liver part, other slices are not taken into account. The interactive time and running time of the method was listed in Table 1.

Table 1.   Experimental results on efficiency

N_{slice}	N_{liver}	Interactive time(s)	Running time(s)
22	22	30	13
22	22	32	17
25	23	36	19
36	32	40	25
87	54	62	59
134	54	67	74
166	54	72	22
298	115	140	59
445	153	133	207

5   Conclusion

In this paper, we proposed a graph-cut based method for intervention in liver CT segmentation. The image is described as a graph, whose optimal cut corresponds to the final segmentation. In order to get the cut, an energy function including prior knowledge on liver is established through fuzzy similarity measure. With the energy minimization, the optimal cut can be computed through the max-flow algorithm. Nine CT images were selected for testing and the experimental results showed satisfied performances. We can conclude that our method gives out an effective and efficient performance for liver segmentation.

Future work will focus on improving the method efficiency. For example, the similarity measure can take more information on the liver's location, intensity and spatial connectivity. Also, fitting the curve of abdominal wall according to the rib information, all the voxels outside the curve can be eliminated directly from the computing space.

Acknowledgments. This work was supported by National Natural Science Foundation of China (No.61103070).

References

1. Casiraghi, E., Lombardi, G., Pratissoli, S., Rizzi, S.: 3D α-Expansion and Graph Cut Algorithms for Automatic Liver Segmentation from CT Images. In: Apolloni, B., Howlett, R.J., Jain, L. (eds.) KES 2007, Part I. LNCS (LNAI), vol. 4692, pp. 421–428. Springer, Heidelberg (2007)
2. Heimann, T., van Ginneken, B., Styner, M., et al.: Comparison and Evaluation of Methods for Liver Segmentation from CT Datasets. IEEE Trans. Med. Imaging 28, 1251–1265 (2009)
3. Esneault, S., Hraiech, N., Delabrousse, E., Dillenseger, J.L.: Graph Cut Liver Segmentation for Interstitial Ultrasound Therapy. In: IEEE Conference on Engineering in Medicine and Biology Society, pp. 5247–5250. IEEE Press, Lyon (2007)
4. Massoptier, L., Casciaro, S.: Fully Automatic Liver Segmentation through Graph-Cut Technique. In: IEEE Conference on Engineering in Medicine and Biology Society, pp. 5243–5246. IEEE Press, Lyon (2007)
5. Zhang, X., Tian, J., Deng, K., Wu, Y., Li, X.: Automatic Liver Segmentation Using a Statistical Shape Model with Optimal Surface Detection. IEEE Trans. Biomed. Eng. 57, 2622–2626 (2010)
6. Campadelli, P., Casiraghi, E., Esposito, A.: Liver Segmentation from Computed Tomography Scans: a Survey and a New Algorithm. Artificial Intelligence in Medicine 45, 185–196 (2009)
7. Delong, A., Osokin, A., Isack, H.N., Boykov, Y.: Fast Approximate Energy Minimization with Label Costs. In: IEEE Conference on Computer Vision and Pattern Recognition, pp. 1–8. IEEE Press, San Francisco (2010)
8. Chen, Y., Zhao, W., Wang, Z.: Level Set Segmentation Algorithm Based on Image Entropy and Simulated Annealing. In: International Conference on Bioinformatics and Biomedical Engineering, pp. 999–1003. IEEE Press, Wuhan (2007)
9. Stawiaski, J., Decenciere, E., Bidault, F.: Interactive Liver Tumor Segmentation Using Graph-cuts and Watershed. The MIDAS Journal - Grand Challenge Liver Tumor Segmentation, MICCAI Workshop (2008),
   http://hdl.handle.net/10380/1416
10. Boykov, Y., Kolmogorov, V.: Computing Geodesics and Minimal Surfaces via Graph Cuts. In: IEEE International Conference on Computer Vision, pp. 26–33. IEEE Press, Nice (2003)
11. Boykov, Y., Kolmogorov, V.: An Experimental Comparison of Min-Cut/Max-Flow Algorithms for Energy Minimization in Vision. IEEE Transactions on Pattern Analysis and Machine Intelligence 26, 1124–1137 (2004)
12. Xu, N., Ahuja, N., Bansal, R.: Object Segmentation Using Graph Cuts Based Active Contours. Computer Vision and Image Understanding 107, 210–224 (2007)
13. Chittajallu, D.R., Brunner, G., Kurkure, U., Yalamanchili, R.P., Kakadiaris, I.A.: Fuzzy-cuts: A Knowledge-Driven Graph-Bases Method for Medical Image Segmentation. In: IEEE Conference on Computer Vision and Pattern Recognition, pp. 715–722. IEEE Press, Miami (2009)
14. Boykov, Y., Funka-Lea, G.: Graph Cuts and Efficient N-D Image Segmentation. International Journal of Computer Vision 70, 109–131 (2006)

Anatomical Feature-Guided Mutual Information Registration of Multimodal Prostate MRI

Xin Zhao and Arie Kaufman

Stony Brook University, Stony Brook, NY, 11794, USA
{xinzhao,ari}@cs.stonybrook.edu

Abstract. Radiological imaging of prostate is becoming more popular among researchers and clinicians in searching for diseases, primarily cancer. Scans might be acquired at different times, with patient movement between scans, or with different equipment, resulting in multiple datasets that need to be registered. For this issue, we introduce a registration method using anatomical feature-guided mutual information. Prostate scans of the same patient taken in three different orientations are first aligned for the accurate detection of anatomical features in 3D. Then, our pipeline allows for multiple modalities registration through the use of anatomical features, such as the interior urethra of prostate and gland utricle, in a bijective way. The novelty of this approach is the application of anatomical features as the pre-specified corresponding landmarks for prostate registration. We evaluate the registration results through both artificial and clinical datasets. Registration accuracy is evaluated by performing statistical analysis of local intensity differences or spatial differences of anatomical landmarks between various MR datasets. Evaluation results demonstrate that our method statistics-significantly improves the quality of registration (compared to the non-feature guided registration). Although this strategy is tested for MRI-guided brachytherapy, the preliminary results from our experiments suggest that it can be also applied to other settings such as transrectal ultrasound-guided or CT-guided therapy, where the integration of preoperative MRI may have a significant impact upon treatment planning and guidance.

Keywords: Anatomical feature, MI registration, Multimodal prostate MRI.

1   Introduction

Prostate cancer is the second leading cause of cancer-related mortality among males in the United States, and is the most commonly diagnosed cancer in general [9]. Although it is such a common cancer, diagnosis methods remain primitive and inexact. More recently, Magnetic Resonance Imaging (MRI) has been used for the detection of prostate cancer. MRI provides superior soft-tissue contrast and visualization of tumor invasion of surrounding soft tissues. Moreover, MRI provides images in nonaxial planes (sagittal and coronal), thus allowing better 3D representation of the tumor volume. Standard MR imaging can clearly define the prostate and its sub-structures, as well as the rectum, neurovascular bundles and urethra. Further, several new MR imaging methods have recently shown promise in their ability to detect and characterize prostate cancer. These

H. Yoshida et al. (Eds.): Abdominal Imaging 2011, LNCS 7029, pp. 165–172, 2012.

include MRSI (spectroscopy), diffusion imaging, and MR imaging with dynamic intra-venous contrast enhancement. In this paper, we use a combination of T_2-weighted MR and MRSI image sequences. T_2-weighted MR images are generally of high quality and resolution, while prostate cancer can be accurately detected by MRSI. The acquisition of these MR image sequences is often done with varying orientations and resolutions per sequence. The prostate, being composed of soft tissues, can undergo significant shape changes between different imaging sessions by the procedures [4]. Therefore, registration methods are necessary for multiple MR sequences for different positions or time periods. Meanwhile, it is possible that doctors might want to correlate MR images to histology information in order to confirm results during development and testing of a system. In this paper, we propose a novel volumetric registration framework, which can help register various MR datasets and reduce the work of radiologists, to monitor the progression of abnormalities, and to facilitate the diagnoses of prostate diseases. The pipeline consists of the anatomical feature detection, alignment, and registration. We first detect anatomical features of each prostate dataset as landmarks. Then we use specified feature points to align and register different prostate datasets. Finally, we evaluate our registration results using statistical analysis based on the differences of local intensity or landmark position of prostates.

This paper is organized as follows. In Section 2 we review the previous work on prostate registration methods. Then we introduce our design and algorithm in Section 3. Experimental results and evaluations are shown in Section 4. We conclude our discussion and sketch the future research plan in Section 5.

2   Related Work

Registration of multimodal prostate images is important for the planning, guidance, and retrospective evaluation of radiotherapy procedures; and the fusion of diagnostic images for improved CaP detection accuracy. Intra-modality prostate image registration has been utilized by Bharatha et al. [1] for image-guided prostate surgery via elastic registration of preoperative and intraoperative prostate MRI. Lee et al. [6] have investigated the use of multimodal prostate images (MRI, CT, and SPECT) to characterize CaP, performing automated multimodal registration of MRI to SPECT via manual registration of MRI to CT using a graphical user interface. Manually identified control points (anatomical landmarks), placed primarily along the gland boundary, are used to define a thin plate spline interpolant. Automated rigid registration of MRI to CT has been addressed by several groups [13]. Park et al. [7] have addressed an automated elastic registration using a spatially constrained B-spline. For registration of MRI to histology information, Zhan et al. [14] have first applied anatomical structures as landmarks for the prostate data. However, their anatomical structures vary in different patient cases and the feature detection is extremely time consuming. By comparison, our method has automatic performance by the application of consistent feature points for the registra-tion of various MRI and MRSI datasets.

Multi-protocol MR imaging is part of standard clinical practice at a number of medical centers for disease diagnosis and treatment [5]. Traditional intensity-based similarity measures, such as mutual information (MI), are typically inadequate to robustly and automatically register images from these significantly dissimilar modalities. There have been several efforts to complement intensity information with alternative image information, including image gradients [8] and image segmentations [11] in conjunction with MI variants, specifically adapted to incorporate these additional channels of information. Inspired by the application of additional image information, our paper has the following contributions: (1) we develop a registration framework using the anatomical feature-guided mutual information to automatically map spatial extent of corresponding MRI datasets; and (2) our method improves over intensity-based similarity metrics by incorporating unique feature landmarks that are relatively robust and accurate to register the target and template images. Our framework allows for the incorporation of multiple modalities, protocols, or even feature images in an automated registration scheme, facilitated by the use of MI. Additionally, the application of MI involves a simple optimization procedure without any pre-segmentation.

3   Design Methods

In this section, we focus on the anatomical feature detection, and the design of feature-guided registration of various prostate MR datasets.

3.1   Anatomical Feature Detection of Prostate

The prostate gland, which surrounds the urethra, is located in front of the rectum, and just below the bladder. MRI provides images with excellent anatomical detail and soft-tissue contrast. We analyze T_2-weighted datasets along the axial, sagittal and coronal view in 3D, as shown in Figure 1(a). The seminal vesicles are tucked between the rectum and the bladder, and attached to the prostate. The urethra goes through entire prostate and joins with two seminal vesicles at the ejaculatory ducts. Therefore, some distinctive anatomical structures, such as ejaculatory ducts, urethra, and dilated gland with prostatic utricle, can be applied for the accurate registration between different datasets or modalities. Specifically, three identified interior anatomical feature points (prostatic utricle points) are detected and marked for the alignment, as represented in Figure 1(b), while Figure 1(c) shows the anatomical feature points as landmarks used for the evaluation. Three exterior feature points are detected based on the structure information of prostatic urethra and seminal vesicles: two surface feature points exactly located at the entrance and exit points of the urethra are manually picked. The third surface point is manually marked at the intersection point between a seminal vesicle and the prostate gland with respect to the fact that seminal vesicles attach to the surface of prostate and merge with the urethra at ejaculatory ducts. A set of interior feature points are marked along the urethra following the user defined criteria (e.g., equidistant sampling), beginning with the entrance surface feature point and ending with the exit one.

On each MRI or MRSI prostate view direction, all corresponding feature points can manually marked with predefined index numbers through the user interface, which can be considered as ground truth references for the automatic feature detection (e.g., a corresponding urethral feature point is marked in three direction views, as shown in Figure 2).

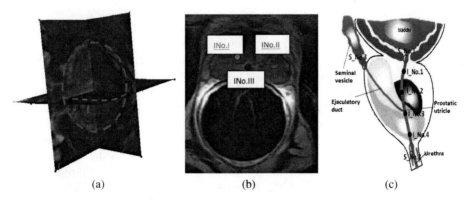

(a)   (b)   (c)

Fig. 1. Anatomical feature points of prostate. (a) Multi-view of prostate MR images along three view directions. (b) An axis slice shows the identified interior anatomical feature points (prostatic utricle) used for the alignment. (c) The illustration of anatomical feature points as landmarks used for the evaluation. Each feature point is marked with a pre-defined index number. S_Nos are the surface feature points, while I_Nos are the interior feature points.

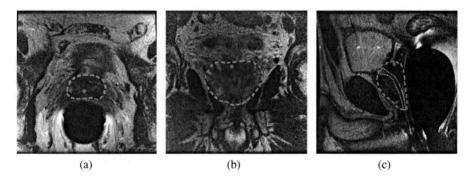

(a)   (b)   (c)

Fig. 2. Illustration of manually marked feature points on the MRI slices using the (a) axial, (b) coronal and (c) sagittal views of the same prostate dataset. Red circles highlight the boundary of prostate and green points show the corresponding feature point in three directions. The entire urethra is marked in the sagittal view by a yellow contour.

Automatic Anatomical Feature Detection. In order to effectively process a large number of datasets, several automatic feature detection methods are embedded into our framework. Corner detection or the more general terminology interest point detection is an approach used within computer vision systems to extract certain kinds of features of an image. We apply the fast corner and blobs detection method [10] to automatically recognize the prostatic utricle points as the identified interior feature points on the axial MR images. Several false positive feature points may be detected by this algorithm, but our system allows the user to interactively mark and highlight accurate anatomical features, by deleting all the false positive points. We also apply the Hough transform [2] for the detection of entire urethra on the sagittal MR images. The Hough transform can find instances of objects within a certain class of shapes by a voting procedure in a parameter space, but will generate some false positive line segments. In order to solve this problem, Grey-Level Co-occurrence Matrices (GLCM) defined in [3] are further used as local texture features to refine the urethra detection based on the pre-defined reference-texture (manually marked by the user). Figure 3 shows the automatic feature detection results on MR images.

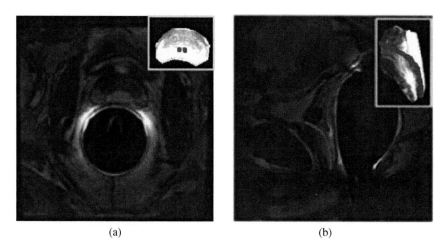

(a)   (b)

Fig. 3. Results of our automatic feature detection design for (a) the axis and (b) the sagittal MR images. The small images highlighted by yellow frames show detected feature structures (red points or line) in the prostate region.

3.2 Anatomical Feature-Guided Registration

For the volumetric alignment, we need to match three identical interior anatomical features (the prostatic utricle points shown in Figure 1(b)) within the MR images of different datasets or modalities to obtain the accurate and reliable registration results. For the volumetric registration, we apply a commonly used similarity measure as the mutual information [12], due to the robustness of the MI measure to differences in intensity patterns between image modalities and protocols. Our framework provides an effective approach to exploit all the information acquired from prior alignment steps to drive the subsequent registration operations, which is fast and accurate.

4 Experimental Results and Evaluation

In this section, we register different prostate MR datasets and modalities using both intensity information and anatomical feature points. Then, we test our framework using both artificially deformed and clinical MR datasets and evaluate the registration results.

Artificial Deformation Datasets. We firstly evaluate the registration algorithm by artificially deforming a dataset by the linear transformation, and then register back to itself. The linear deformation approximation is well-deformed, and the image intensities of the deformed volume are interpolated from the original dataset, which provides an accurate estimation. Therefore, with the known ground truth, the mean squared difference (MSD) between the registered voxels could directly give us a good understanding of the performance of our anatomical feature based registration method. We apply our framework to 5 T_2-weighted MR cases. The MSD of intensity between the registered volume and the original volume using or without using the anatomical feature based landmarks, is calculated for each deformation case. Figure 4 shows the voxel-wise MSD of intensity for all the test cases.

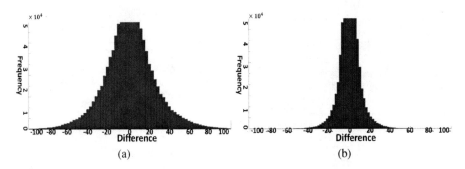

(a)   (b)

Fig. 4. Registration results of artificial deformation T_2-weighted MR datasets. The MSD of image intensity values (a) without using anatomical feature points, and (b) using anatomical feature points. Histograms show that differences are much smaller using our feature-guided framework for registration.

Clinical MRI Datasets. In cases where considerable image differences between modalities (e.g. MRI and histology) exist, and when imaging artifacts (e.g. bias field inhomogeneity in MRI) are present, the MSD of voxel intensity is not adequate and accurate as a good criterion for the evaluation in the multimodal situation. Therefore, we use the average prostate boundary (manually drawn after the registration of each test case) as a measure. In addition, we notice that identical feature points are consistent in world coordinate space, which inspires us to use the voxel-wise difference of their world coordinates as another criterion. In fact, if the volumes are registered, the differences of world coordinates have a correlation among voxels. Thus, we can use both interior (set I_No) and exterior (set S_No) feature points (as shown in Figure 1(c)) as landmarks to compare the spatial distance differences between registered multimodal datasets without and with anatomical features. We test our design using 5 cases of two modalities: T_2-weighted MRI and MRSI. Figure 5 shows the average prostate boundary of two modalities from all test cases. In addition, for each test case, Table 1 lists the average voxel-wise spatial distance differences of all the feature points marked in the world coordinates without or with interior anatomical features as alignment landmarks for registration.

Statistical Analysis. The statistical analysis is performed using the SPSS software (version 10.0). One-way ANOVA (Analysis of Variance) is used to analyze the differences between MI registration without and with anatomical features as landmarks. A

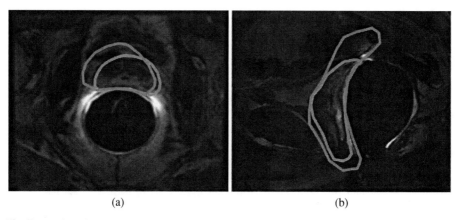

| (a) | (b) |

Fig. 5. Registration results of clinic datasets with two modalities: MRI and MRSI. The average prostate boundary detected without using anatomical feature points (red curve), and using anatomical feature points (green curve) in the (a) axis and (b) sagittal directions. The results show that our framework is able to register various modalities consistently and accurately.

two-tailed $p < 0.05$ is considered statistically significant in all the cases. All the results in both situations (artificial and clinical datasets) show the statistically significant improvement by the use of anatomical features for prostate registration.

Table 1. Average voxel-wise spatial distance differences of all the features points for all 5 registration cases without or with the interior anatomical features as alignment landmarks

Case #	1	2	3	4	5
Without	18.3	17.7	15.8	21.7	16.0
With	7.3	7.8	5.2	8.0	6.7

5   Conclusions

In this paper, we perform a registration method of volumetric MRI prostate using anatomical feature-guided mutual information. The evaluation, using the differences of local intensity and Euclidean distance of anatomical feature points as metrics for the statistical analysis, shows that our anatomical feature-guided MI registration framework has a significant improvement over the traditional MI registration method. Our framework is able to provide the physician with an integrated view of the intra-operative and high quality pre-operative imaging during the biopsy procedure. Although presented here for MR imaging, our pipeline has the potential applicability to other less discriminating but widely used intra-operative imaging modalities such as CT and ultrasound, although our design may be affected by different scanning protocols for the target gland. We plan to test our framework for these modalities in the future. In addition, potential use of our method includes the registration of other organs, such as the liver and kidney.

Acknowledgements. This paper has been supported by NSF grants IIS0916235, CCF0702699 and CNS0959979 and NIH grant R01EB7530.

References

1. Bharatha, A., Hirose, M., Hata, N., Warfield, S., Ferrant, M., Zou, K., Suarez-Santana, E., Ruiz-Alzola, J., D'Amico, A., Cormack, R., Kikinis, R., Jolesz, F., Tempany, C.: Evaluation of Three-Dimensional Finite Element-Based Deformable Registration of Pre- and Intra-Operative Prostate Imaging. Med. Phys. 28, 2551–2560 (2001)
2. Duda, R.O., Hart, P.E.: Use of the Hough Transformation to Detect Lines and Curves in Pictures. Comm. ACM 15, 11–15 (1972)
3. Haralick, R., Shanmugam, K., Dinstein, I.: Textural Features for Image Classification. IEEE Trans. Syst. Man Cybern. 3, 269–285 (1973)
4. Hirose, M., Bharatha, A., Hata, N., Zou, K., Warfield, S., Cormack, R., DiAmico, A., Kikinis, R., Jolesz, F., Tempany, C.: Quantitative MR Imaging Assessment of Prostate Gland Deformation Before and During MR Imaging-Guided Brachytherapy. Acad. Rad. 9(8), 906–912 (2002)
5. Kurhanewicz, J., Swanson, M.G., Nelson, S.J., Vigneron, D.B.: Combined Magnetic Resonance Imaging and Spectroscopic Imaging Approach to Molecular Imaging of Prostate Cancer. J. Magn. Reson. Imaging 16, 451–463 (2002)
6. Lee, Z., Sodee, D.B., Resnick, M., Maclennan, G.T.: Multimodal and 3D Imaging of Prostate Cancer. Comput. Med. Imaging Graph. 29, 477–486 (2005)
7. Park, S.B., Rhee, F.C., Monroe, J.I., Sohn, J.W.: Spatially Weighted Mutual Information Image Registration for Image Guided Radiation Therapy. Med. Phys. 37, 4590–4601 (2010)
8. Pluim, J., Maintz, J., Viergever, M.A.: Image Registration by Maximization of Combined Mutual Information and Gradient Information. IEEE Trans. Med. Imaging 19, 809–814 (2000)
9. Ries, L.A.G., Melbert, D., Krapcho, M., Stinchcomb, D.G., Howlader, N., Horner, M.J., Mariotto, A., Miller, B.A., Feuer, E.J., Altekruse, S.F., Leqis, D.R., Clegg, L., Eisner, M.P., Reichman, M., Edwards, B.K.: SEER Cancer Statistics Review. National Cancer Institute, http://seer.cancer.gov/csr/19752005/
10. Rosten, E., Porter, R., Drummond, T.: Faster and Better: a Machine Learning Approach to Corner Detection. IEEE Trans. Pattern Anal. Machine Intell. 32(1), 105–119 (2010)
11. Studholme, C., Hill, D., Hawkes, D.J.: Incorporating Connected Region Labeling into Automatic Image Registration Using Mutual Information. Mathematical Methods in Biomedical Image Analysis 3979, 23–31 (1996)
12. Thevenaz, P., Unser, M.: Optimization of Mutual Information for Multiresolution Image Registration. IEEE Trans. Image Process 9(12), 2088–2099 (2000)
13. Vidakovic, S., Jans, H.S., Alexander, A., Sloboda, R.S.: Post-Implant Computed Tomographylmagnetic Resonance Prostate Image Registration Using Feature Line Parallelization and Normalized Mutual Information. J. Appl. Clin. Med. Phys. 8(1), 21–32 (2007)
14. Zhan, Y., Ou, Y., Feldman, M., Tomaszeweski, J., Davatzikos, C., Shen, D.: Registering Histologic and MR Images of Prostate for Image-Based Cancer Detection. Acad. Radiol. 14(11), 1367–1381 (2007)

Abdominal Multi-Organ Segmentation of CT Images Based on Hierarchical Spatial Modeling of Organ Interrelations

Toshiyuki Okada[1], Marius George Linguraru[2], Yasuhide Yoshida[3],
Masatoshi Hori[1], Ronald M. Summers[4], Yen-Wei Chen[3], Noriyuki Tomiyama[1],
and Yoshinobu Sato[1]

[1] Department of Radiology, Graduate School of Medicine Osaka University, 2-2
Yamadaoka, Suita, Osaka 565-0871, Japan
toshi@image.med.osaka-u.ac.jp
[2] Children's National Medical Center, 111 Michigan Ave., N.W Washington, D.C
20010, USA
[3] Graduate School of Information Science and Engineering, Ritsumeikan University,
1-1-1, Nojihigashi, Kusatsu, Shiga, Japan
[4] National Institutes of Health, Clinical Center, Radiology and Imaging Sciences, 10
Center Drive Bethesda, MD 20892, USA

Abstract. The automated segmentation of multiple organs in CT data
of the upper abdomen is addressed. In order to explicitly incorporate
the spatial interrelations among organs, we propose a method for finding and representing the interrelations based on canonical correlation
analysis. Furthermore, methods are developed for constructing and utilizing the statistical atlas in which inter-organ constraints are explicitly
incorporated to improve accuracy of multi-organ segmentation. The proposed methods were tested to perform segmentation of seven abdominal
organs (liver, spleen, kidneys, pancreas, gallbladder and inferior vena
cava) from contrast-enhanced CT datasets and was compared to a previous approach. 28 datasets acquired at two institutions were used for
the validation. Significant accuracy improvement was observed for the
segmentation of pancreas and gallbladder while there was no accuracy
reduction for any organ.

Keywords: statistical shape prediction, statistical shape model, probabilistic atlas.

1 Introduction

In the abdomen, anatomical structures are spatially interrelated. Constraints on
the interrelations among the organs as well as individual positions and shapes
in the standardized space would be useful to perform their segmentation from
3D images. Several general approaches for multi-organ segmentation have been
proposed [7,4,9]. Although these works provide unified frameworks for statistical multi-organ modeling and segmentation, the hierarchical nature of organ

H. Yoshida et al. (Eds.): Abdominal Imaging 2011, LNCS 7029, pp. 173–180, 2012.
© Springer-Verlag Berlin Heidelberg 2012

relations was not explicitly considered. Our assumption is that some organs are constrained in their shapes and locations by other organs whose segmentation is relatively stable and accurate. Such a hierarchical relation can be utilized for effectively constraining the search space to improve the segmentation accuracy and stability. In previous work [10], the hierarchical modeling of multiple organs has been addressed in the pelvic area. However, they tested it for only a small number of organs. More recently, a method for pancreas segmentation was developed by fully utilizing the constraints from surrounding structured [8]. However, the method is not general-purpose but specifically focused on the pancreas.

In this paper, we describe our recent developments towards a general framework of multi-organ segmentation in which hierarchy and interrelations among organs are explicitly incorporated. We describe the key components of the overall framework to identify significant interrelations among organs, derive the constraints on organ shapes and locations from the interrelation, and utilize the constraints for the segmentation of multiple interrelated organs. These components are incorporated into a segmentation of seven upper abdominal organs from CT images.

2   Methods

2.1   Overview

The basic idea is to incorporate inter-organ spatial relations to attain stable and accurate segmentation of multiple organs. To do so, we firstly perform segmentation of relatively stable organs in their position, shape, and contrast, and then segment other organs which are expected to be well-constrained in their position and shape by the stable organs segmented during the first step.

We use two types of multi-organ atlas representation schemes. One is a prediction-based statistical atlas. Given the segmented interrelated organ regions, the target organ position and shape are predicted from them and the remaining ambiguity is represented in the form of the probabilistic atlas (PA) and statistical shape model (SSM), which we call prediction-based PA and SSM (P-PA & P-SSM). The other is a conventional multi-organ SSM (MO-SSM), in which multiple organ shapes are modeled as one SSM [3,10] in addition to single-organ SSMs corresponding to the individual organs. P-SSM and MO-SSM are combined with multi-level SSM (ML-SSM) where the whole organ shape is hierarchically divided into sub-shapes to attain higher representation accuracy while maintain the organ-specific shape constraints [6].

2.2   Basic Method

In this paper, we deal with seven organs, that is, the liver, spleen, left and right kidneys, gallbladder, inferior vena cava (IVC), and pancreas. The basic method is a modified version of a method for liver segmentation using PA and ML-SSM [6]. The modification has been made on modeling the distribution of CT value (which we call intensity hereafter) of each organ. While it was originally modeled

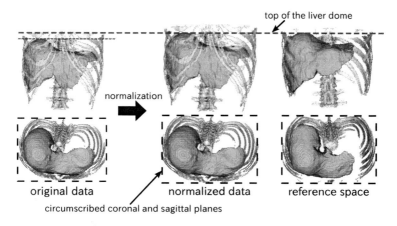

Fig. 1. Abdominal normalization using top of live dome and bone tissue regions. The image shows the liver in orange and the ribs and vertebral bodies in white.

by a single Gaussian fitted to the patient-specific histogram of the liver in each patient CT dataset estimated from the region having high probability values in PA [6], a Gaussian mixture model is fitted to the average intensity distribution obtained from the training datasets in order to adapt to various organs which may have multi-peak intensity distributions and may be too variable in position to have the high probability region in PA. Because the intensity distribution depends on a contrast enhanced CT protocol, its Gaussian mixture model is assumed to be prepared for each protocol.

A brief summary of the modified basic method is described below. Given an abdominal CT patient dataset, the abdominal normalized space is determined using the top of the liver dome (determining the height of the reference axial plane) and bone tissue regions (determining the circumscribed coronal and sagittal planes) as shown in Fig. 1. The liver dome top and bone tissue regions are automatically extracted [6] and used to align the patient dataset to the normalized space, in which the PAs and ML-SSMs of all the seven organs are defined. The PA and the intensity model of each organ are used to convert the voxel position and its intensity value to the likelihood of the organ existence, by which the likelihood image is generated. After obtaining the initial region by thresholding the likelihood image, the SSM is fitted to the initial region and then ML-SSM is further fitted to the original CT image to segment the organ region. Finally, a graph-cut-based refinement is performed [5], which was not included in the original basic method [6].

2.3   Organ Classification, Correlation Analysis, and Atlas Construction

The modified basic method described above was performed for the seven abdominal organs (see Section 3 for the datasets used for experiments). Based on the resulted segmentation accuracy, we classify them into two categories; stable and

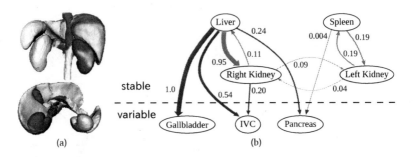

Fig. 2. Correlation analysis of inter-organ relations. (a) Organ surfaces influenced by the liver. Yellow surface indicates organ Y (=“liver”). Red indicates the region where $p_Y(x_i') < \alpha$. (b) Organ interrelation graph for liver, spleen, left and right kidneys, gallbladder, IVC, and pancreas.

variable organs. The volume overlap (VO) was used as a measure of segmentation accuracy, which is defined by $|A \cap B|/|A \cup B|$, where A and B denote the ground truth and automatically segmented region, respectively. If the average volume overlap was larger (smaller) than 70 %, we regarded it as “stable” (“variable”). As a result, the liver, spleen, left and right kidneys were regarded as “stable”, and the gallbladder, IVC, and pancreas as “variable”. We first segment “stable” organs and then segment “variable” organs assuming that “stable” organs have already been segmented.

In order to find the organ interrelations, canonical correlation analysis (CCA) is applied. In previous work [2], a p-value to test the significance of correlation between two points was derived using CCA to find intra-organ relations in the brain surface, where small p-values denote strong correlations. We extend this CCA-based method so as to deal with multiple organs. Given organ surfaces X and Y, we define the p-value of point $x_i(x_i \in X)$ representing correlation with Y by $p_Y(x_i) = \min_j p(x_i, y_j)$, where $y_j \in Y$ and $p(x, y)$ is the p-value between points x and y. We define the inter-organ correlation as $C(X|Y) = |X_Y|/|X|$ where $X_Y = \{x_i'|x_i' \in X \wedge p_Y(x_i') < \alpha\}$ in which α is the significance level. Intuitively, $C(X|Y)$ denotes a degree of influence of organ Y on organ X. $C(X|Y)$ is not commutative. That is, $C(X|Y) \neq C(Y|X)$. For example, when X =“gallbladder” and Y =“liver”, $C(X|Y) = 1.0$ and $C(Y|X) = 0.36$ at $\alpha = 10^{-10}$, which means that the whole gallbladder surface is influenced by the liver while 36 % of the liver surface by the gallbladder. Figure 2 (a) shows X_Y of the spleen, left and right kidneys, gallbladder, IVC, and pancreas when Y =“liver” and $\alpha = 10^{-10}$.

Based on the classification and correlation analysis, we represent the organ interrelations as a directed graph, which we call the organ interrelation graph (Fig. 2 (b)). In the graph, an edge is directed from node Y to node X when Y is a “stable” organ and $C(X|Y)$ is larger than a threshold (the threshold was zero in Fig. 2 (b)).

Based on the graph, statistical atlases are constructed. Among the “stable” organs, MO-SSM is constructed for organ pairs which have strong correlation.

Because the correlation is relatively weak between the left and right kidneys, two MO-SSMs were constructed for the liver and right kidney and for the spleen and left kidney. For the "variable organs", prediction-based PA (P-PA) and prediction-based SSM (P-SSM) were constructed based on the prediction from the "stable" organs which have high correlation (represented as arcs in the graph). The prediction-based statistical atlas is described in the next subsection.

2.4 Prediction-Based Statistical Atlas

The "variable" organ shape $\mathbf{v}$ is predicted from the "stable" organs ($\mathbf{s} = \{\mathbf{s}_1, \mathbf{s}_2, \cdots, \mathbf{s}_{n-1}\}$) having high correlation with the "variable" organ using principal component analysis (PCA). The organ surface shape is assumed to be represented by a point distribution, that is, a vector consisting of the sequence of 3D point coordinates. Let $\boldsymbol{q}$ denote the concatenation of the vector of the "variable" organ, $\mathbf{v}$, and those of "stable" organs, $\mathbf{s}$, that is, $\mathbf{q} = [\mathbf{v}; \mathbf{s}]$. SSM of the n organs is given by $\mathbf{q}(\mathbf{b}) = \mathbf{q}_{\text{ave}} + \Phi \mathbf{b}$ where $\mathbf{q}_{\text{ave}}$ is the average of $\mathbf{q}$, Φ the principal components obtained by PCA, and $\mathbf{b}$ the coefficients for the components. Given the segmented region boundaries B_s of the "stable" organs, we estimate $\mathbf{b}^*$ by $\mathbf{b}^* = \text{argmin}_{\mathbf{b}}\{C_D(\mathbf{q}(\mathbf{b}), B_s) + \lambda C_R(\mathbf{b})\}$ where C_D denotes the data term (the average of squared distances between $\mathbf{q}(\mathbf{b})$ and B_s), C_R the regularization term that $\mathbf{q}(\mathbf{b})$ should be close to the average shape $\mathbf{q}_{\text{ave}}$, and λ the weight parameter. The predicted "variable" organ shape $\mathbf{v}^*$ is obtained by extracting the $\mathbf{v}$ component from $\mathbf{q}(\mathbf{b})$. In the prediction, the number of principal components, N_c, as well as the weight parameter, λ, should be adjusted. This adjustment is performed by cross-validation using the training dataset. The prediction equation is given by $\mathbf{v} = P(B_s; N_c, \lambda) + \mathbf{r}$, where $\mathbf{v}$ is the true shape, $P(B_s; N_c, \lambda)$ denotes the prediction function described above, which is written as $\mathbf{v}^* = P(B_s; N_c, \lambda)$, and $\mathbf{r}$ denotes the residual after the prediction which represents the difference between the predicted and true shapes. Here, $\mathbf{r}$ is represented using PA and SSM.

To obtain PA and SSM of $\mathbf{r}$, we consider a reference shape $\mathbf{v}_0'$ in the reference dataset. The dense 3D deformation field $\mathbf{d}(\mathbf{x}; \mathbf{v}^*, \mathbf{v}_0')$ from the original space to the reference space is determined by thin-plate spline interpolation using correspondences from $\mathbf{v}^*$ to $\mathbf{v}_0'$, where $\mathbf{x}$ denotes the 3D position in the original space. The correspondences between $\mathbf{v}^*$ and $\mathbf{v}_0'$ are known because they are represented by the same SSM. The true shape $\mathbf{v}$ in the original space is mapped to the reference space using $\mathbf{d}(\mathbf{x}; \mathbf{v}^*, \mathbf{v}_0')$ and the mapped version $\mathbf{v}'$ is given by $\mathbf{v}' = \mathbf{v} + \mathbf{d}(\mathbf{x}; \mathbf{v}^*, \mathbf{v}_0')$.

Now, the residual $\mathbf{r}'$ in the reference space is given by $\mathbf{r}' = \mathbf{v}' - \mathbf{v}_0'$, which is obtained in each training dataset. In the reference space, SSM and PA of $\mathbf{r}'$ are constructed. The SSM in the reference space is represented as $\mathbf{q}'(\mathbf{b}_r) = \mathbf{v}_0' + \mathbf{r}'(\mathbf{b}_r)$, where $\mathbf{r}'(\mathbf{b}_r) = \Phi_r \mathbf{b}_r$, in which Φ_r are the principal components of the residual and $\mathbf{b}_r$ their coefficients. The SSM in the original space is obtained by $\mathbf{q}(\mathbf{b}_r) = \mathbf{q}'(\mathbf{b}_r) + \mathbf{d}^{-1}(\mathbf{x}'; \mathbf{v}^*, \mathbf{v}_0')$, where $\mathbf{d}^{-1}(\mathbf{x}'; \mathbf{v}^*, \mathbf{v}_0')$ is the inverse deformation filed of $\mathbf{d}(\mathbf{x}; \mathbf{v}^*, \mathbf{v}_0')$ and $\mathbf{x}'$ 3D positions in the reference space. The extension of the SSM defined here to ML-SSM is straight forward and it is used for segmentation described in the next section. Similarly, PA is constructing by adding 3D

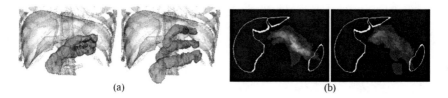

(a)   (b)

Fig. 3. Constructed prediction-based SSM and PA (left) and those without prediction (right). (a) SSM. (b) PA. In SSM, average (green) and $\pm 2\sigma$ (blue) of the first mode are shown. The color-scheme of PA shows probability from cold (low) to hot (high).

binary images of the true regions $\mathbf{v}'$ in the reference space, and mapped inversely to the original space using $\mathbf{d}^{-1}(\mathbf{x}'; \mathbf{v}^*, \mathbf{v}'_0)$. Figure 3 shows prediction-based PA and SSM for the pancreas (in comparison with the conventional ones).

2.5   Segmentation Procedure

The additional components which differ from the basic method described in 2.2 are described. The "stable" organs, the liver, spleen, and left and right kidneys are first segmented. After extracting the initial regions using PA as described in 2.2, MO-SSM of the liver and right kidney is fitted to their initial regions, and then individual ML-SSMs of the liver and right kidney are fitted to the CT images to segment them followed by graph-cut refinement. The spleen and left kidney were segmented in the same manner.

Given segmented "stable" organs, the "variable" organs, gallbladder, IVC, and pancreas, are segmented. Instead of conventional PA and SSM, P-PA and P-SSM described in 2.4 are used in the basic method in 2.2, followed by ML-SSM fitting and graph-cut refinement.

3   Results

The methods were applied to 28 abdominal contrast-enhanced CT scans of patients from two institutions, of which 18 scans from one institution 10 from the other. The CT scans showed different tissue contrasts between the two institutions. Data were collected with a Light Speed Ultra scanner (GE Healthcare). The slice thickness was 1 mm and the in-slice resolution varied from 0.54 mm to 0.77 mm. In all images, the seven organs (liver, spleen, left and right kidneys, gallbladder, IVC, and pancreas) were manually segmented by two fellows and supervised by a radiologist. Leave-one-out cross validation was performed for evaluation of segmentation accuracy.

Table 1 shows the quantitative evaluation of the segmentation results of the proposed method in comparison with the basic method described in 2.2, in which organ interrelation is not explicitly utilized. Figure 4 shows typical segmentation results. Both methods were fully automated. Segmentation accuracy was evaluated using VO. Among the "stable" organs, VO was improved for the left kidney from 83.6 % (in the basic method) to 87.4 % (in the proposed method)

Table 1. Volume overlap of segmentation results by proposed and basic methods

	Liver	Spleen	Right kidney	Left kidney	Pancreas	Gallbladder	IVC
proposed	89.1 %	82.5 %	88.2 %	87.4 %	46.6 %	63.4 %	54.8 %
basic	89.2 %	83.6 %	88.0 %	83.6 %	34.8 %	53.0 %	54.5 %
signicance	-	-	-	-	$p < 0.05$	$p < 0.05$	-

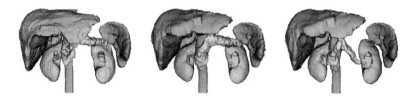

Fig. 4. Manual segmentation (left) and typical segmentation results of proposed (middle) and basic (right) methods. Orange, purple, pink, yellow, green, and cyan surfaces indicate the liver, spleen, kidneys, pancreas, gallbladder, and IVC, respectively.

although it was not statistical significant. For other "stable" organs, differences in VO were not observed. Regarding the "variable organs", VO of the gallbladder and pancreas improved around 10 % compared with the basic method and statistical significance was observed for the both organs while improvement was not observed in IVC.

4   Discussion and Conclusion

This paper has described methods for finding multi-organ spatial interrelations and their incorporation into segmentation via statistical atlas. The methods were applied to the abdominal organs and experimental results showed significant improvement of the segmentation accuracy for the gallbladder and pancreas, whose shape and position are largely influenced by other organs. Other abdominal organs will be added in a straightforward manner.

The prediction-based atlas described in 2.4 was newly proposed in this paper. This is an atlas representation whose variability is constrained by interrelated other organs. A conditional (statistical) shape model was proposed as a similar representation [1]. The prediction-based atlas would be replaced by the conditional model. However, the conditional PA will need to be constructed for each patient and organ by generating instances of the conditional SSM by Gaussian random numbers during the segmentation processes after segmentation of the interrelated organs while prediction-based PA is adapted for each patient by only the nonrigid transform of PA in the reference space with known correspondences. In our experiments, the prediction-based PA was shown to improve the segmentation accuracy. The easier use of PA is an additional advantage of the prediction-based atlas.

The proposed methods are generally applicable to various domains, when multiple organs are interrelated and some of them are more stable in segmentation. One feature of the proposed methods is to find organ interrelations systematically based on CCA. Given the ground truth segmentation of multiple organs, the organ interrelation graph is automatically constructed to provide a guideline for multi-organ and prediction-based atlas construction.

Acknowledgements. This work was partly supported by the Intramural Research Program of the National Institutes of Health, Clinical Center. The PLUTO system developed at Nagoya University was partly used to generate the ground truth datasets from CT images.

References

1. de Bruijne, M., et al.: Quantitative vertebral morphometry using neighbor-conditional shape models. Medical Image Analysis 11(5), 503–512 (2007)
2. Fillard, P., et al.: Evaluating brain anatomical correlations via canonical correlation analysis of sulcal lines. In: MICCAI 2007 Workshop: Statistical Registration, HAL - CCSD (2007)
3. Frangi, A.F., et al.: Automatic construction of multiple-object three-dimensional statistical shape models: Application to cardiac modelling. IEEE Trans. Med. Imaging 21(9), 1151–1166 (2002)
4. Linguraru, M.G., Pura, J.A., Chowdhury, A.S., Summers, R.M.: Multi-Organ Segmentation from Multi-Phase Abdominal CT Via 4D Graphs Using Enhancement, Shape and Location Optimization. In: Jiang, T., Navab, N., Pluim, J.P.W., Viergever, M.A. (eds.) MICCAI 2010, Part III. LNCS, vol. 6363, pp. 89–96. Springer, Heidelberg (2010)
5. Massoptier, L., et al.: Fully automatic liver segmentation through graph-cut technique. In: 29th Annual International Conference of the IEEE Engineering in Medicine and Biology Society, EMBS 2007, pp. 5243–5246 (August 2007)
6. Okada, T., et al.: Automated segmentation of the liver from 3D CT images using probabilistic atlas and multilevel statistical shape model. Academic Radiology 15(11), 1390–1403 (2008)
7. Park, H., Bland, P.H., Meyer, C.R.: Construction of an abdominal probabilistic atlas and its application in segmentation. IEEE Transactions on Medical Imaging 22(4), 483–492 (2003)
8. Shimizu, A., et al.: Automated pancreas segmentation from three-dimensional contrast-enhanced computed tomography. International Journal of Computer Assisted Radiology and Surgery 5(1), 85–98 (2010)
9. Liu, X., Linguraru, M.G., Yao, J., Summers, R.M.: Organ Pose Distribution Model and an MAP Framework for Automated Abdominal Multi-organ Localization. In: Liao, H., Edwards, P.J., Pan, X., Fan, Y., Yang, G.-Z. (eds.) MIAR 2010. LNCS, vol. 6326, pp. 393–402. Springer, Heidelberg (2010)
10. Yokota, F., Okada, T., Takao, M., Sugano, N., Tada, Y., Sato, Y.: Automated Segmentation of the Femur and Pelvis from 3D CT Data of Diseased Hip Using Hierarchical Statistical Shape Model of Joint Structure. In: Yang, G.-Z., Hawkes, D., Rueckert, D., Noble, A., Taylor, C. (eds.) MICCAI 2009, Part II. LNCS, vol. 5762, pp. 811–818. Springer, Heidelberg (2009)

Organ Segmentation from 3D Abdominal CT Images Based on Atlas Selection and Graph Cut

Masahiro Oda[1], Teruhisa Nakaoka[2], Takayuki Kitasaka[3],
Kazuhiro Furukawa[4], Kazunari Misawa[5],
Michitaka Fujiwara[4], and Kensaku Mori[1,2]

[1] Information Planning Office, Information and Communications Headquarters,
Nagoya University, Furo-cho, Chikusa-ku, Nagoya, Aichi, 464-8601, Japan
[2] Graduate School of Information Science, Nagoya University,
Furo-cho, Chikusa-ku, Nagoya, Aichi, 464-8603, Japan
moda@mori.m.is.nagoya-u.ac.jp
[3] Faculty of Information Science, Aichi Institute of Technology,
1247 Yachigusa, Yagusa-cho, Toyota, Aichi, 470-0392, Japan
[4] Graduate School of Medicine, Nagoya University,
65 Tsurumai-cho, Syouwa-ku, Nagoya, Aichi, 466-8550, Japan
[5] Aichi Cancer Center,
1-1 Kanokoden, Chikusa-ku, Nagoya, Aichi, 464-8681, Japan

Abstract. This paper presents a method for segmenting abdominal organs from 3D abdominal CT images based on atlas selection and graph cut. The training samples are divided into multiple clusters based on the image similarity. The average image and atlas for each cluster are created. For an input image, we select the most similar atlas to the input image by measuring the image similarity between the input and average images. Segmentation of organs based on the MAP estimation using the selected atlas is then performed, followed by the precise segmentation by the graph cut algorithm. We applied the proposed method to a hundred cases of CT images. The experimental results showed that the extraction accuracy could be improved using multiple atlases, achieving more than 90% of the precision rate except for the pancreas.

1 Introduction

Segmentation is one of the most important functions in computer-aided diagnosis systems. To understand the human anatomy by computers, organs should be segmented accurately. Recognition of the human anatomy is also indispensable for computer-assisted surgery systems. So far as segmentation of organs, one of most promising approaches is an atlas-based segmentation. The atlas tells us a priori information of organs such as the relative position in a body and shape. Park et al.[1] proposed an atlas-based segmentation method of abdominal organs. They constructed the probability map of organ existence as the atlas. Okada et al.[2] analyzed the shape of organs statistically and constructed hierarchical multi-organ statistical atlases. Recently, segmentation methods based on the

H. Yoshida et al. (Eds.): Abdominal Imaging 2011, LNCS 7029, pp. 181–188, 2012.

graph cut[3,4], which can solve global optimization problems, have been paid to attention. Shimizu et al.[5] proposed an automated segmentation method of the pancreas using the probabilistic atlas and graph cut.

Aljabar et al.[6] also proposed a multi-atlas based segmentation of brain images. They constructed multiple atlases and select an appropriate atlas for segmentation. This approach would have the benefit for segmenting organs that the topology or positional relationship between adjacent objects can change drastically such as the brain and abdominal organs. In the atlas construction, samples whose properties are quite different from others should be separated because these can be the causes of the fade of the atlas and deterioration of the segmentation accuracy. Therefore, we divide the training samples into multiple clusters and construct multiple atlases for abdominal organ segmentation. In the extraction process of organs, we select an appropriate atlas and extract abdominal organs precisely by the graph cut algorithm. In the section 2, details of multi-atlas based graph cut segmentation method are provided. The sections 3 and 4 shows the experimental results and discussion.

2   Method

2.1   Overview

The proposed method extracts abdominal organs; the liver, spleen, pancreas and kidneys, by utilizing multiple atlases that represent the probability map of organ existence. Figure 1 shows the flow chart of the proposed method. Before executing the extraction process, we construct multiple atlases. we perform the clustering of the training samples based on an image similarity. The average image and probability map of organ existence for each cluster are calculated. In the extraction process, the most similar atlas is selected by comparing an input image with average images of all clusters. The selected atlas is used for the MAP estimation to extract rough organ regions. At last, the precise organ regions are obtained by performing the graph cut algorithm, in which the rough organ regions are set to the foreground. The detail procedures are given as follows.

2.2   Image Regularization

All samples in the training dataset as well as an input image are regularized based on the size of the lung to reduce the individual change with respect to the body size. First, the lung regions are extracted from each image by the thresholding and connected component analysis. The bounding box of the lung regions are then calculated. The image is translated so that the bottom of the lung becomes the middle of the image. The size of the image is scale-up (or down) so that the size of the lung becomes 150[mm] × 150[mm] and the resolution in z-axis becomes 1[mm].

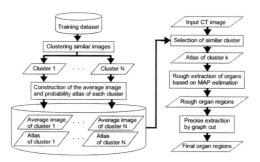

Fig. 1. The flow chart of the proposed method

2.3   Clustering of Training Samples

All samples in the training dataset are divided into clusters based on an image similarity. Here, the normalized cross correlation (NCC) is used as the image similarity(Eq. 2.3).

$$R_{NCC}(S,T) = \frac{\sum\limits_{k=0}^{N-1}\sum\limits_{j=0}^{M-1}\sum\limits_{i=0}^{L-1}\left(S(i,j,k) - \bar{S}\right)\left(T(i,j,k) - \bar{T}\right)}{\sqrt{\sum\limits_{k=0}^{N-1}\sum\limits_{j=0}^{M-1}\sum\limits_{i=0}^{L-1}\left(S(i,j,k) - \bar{S}\right)^2 \times \sum\limits_{k=0}^{N-1}\sum\limits_{j=0}^{M-1}\sum\limits_{i=0}^{L-1}\left(T(i,j,k) - \bar{T}\right)^2}} \quad (1)$$

Where, N, M and L are the size of x-, y- and z-axes, respectively. S and T represent images and $\bar{S}$ and $\bar{T}$ are the mean of intensity in S and T. $S(i,j,k)$ is the intensity of S at a point (x,y,z). Images in the training dataset have been transformed by a non-rigid image registration[7].

After registration of all images, we construct a similarity graph, calculating the similarity $R_{NCC}(I^i, I^j)$ between I^i and I^j. The image clustering is done by the normalized cut[8] using the similarity graph, which is a clustering algorithm based on a graph. This algorithm treats the problem of dividing a graph $\mathbf{G} = (\mathbf{V}, \mathbf{E})$ into two independent sets of vertices, $\mathbf{A}$ and $\mathbf{B}$, where $\mathbf{A} \cup \mathbf{B} = \mathbf{V}$ and $\mathbf{A} \cap \mathbf{B} = \emptyset$. The edges $\mathbf{E}$ of the graph $\mathbf{G}$ have weights $w(i,j)$. In the normalized cut, $\mathbf{G}$ is divided into clusters $\mathbf{A}$ and $\mathbf{B}$ by minimizing the cost

$$\text{Ncut}(\mathbf{A}, \mathbf{B}) = \frac{\sum\limits_{u \in \mathbf{A}, v \in \mathbf{B}} w(u,v)}{\sum\limits_{u \in \mathbf{A}, t \in \mathbf{V}} w(u,t)} + \frac{\sum\limits_{u \in \mathbf{A}, v \in \mathbf{B}} w(u,v)}{\sum\limits_{v \in \mathbf{B}, t \in \mathbf{V}} w(v,t)}. \quad (2)$$

We divide all images into four clusters by applying the normalized cut recursively. The weight between vertices i and j is defined by

$$w(i,j) = 1 + R_{NCC}(I^i, I^j). \quad (3)$$

2.4   Construction of Probability Atlases of Organ Existence

The probability map of organ existence is created for each cluster obtained above. First, we calculate the average image M^j of each cluster j[9]. All images in a cluster are registered to the average image. The probability map of organ existence is calculated by

$$A_p^j(l) = \frac{\sum_{L^{j,i} \in D^j} S(L_p^{j,i}, l)}{|D^j|}, \tag{4}$$

$$S(l, l') = \begin{cases} 1 \text{ if } l = l' \\ 0 \text{ otherwise} \end{cases} \tag{5}$$

where D^j is a set of label images in the cluster j. The i-th label image $L_p^{j,i}$ of the cluster j contains the organ label l at a voxel p. Here, the labels of the liver, spleen, pancreas and kidneys are 1, 2, 3 and 4, respectively. $|D^j|$ indicates the number of label images belonging to the cluster j.

2.5   Selection of Most Similar Atlas

To extract organ regions accurately, we select the most similar atlas to the input image I. The atlas of the cluster c is selected when the similarity $R_{NCC}(M^c, I)$ is the largest.

2.6   Rough Extraction by MAP Estimation

We extract organ regions roughly by using selected atlas $A_p^c(l)$. Assuming that the intensity distribution of each organ is a normal and that the intensity distribution of an input image is a mixture of normals, the mean μ_l and variance σ_l^2 of the normal corresponding to the organ label l are estimated by the EM-algorithm[10]. The conditional probability $\text{Pr}_p(I_p|l)$ is expressed by a normal distribution with μ_l and σ_l^2

$$\text{Pr}_p(I_p|l) = \text{Pr}(I_p|\mu_l, \sigma_l^2). \tag{6}$$

The prior probability $\text{Pr}_p(l)$ of the organ existence is given by the atlas

$$\text{Pr}_p(l) = A_p^c(l). \tag{7}$$

The posterior probability $\text{Pr}_p(l|I_p)$ is calculated by

$$\text{Pr}_p(l|I_p) = \frac{\text{Pr}_p(I_p|l)\text{Pr}_p(l)}{\text{Pr}_\mu(I_\mu)}. \tag{8}$$

Hence, the rough extraction result C is obtained by

$$C_p = \arg \max_l \text{Pr}_p(l|I_p). \tag{9}$$

2.7   Precise Extraction by Graph Cut

Using the rough extraction result C, we extract the precise organ regions based on the graph cut algorithm[3]. We minimize the following cost

$$E(L) = \sum_{p \in P} R_p(L_p) + \sum_{(p,q) \in N} B_{p,q}(L_p, L_q), \tag{10}$$

where L is the label image whose voxels take each of 0 to 4 (0 is the background). P represents the set of voxels of the input image. $N = \{(p, q) | p \in P, q \in N^p\}$, N^p is the set of neighbors of a voxel p.

In the proposed method, R_p is defined using the rough extraction result C as follows.

$$R_p(l) = \begin{cases} 0 \text{ if } C_p = l \\ 1 \text{ otherwise.} \end{cases} \tag{11}$$

$B_{p,q}$ is expressed by

$$B_{p,q}(l, l') = \begin{cases} 0 & \text{if } l = l' \\ \lambda \frac{1}{(1+|I_p - I_q|)\text{dist}(p,q)} & \text{otherwise,} \end{cases} \tag{12}$$

where λ is the weight and $\text{dist}(p, q)$ represents the Euclidean distance between voxels p and q. $B_{p,q}$ becomes larger when the intensity difference and distance between p and q are smaller and closer.

3   Experiments

We applied the proposed method to a hundred cases of 3D abdominal CT images. The acquisition parameters of the images are; 512×512 pixels, 263-538 slices, 0.546-0.820[mm] in pixel spacing, and 0.400-0.800[mm] in slice spacing. We conducted the ten-folds cross validation. The recall and precision rates were used for evaluation criteria. The ground truth data was constructed by authors, which was also checked by a physician.

$$\text{Recall rate} = \frac{TP}{TP + FN} \times 100 \ (\%), \tag{13}$$

$$\text{Precision rate} = \frac{TP}{TP + FP} \times 100 \ (\%), \tag{14}$$

where TP, FP and FN represent the number of voxels coincided with the ground truth, the number of voxels not overlapped with the ground truth, and the number of voxels overlooked from the ground truth. The computation time was about 15 hours for clustering, 5 hours for construction of atlases, and 10 minutes/case for the extraction process by Intel(R) Xeon(R) W5590 3.33GHz × 2 processors. The extraction parameter λ in Section 2.7 was set to 25, relatively large value

Table 1. Average extraction accuracy of abdominal organs

	Single atlas		Two atlases		Four atlases	
	Recall	Precision	Recall	Precision	Recall	Precision
Liver	93.7%	95.6%	93.3%	95.5%	93.3%	95.6%
Spleen	82.9%	89.9%	82.9%	88.3%	85.1%	91.0%
Pancreas	64.3%	59.1%	60.1%	58.8%	55.7%	57.3%
Kidney	87.6%	90.4%	87.3%	90.2%	88.4%	90.7%

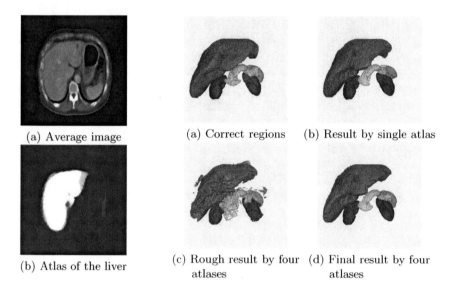

(a) Average image

(a) Correct regions   (b) Result by single atlas

(b) Atlas of the liver

(c) Rough result by four atlases   (d) Final result by four atlases

Fig. 2. An example of average images and atlases

Fig. 3. Examples of extraction results. The pancreas could be extracted better by using four atlases than single atlas.

so that the boundary term $B_{p,q}$ dominantly contributed to optimization, since the rough extraction result includes FPs and FNs as well. Figure 2 shows an example of average images and atlases.

Table 1 shows the comparison of the extraction accuracy using four atlases, two atlases and single atlas. Examples of the extraction results are shown in Figs. 3 and 4. Figure 3 indicates an example of extraction results by single and four atlases. Figure 4 indicates a successful result that the atlas selection can reduce FPs.

4 Discussion

From Table 1, the precision rate of all organs except for the pancreas by the proposed method with four atlases was able to achieve 90% or more. The extraction accuracy of the spleen becomes better as the number of atlases increases. Also, as shown in Fig. 4, FPs could be reduced by the atlas selection. Since the single

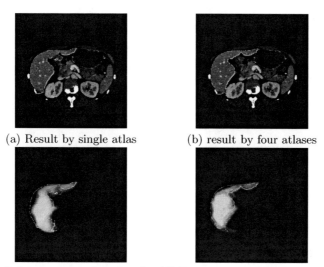

(a) Result by single atlas   (b) result by four atlases

(c) Existence map of single atlas (d) Existence map of selected atlas

Fig. 4. Example of FP reduction by multiple atlases. FPs in the right kidney were reduced by selecting an appropriate atlas.

atlas has high probability of the liver existence in the right kidney (Fig. 4(c)), FPs were detected in the right kidney by the MAP estimation, and the graph cut could not modify them (Fig. 4(a)). By selecting an appropriate atlas, more suitable probability map for the input image was used in the MAP estimation (Fig. 4(d)). Thus, FPs in the right kidney were not detected in the final extraction result (Fig. 4(b)). The clustering of the training samples and selection of atlases can improve the extraction accuracy.

However, the extraction accuracy of the pancreas becomes worse. This is because the number of training samples for each cluster becomes less as the number of clusters increases. Since individual differences of the pancreas with respect to the position and shape vary wider than those of other organs, the training was not sufficient due to the lack of training samples. The proposed method should be tested by much larger number of the training samples.

5   Conclusions

This paper proposed a method for segmenting abdominal organs from 3D abdominal CT images based on atlas selection and graph cut. The training samples were divided into multiple clusters based on the image similarity and multiple atlases were constructed. For an input image, we selected the most similar atlas to the input image. Segmentation of organs based on the MAP estimation using the selected atlas was then performed, followed by the precise segmentation by the graph cut algorithm. We applied the proposed method to a hundred cases of CT images. The experimental results showed that the extraction accuracy could be improved using multiple atlases, achieving more than 90% of the precision rate except for the pancreas. Future work includes the improvement of the clustering method of the training dataset and the selection method of atlases, testing for much larger number of cases.

Acknowledgements. The authors thank our colleagues for suggestions and advices. Parts of this research were supported by the Grant-in-Aid for Scientific Research from the Ministry of Education (MEXT), Japan Society for the Promotion of Science (JSPS), the Fund for Cancer Research and Development from the National Cancer Center, the Center of Excellence in Aichi Prefecture, and the Kayamori Foundation of Informational Science Advancement.

References

1. Park, H., Bland, P.H., Meyer, C.R.: Construction of an abdominal probabilistic atlas and its application. IEEE Transactions on Medical Imaging 22(4), 483–492 (2003)
2. Okada, T., Yokota, K., Hori, M., Nakamoto, M., Nakamura, H., Sato, Y.: Construction of Hierarchical Multi-Organ Statistical Atlases and Their Application to Multi-Organ Segmentation from CT Images. In: Metaxas, D., Axel, L., Fichtinger, G., Székely, G. (eds.) MICCAI 2008, Part I. LNCS, vol. 5241, pp. 502–509. Springer, Heidelberg (2008)
3. Boykov, Y., Jolly, M.P.: Interactive graph cuts for optimal boundary and region segmentation of objects in n-d images. In: ICCV, pp. 105–112 (2001)
4. Boykov, Y., Veksler, O., Zabih, R.: Efficient approximate energy minimization via graph cuts. IEEE Transactions on PAMI 20(12), 1222–1239 (2001)
5. Shimizu, A., Kimoto, T., Kobatake, H., Nawano, S., Shinozaki, K.: Automated pancreas segmentation from three-dimensional contrast-enhanced computed tomography. International Journal of Computer Assisted Radiology and Surgery 5(1), 85–98 (2010)
6. Aljabar, P., Heckemann, R.A., Hammers, A., Hajnal, J.V., Rueckert, D.: Multi-atlas based segmentation of brain images: Atlas selection and its effect on accuracy. NeuroImage 46, 726–738 (2009)
7. Glocker, B., Komodakis, N., Tziritas, G., Navab, N., Paragios, N.: Dense image registration through MRFs and efficient linear programming. Medical Image Analysis 12(6), 731–741 (2008)
8. Shi, J., Malik, J.: Normalized cuts and image segmentation. IEEE Transactions on PAMI 22, 888–905 (1997)
9. Guimond, A., Meunier, J., Thirion, J.P.: Average brain models: A convergence study. Computer Vision and Image Understanding 77(77), 192–210 (1999)
10. Dempster, A.P., Laird, N.M., Rubin, D.B.: Maximum likelihood from incomplete data via the EM algorithm. Journal of the Royal Statistical Society, B 39(1), 1–38 (1977)

Liver Segmental Anatomy and Analysis from Vessel and Tumor Segmentation via Optimized Graph Cuts

Vivek Pamulapati, Aradhana Venkatesan, Bradford J. Wood,
and Marius George Linguraru

Radiology and Imaging Sciences, Clinical Center, National Institutes
of Health,Bethesda, MD
{pamulapativ,lingurarum}@mail.nih.gov

Abstract. The segmentation and classification of the major intra-hepatic blood vessels along with the segmentation and analysis of hepatic tumors are critical for patient specific models of the diseased liver. Additionally, the accurate identification of liver anatomical segments can assist in the clinical assessment of the risks and benefits of hepatic interventions. We propose a novel 4D graph-based method to segment hepatic vasculature and tumors. The algorithm uses multi-phase CT images to model the differential enhancement of the liver structures and Hessian-based shape likelihoods to avoid the common pitfalls of graph cuts with undersegmentation and intensity heterogeneity. A hybrid classification step based on post-order walks of a graph identifies the right, middle and left hepatic, and portal veins. Veins are tracked using the graph representation and planes fitted to the vessel segments. The method allows the detection of all hepatic tumors and identification of the liver segments with 87.8% accuracy.

Keywords: contrast-enhanced CT, liver, vein, tumor, segmental anatomy.

1   Introduction

Patient specific knowledge of hepatic segmental anatomy is essential to liver therapy and surgical planning. Contrast enhanced computed tomography (CT) is the predominant 3D imaging modality for non-invasive hepatic analysis and surgical planning due to its ability to highlight the intra-hepatic vascular network and distinguish tumor from normal parenchyma. In this clinical context, computer-aided tools can assist diagnostic and therapeutic planning for liver diseases.

Information about the proximity of tumors to the major branches of the hepatic and portal veins, and therefore the liver segments, is a key determinant of a patient's suitability for surgical resection of hepatocellular carcinomas [1]. Similarly, the advanced planning of living donor liver transplantation must ensure that the grafted liver volume is independently functional [2]. The Couinaud atlas is the most widely accepted classification for liver segmental anatomy [3] and divides the liver into eight segments with independent vascular circulation and biliary drainage.

H. Yoshida et al. (Eds.): Abdominal Imaging 2011, LNCS 7029, pp. 189–197, 2012.
© Springer-Verlag Berlin Heidelberg 2012

Previous attempts to develop (semi-)automated computer tools for identifying the segments specified by the Couinaud atlas in CT data had varying degrees of success, but all are highly dependent on the quality of segmentation and classification of the major intra-hepatic veins [2, 4-6]. Image intensity analysis was key in [6] and liver segments were found solely from the portal vein, despite the fact that the hepatic veins are the other main anatomical landmarks defining the segments [3]. Similarly, an interactive technique was used in [4]. These techniques are sensitive to image acquisition and local variations in enhancement. Additional challenges are the high degree of inter-patient liver variability and the presence of hepatic tumors.

Graph-based image analysis has gained increasing attention in image analysis due to the ability to find a globally optimal fast solution to segmentation problems [7]. In its basic form, the graph cuts algorithm suffers from the shrinking bias problem [8]. This is particularly ill-suited for the segmentation of small and elongated objects, such as certain types of tumors and blood vessels. Graph cuts applications for liver analysis were presented in [9,10,11], but did not perform a holistic analysis of the liver.

In this study, we propose a novel extension of 4D graph cuts to first segment and classify the major intra-hepatic vasculature. Secondly, hepatic tumors are detected and segmented using the same framework. The segmentation incorporates constraints for differential enhancement from 4D multi-phase CT images and Hessian-based shape constraints to provide new cost terms adapted to the shape of vessels and tumors. The hepatic and portal veins are identified and labeled using a hybrid process that incorporates anatomical information and post-order walks of the graph representation of the vasculature. Finally, the liver volume is divided into anatomical segments by fitting planes to the trajectories of the hepatic and portal veins. The technique allows the visualization of liver tumors and vasculature in relation to the liver segmental anatomy.

2   Methods and Materials

The liver vessel segmentation and classification method was tested on 13 patient multi-phase CT data sets with normal and abnormal liver anatomy; tumors were present in four cases. CT images were acquired at two temporal phases, a non-contrast phase image (NCP) and a contrast-enhanced phase image (CEP), ideally at portal venous enhancement, captured at a fixed delay on a variety of scanners. Image slice thickness was 1mm with in slice resolutions from 0.59-0.82mm.

Liver masks were obtained using the segmentation method in [11]. NCP images were registered to CEP images using the non-linear registration algorithm in [12] (Fig. 1). 4D data were smoothed using anisotropic diffusion [13]. To validate the segmentation of tumors, an additional set of 14 CT cases (79 tumors, 5mm slice thickness) from patients with liver cancer and manually segmented tumors was used.

The graph cuts segmentation finds a globally optimal cut through the graph based on the input data. In this case, the input is represented by 4D CT composed of NCP and CEP images. For each voxel p, there are two associated intensity values, I^p_{NCP} and I^p_{CEP}. Seed points were generated automatically by finding optimal thresholds in the

CEP data for vessels and tumors [4]. Additionally, the object seed points are further constrained to have non-zero Hessian-based shape response, as described below.

The t-link costs in graph cuts traditionally correspond to regional information in log-likelihood form [7]. Similarly, n-links are placed between adjacent voxels in a connected grid. In our application, the cost function of the graph E for a binary vector $A = \{A_1, A_2,..., A_p\}$ can be written as

$$E(A) = E_{data}(A) + E_{enhance}(A) + E_{shape}(A) + E_{boundary}(A),$$

where the first three terms represent the t-links and $E_{boundary}$ represents the n-links.

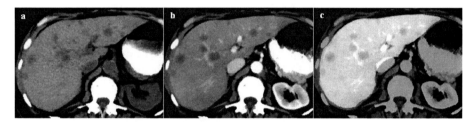

Fig. 1. Multi-phase liver CT; a) the registered NCP image; b) the CEP image; and c) the liver mask on   CEP. Veins appear dark in a) and bright in b); tumors are darker at both phases.

Intensity histograms for the object (O) and background (B) were built from the seed voxels in NCP and CEP images. E_{data} becomes a regional term that computes penalties based on the 4D histograms of O and B.

$E_{enhance}$ is the regional term that penalizes voxels that do not follow the correct multi-phase (MP) enhancement distribution between CEP and NCP, where P_{MP} is the probability. The vessels should enhance significantly more than the parenchyma, while tumors less (Fig. 1).

$$E_{enhance}(A) = \delta \sum_{p \in O} R_{pMP}(O) + (1-\delta) \sum_{p \in B} R_{pMP}(B); \text{ with } I^p_{MP} = \left| I^p_{CEP} - I^p_{NCP} \right|; \text{ and}$$

$$R_{pMP}(O) = -\ln \left(\frac{P_{MP}(I^p_{MP} \mid O)}{P_{MP}(I^p_{MP} \mid O) + P_{MP}(I^p_{MP} \mid B)} \right).$$

E_{shape} has distinct forms for vessels and tumors. Hessian-based vesselness V likelihoods were generated from the CEP image data using an implementation of the multi-scale curvilinear structure enhancing filter in. [14].

$$E_{vesselness} = -\ln \max_{\sigma}\left(\sigma^2 v(p, \sigma)\right); \text{ with } v = \begin{cases} |\lambda_2| + \lambda_1, & if \lambda_3 < \lambda_2 < \lambda_1 < 0 \\ |\lambda_2| - \dfrac{\lambda_1}{4}, & if \lambda_3 < \lambda_2 < 0 < \lambda_1 < 4|\lambda_2|; \\ 0 & ,otherwise \end{cases}$$

where σ is the scale of the Gaussian convolution used to calculate the discrete Hessian, and $\lambda_1, \lambda_2, \lambda_3$ are the eigenvalues of the Hessian matrix. Alternatively, to emphasize the roundness of tumor, a blobness constraint is defined as

$$E_{blobness} = -\ln\max_{\sigma}(w); \quad with \quad w = \begin{cases} \exp-\left(\dfrac{\lambda_1}{\lambda_3}-1\right), if\lambda_1 > \lambda_2 > \lambda_3 > 0 \\ 0 \qquad\qquad , otherwise \end{cases};$$

The n-link costs w between adjacent voxels p and q are initially symmetric

$$E_{boundary}(A) = \mu \sum_{\{p,q\}\in N_p} w_{\{p\to q\}} + (1-\mu) \sum_{\{p,q\}\in N_p} w_{\{q\to p\}};$$

$$w_{\{p\to q\}} = w_{\{q\to p\}} = \begin{cases} 0 & , if A_p = A_q \\ \exp\left(-\dfrac{\left|I^p_{NCP}-I^q_{NCP}\right|\cdot\left|I^p_{CEP}-I^q_{CEP}\right|}{2\sigma_{NCP}\sigma_{CEP}}\right)\dfrac{1}{dist(p,q)} & , otherwise. \end{cases}$$

However, an additional directional constraint penalizes transitions from bright to dark (for tumors) and dark to bright (for vessles, not shown) in the CEP image and transitions from bright to dark in the non-contrast phase for all objects (see Fig. 1).

$$IF\left(\left(I^p_{CEP}-I^q_{CEP}\right) > \sigma_{CEP} OR\left(I^p_{NCP}-I^q_{NCP}\right) > \sigma_{NCP}\right), \; THEN \; w_{\{p\to q\}} = 1; \; ELSE \; w_{\{q\to p\}} = 1,$$

where σ_{CEP} and σ_{NCP} are the standard deviations of noise in each respective phase.

The 4D graph cuts produce an unlabeled segmentation of the hepatic and portal veins. To generate the Couinaud segments of a liver, it is necessary to identify the three main hepatic vein branches and the portal vein within the initial unlabled vessel segmentation. Due to partial volume effects, the hepatic and portal veins are often connected in this initial segmentation. In addition, the hepatic vein branch roots are not always connected at the inferior vena cava in the graph cuts segmentation due to varying levels of contrast enhancement. Thus, the vessel identification scheme must be robust enough to support this level of variability in the vessel segmentation result.

Our vessel identification algorithm generates a graph representation of the vessel tree to locate the main hepatic and portal venous branches. First, the unlabeled vessel tree is skeletonized using a 3D parallel thinning algorithm [12]. Skeleton voxels with a single neighbor are considered end nodes, voxels with more than two neighbors are considered branching nodes, and finally voxels with two neighbors are grouped into segments that connect the nodes. The diameter of each segment is calculated by taking the mean normal distance from each skeleton voxel in a segment to the boundary of the vessel segmentation. This process results in an undirected graph representation of the vessel tree in which every segment has an estimated diameter.

Next, all valid sub-trees within the undirected vessel graph are identified. A sub-tree is valid if it meets the following criteria: the diameter of the vessel tree must progressively increase from a child node towards the root of the tree and the minimal angle between a child node and a parent node across a branching node must be obtuse. A traversal operation is performed on each end point. The traversal operation is a post-order walk beginning at the end point and following a single valid sub-tree path. A traversal terminates in three cases. If the traversal can no longer continue to a node without violating the criteria of a valid vessel tree, the last node of the traversal is considered the root of a new sub-tree within the graph. If the traversal arrives at a node that has already been traversed, the traversal is merged into the existing sub-tree of the previous traversal. Finally, if the traversal arrives at an untraversed end-point, that traversal represents a new valid sub-tree of the graph with the root node at the untraversed end-point. The algorithm terminates when there are no untraversed end-points remaining in the graph.

The primary sub-trees of the left, middle and right hepatic, and left and right portal veins are identified by exploring all the candidate sub-trees according to their anatomical positions and orientations. For this purpose, statistical shape measures are calculated for each sub tree to identify their primary axes, its bounding box, and centroid. The primary axis of the three hepatic veins run along from the superior to inferior portions of the liver and move outwards from the center of the abdomen. The portal veins are positioned below the hepatic veins and run to the left and right.

Finally, an atlas of the liver segmental anatomy according to the Couinaud nomenclature [3] is generated by fitting a series of planes to the trajectories of the hepatic and portal veins. Anterior and posterior segments of the liver are separated by the left, middle and right hepatic veins; inferior and supperior segments are separated by the portal veins. Thus, piecewise surfaces of planes are generated for each of the three hepatic and two portal veins. In order to fit the planes, the primary path of each hepatic vein sub-tree is tracked from the root of the sub-tree. The same path validity constraints used in the sub-tree construction are used in reverse order to find a primary path with an additional constraint to minimize the angular change between the parent and the child segments moving away from the root. Thus, each of the three hepatic vein paths consists of the root point, all branching points traversed by the path, and the end point. Pairs of branching points starting from the superior root of each hepatic vein form the basis of planes to be fitted to the vein segments. The series of planes forms a piecewise surface for each hepatic vein. Planes are similarly fitted to the left and right portal veins. Below the portal vein (in the inferior lobe), only one additional plane is fitted to each hepatic vein, as vascular information becomes sparse.

The Couinaud segments of the liver are delineated by the surfaces fitted to the hepatic veins [3]. To validate the segmental anatomy, twenty points were randomly places in each test liver. The points were restricted to be at least two centimeters from the edge of the liver, where vascular information is sparse. An experienced radiologist then manually identified the segment that each point was in and the observations were compared to the automatic results. The accuracy of our method was calculated as the number of correctly labeled points over the total number of points.

3   Results

Fig. 2 shows the segmentation and labeling of intra-hepatic veins and tumors in axial slices of 3D CT data. The hepatic vasculature was classified into the major vessel trees in the liver: the portal and right, middle and left hepatic veins. The accuracy of the automated Couinaud segmental anatomy was 87.8±7.9%.

For the detection of tumors larger than 1cm in diameter, the true positives fraction was 100.0% at 3.1 false positives/case. For segmenting tumors the Dice overlap was 74.1% with a volume error of 12.4% respectively. False positives occurred generally near the hepatic ligaments, where there is lack of enhancement and high curvatures.

The 3D visualization of a diseased liver is presented in Fig. 3. The results of our hepatic vessel detecor is ilustrated near the response of the vesselness filter. Similarly, Fig. 3 compares the detection of blobs with the segmentation of tumors using 4D graph cuts. Anatomical liver segments are shown in the 3D renderings in Fig. 4.

4   Discussion

A novel graph-based method for the segmentation of tumors and major intra-hepatic blood vessels was presented to allow visualization and risk analysis for interventional planning. The method avoided the shortcomings of the traditional graph cuts or intensity-based segmentation methods by including 4D enhancement modeling and shape likelihoods. The vessels were correctly classified into right, middle and left hepatic, and right and left portal veins using a hybrid process that incorporates anatomical information and post-order walks of a graph representation of the vessels. All the hepatic tumors were detected and segmented using their differential enhancement and shape with accuracy comparable to the reports from the MICCAI competition [17]. Finally, a vessel tracker allowed fitting planes to the major hepatic vasculature and identified the liver segments according to the Couinaud atlas.

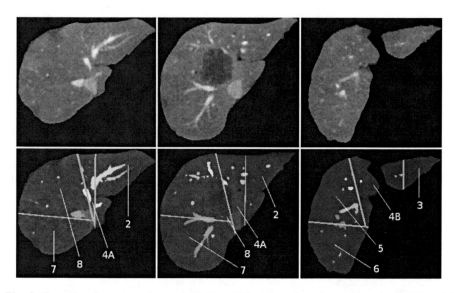

Fig. 2. Example of segmentation and labeling of intra-hepatic veins and tumors on 2D axial slices of 3D CT data; the top row shows the liver in CEP with enhanced vessels and opaque tumors; the bottom row presents the corresponding segmented images with the tumors in dark blue, portal vein in light blue and the right, middle and left hepatic veins in red, yellow and green, respectively. Liver segments are also shown separated by pink planes with numbers referring to the Couinaud classification [3]. As shown, the tumor is encapsulated in segment 8.

As the liver is a large organ, contrast enhancement is heterogeneous and regions that are highly enhanced tend to be labeled incorrectly as vessels by the basic graph cuts [16]. The basic graph cuts segmentation is equally sensitive to local minima in the image intensity in the liver and erroneously identifies tumors. Similar errors arise in methods using just histogram analysis to detect vessels and tumors as intensity outliers. These techniques struggle in particular when analyzing difficult cases from diseased patients. For instance, the optimal thresholding in [4] is affected by image appearance and quality, but is sufficient to initialize our algorithm.

The Hessian-based analysis is less sensitive to uneven contrast enhancement if the shape of a structure is preserved, but is affected by noise and artifacts, which results in discontinuous segmentations of vessels. This measure used alone misses branching regions of the vessels where the local shape is not tubular. Similarly, spurious detections are marked as tumors around less enhanced areas near the liver surface.

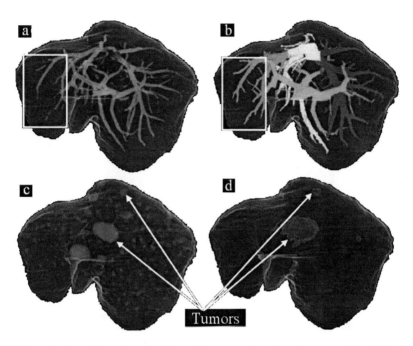

Fig. 3. 3D rendering of intra-hepatic veins and tumors using the color map in Fig. 2 a) using the vesselness filter [14]; b) vessels segmented by our technique with labels; c) using the blobness filter; d)   tumors segmented by our technique; true tumor detections are highlighted

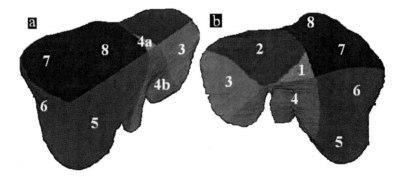

Fig. 4. 3D visualization of a diseased liver according to the antomical atlas in [3]. (a) is the anterior and (b) the posterior view. Liver segments are identified/numbered by our method.

The proposed technique performs vasculature labeling, an essential step for the identification of liver segments. According to [3], the liver has eight functionally independent segment with distinct vasculature and biliary drainage. The middle hepatic vein divides the liver into left end right lobes; each of these lobes is further divided by the left and right hepatic veins respectively. The portal vein separates the upper and lower segments of the liver. The accurate identification of these segments is essential in assessing the risks and benefits of hepatic interventions.

Techniques (many commercial) to identify the liver segments are interactive [4,19,20,21], not surprising given the difficulty of the task. Our automated method for liver analysis promises to assist in a robust and reproducible fashion the development of image-based minimally invasive tools for interventional and surgical planning.

Acknowledgments. This work was supported by the Intramural Research Program of the National Institutes of Health, Clinical Center.

References

1. Foley, W.: Liver: Surgical Planning. European Rad Supplements 15(4), d89–d95 (2005)
2. Huang, S., et al.: The Use of a Projection Method to Simplify Portal and Hepatic Vein Segmentation in Liver Anatomy. Comp. Meth. Programs Biomed. 92(3), 274–278 (2008)
3. Couinaud, C.: Liver Anatomy: Portal (and Suprahepatic) or Biliary Segmentation. Digestive Surgery 16(6), 459–467 (2000)
4. Selle, D., et al.: Analysis of Vasculature for Liver Surgical Planning. IEEE Trans. Med. Imaging 21(11), 1344–1357 (2002)
5. Beichel, R., et al.: Liver Segment Approximation in CT Data for Surgical Resection Planning. In: SPIE Med. Imaging (2004)
6. Soler, L., et al.: Fully Automatic Anatomical, Pathological, and Functional Segmentation from CT Scans for Hepatic Surgery. Computer Aided Surgery 6(3), 131–142 (2001)
7. Boykov, Y., Kolmogorov, V.: An Experimental Comparison of Min-Cut/Max-Flow Algorithms for Energy Minimization in Vision. IEEE Trans. PAMI 26(9), 1124–1137 (2004)
8. Kolmogorov, V., Boykov, Y.: What Metrics Can Be Approximated by Geo-Cuts, or Global Optimization of Length/Area and Flux. In: IEEE Int. Conf. Comp. Vis., pp. 564–571 (2005)
9. Esneault, S., Lafon, C., Dillenseger, J.L.: Liver Vessels Segmentation Using a Hybrid Geometrical Moments/Graph Cuts Method. IEEE Trans. Biomed. Eng. 57(2), 276–283 (2009)
10. Kaftan, J.N., Tek, H., Aach, T.: A Two-Stage Approach for Fully Automatic Segmentation of Venous Vascular Structures in Liver CT Images. In: SPIE Med. Imaging (2009)
11. Linguraru, M.G., Pura, J.A., Chowdhury, A.S., Summers, R.M.: Multi-Organ Segmentation from Multi-Phase Abdominal CT via 4D Graphs Using Enhancement, Shape and Location Optimization. In: Jiang, T., Navab, N., Pluim, J.P.W., Viergever, M.A. (eds.) MICCAI 2010, Part III. LNCS, vol. 6363, pp. 89–96. Springer, Heidelberg (2010)
12. Thirion, J.: Image Matching as a Diffusion Process; An Analogy with Maxwell's Demons. Med. Image Anal. 2(3), 243–260 (1998)
13. Perona, P., Malik, J.: Scale-Space and Edge Detection Using Anisotropic Diffusion. IEEE Trans. PAMI 12(7), 629–639 (1990)

14. Sato, Y., et al.: 3D Multi-Scale Line Filter for Segmentation and Visualization of Curvilinear Structures in Medical Images. In: Troccaz, J., Mösges, R., Grimson, W.E.L. (eds.) CVRMed-MRCAS 1997, CVRMed 1997, and MRCAS 1997. LNCS, vol. 1205, pp. 213–222. Springer, Heidelberg (1997)

15. Lee, T., Kashyap, R., Chu, C.: Building Skeleton Models via 3-D Medial Surface/Axis Thinning Algorithms. Graphical Models and Image Processing 56(6), 462–478 (1994)

16. Pamulapati, V., Wood, B.J., Linguraru, M.G.: Intra-Hepatic Vessel Segmentation and Classification in Multi-Phase CT Using Optimized Graph Cuts. In: ISBI, pp. 1982–1985 (2011)

17. Deng, X., Du, G.: Editorial: 3D Segmentation in the Clinic: A Grand Challenge II - Liver Tumor Segmentation. In: MICCAI Workshop (2008)

18. http://www.mevismedical.com/

19. http://www.liversuite.com/

20. http://www.ircad.fr/

Liver and Tumor Segmentation and Analysis from CT of Diseased Patients via a Generic Affine Invariant Shape Parameterization and Graph Cuts

Marius George Linguraru, William J. Richbourg, Jeremy M. Watt,
Vivek Pamulapati, and Ronald M. Summers

Imaging Biomarkers and Computer Aided Laboratory, Radiology and Imaging Sciences,
Clinical Center, National Institutes of Health, Bethesda, MD
lingurarum@mail.nih.gov

Abstract. The paper presents the automated segmentation of livers from abdominal CT images of diseased populations from images with inconsistent enhancement. A novel three-dimensional (3D) affine invariant shape parameterization is employed to compare local shape across organs. By generating a regular sampling of the organ's surface, this parameterization can be effectively used to compare features of a set of closed 3D surfaces point-to-point while avoiding common problems with the parameterization of concave surfaces. From an initial segmentation, the areas of atypical local shape are determined using training sets. A geodesic active contour corrects locally the segmentations of organs in abnormal images and optimized graph cuts segment the vasculature and hepatic tumors using shape and enhancement constraints. Liver segmentation errors are reduced significantly, all tumors are detected and the tumor burden is estimated with 0.9% error. Results from test data demonstrate the method's robustness to analyze livers from difficult clinical cases to allow temporal monitoring of patients with hepatic cancer.

Keywords: Contrast-enhanced CT, segmentation, liver, tumor, shape, 3D parameterization, monitoring.

1   Introduction

Computed tomography (CT) is commonly adopted for imaging abdominal organs for diagnosis and pre-operative planning. The volumes, shapes and enhancement of abdominal organs, such as the liver, are common indicators of disorders [5]. In addition, the tumor burden in the liver is used to monitor the evolution of disease in patients with hepatic cancer, while the spatial relationship between vasculature and cancerous tissues is an indicator of risk in hepatic surgery [7].

The automated segmentation of livers from medical scans can provide quantitative data, but computer-aided diagnosis (CAD) techniques generally struggle in the presence of abnormal anatomical and/or physiological features. Imaging artifacts are an additional challenge. It is beneficial to compare the shapes of analyzed patient organs to those of a training set to guide the segmentation. [22]

H. Yoshida et al. (Eds.): Abdominal Imaging 2011, LNCS 7029, pp. 198–206, 2012.

To identify subtle shape differences between two objects, a robust parameterization of their surfaces is required in combination with an invariant shape descriptor and a point-to-point correspondence. Previous methods for 3D surface analysis have been proposed in medical applications [6]. In particular, the method in [2] involves generating a bijective mapping from the 3D surface to the unit sphere, while in [9] spherical harmonics-based parameterizations divide a given surface into a set of basis functions. For the liver, corresponding points were initialized by the user in [11].

A variety of methods have been proposed to segment the liver or to segment liver tumors in recent years. In 2007-8, liver and liver tumor segmentation competitions from CT data were held in conjunction with MICCAI [4,8]. Statistical shape models were the best fully automated liver segmentation methods and performed competitively with the semi-automatic techniques. Tumors were best automatically segmented via machine learning and classification techniques. A shape-constrained graph-cut approach segmented the liver in [13]. CAD and surgical planning would benefit from fully automated 3D segmentation of both the liver and liver tumors, as well as the organ's vasculature [20]. Methods for the concurrent segmentations of liver structures are mainly interactive [17]. Commercial applications are also available, but less flexible in the clinical environment.

We present a novel automated technique to segment diseased livers from everyday CT data with inconsistent contrast-enhancement and spurious imaging artifacts. A robust parameterization of 3D surfaces, like those of abdominal organs, is proposed for the comparison of objects by point-to-point correspondence. 3D objects are represented by parallel planes that intersect the surface of objects in closed planar curves. This spatial representation avoids common problems with the surface parameterization of concave objects. To compare local shape features of two organs we employ a shape descriptor invariant under rotation, scale, and noise. Once shape ambiguities are detected on an initial segmentation of the liver, a geodesic active contour improves the segmentation significantly even in severe cases. From the segmented liver, optimized graph cuts are employed to segment hepatic blood vessels and tumors using shape and enhancement constraints. The automated liver analysis technique allows monitoring and diagnosing patients with abnormal livers under poor image quality and inconsistent enhancement, and provides assessments for treatment and disease evolution.

2   Methods and Materials

Fifty-eight abdominal CT scans were collected from 23 patients with prostate cancer at single/multiple time-points on five different scanners. Image resolution was 0.63 to 0.92 mm in the axial view with 5 mm slice thickness. Images were acquired with/out constrast; contrast data were obtained at varying enhacement times from early-arterial to late portal venous. Additional to the inconsistent enhancement, cases with imaging and movement artifacts were present in the database. Livers from eight cases without artifacts were manually segmented and used as the shape training set. The volumes of the other 50 livers (test cases) were clinically estimated by two technologists supervised by an experienced radiologist, but no manually segmented volumes were available. The images were cropped at the first slice containing the liver, identified through histogram analysis and image parsing in the cranio-caudal direction.

Livers were automatically segmented from the 50 CT cases using a technique previously designed for the analysis of hepatic artifact-free CT data acquired at portal-venous enhancement from patients without tumors [12]. Twenty-two cases presented tumors of highly variable size. Nighteen cases had severe liver segmentation errors (>10% volume error) and the other 31 livers needed only minor to moderate corrections. Tumors were manually segmented in 14 cases (79 tumors) with liver cancer by a research fellow supervised by an experienced radiologist. Tumor size varied from 10.0 to 206.4 mm in the largest diameter.

Additionally, 20 cases, mainly pathological but less severe, with manual liver segmentations from the MICCAI challenge held in 2007 [8] were used for testing (www.sliver07.org). The MICCAI cases had contrast enhancement and no artifacts.

2.1   Shape Analysis and Surface Parameterization

To detect shape ambiguities, a 3D-analogue of a curvature-feature [14] was used as shape feature S for comparing closed planar curves [21]. Specificaly, at a given point p on a planar curve, S is the area of intersection of the interior of the curve and a 'seed' (a sphere centered at p). S of a curve C can be used for both local (at every corresponding point on two matched curves) and global comparison of two curves, given an adequate simultaneous parameterization of the two curves.

$$S(p) = \frac{\int_C V_r(p, x)dx}{\int_{\mathfrak{R}^3} V_r(p, x)dx};$$

V_r is the volume of the intersection of C and the seed sphere of radius r proportional to the size of C. A compensation function accounted for the pixilation of digital objects. The shape descriptor is rotation and scale invariant by design and robust to noise [14].

To allow point-to-point comparisons across multiple surfaces, our method uses the structure of a general class of objects we call 'planar-convex'. We assume that livers fall under this category. We define a planar-convex object O in $\mathfrak{R}^n$ to be a closed surface for which a set of parallel hyper-planes P exists, such that every intersection of a plane in P with O results in a singular closed planar curve. We call each set of parallel hyper-planes which intersects with O in this way 'convexity planes'[21].

To match two objects, we align their principal components and then orient about the object's largest principal component a set of symmetric points comprising the vertices of a pentakis dodecahedron. This allows us to find multiple sets of parallel planes that intersect the object with normals ranging uniformly over a hemisphere; we sampled over a 32-vertice dodecahedron. Then we determine which primary plane (x, y or z plane) maps injectively to the parallel planes. Each intersection of the planes with the liver is then analyzed and the average number of connected components is found. The minimum sum of average components across the corresponding axes/planes of the two compared objects is then computed. This defines the set of matched convexity planes P (as defined above) between the two compared objects.

The surface of each convexity plane is uniformly sampled by a user-defined number of partitions, with points at these partitions being projected onto the object surface [21]. An example of liver parameterization is shown in Fig. 1. These projections or 'parameterization points' have point-to-point correspondence between the compared objects/livers. At each parameterization point we then compute the shape feature S and its value is mapped onto both objects' surfaces to allow the visualization of results. S is computed from matched training surfaces, averaged at every point, and normalized between 0 and 1.

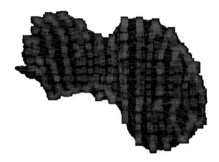

Fig. 1. Parameterization points are highlighted as small cubes on the surface of a liver with irregular shape. These points allow point-to-point correspondence between two shapes.

2.2   Segmentation of Liver, Blood Vessels and Tumors

From the initial liver segmentation, the shape analysis on matched surface points with training data identifies areas on the surface of the liver that have ambiguous shape. To allow some level of intra-patient variability, S is thresholded at 0.5 and component analysis used to assign inidvidual labels to each ambiguous area. As livers were primarily undersegmented by the initial method [12], seeds are placed at the centroid of these labels and a fast marching level set [19] employed to "grow" the segmentation based on the sigmoid of the gradient of the CT image. A geodesic active contour [3] refines the segmentation. The process is iterated until $S < 0.5$ or the volume change between iterations becomes insignificant.

With the liver segmented, a graph-cut approach [1] is applied to find tumorous hepatic masses. In the basic form, graph cuts suffer from the shrinking bias problem, particularly for segmenting elongated and small structures, such as the blood vessels and certain types of tumors [10]. Graph-cuts were shown to improve the segmentation of abdominal organs in [13] using training shapes, but tumors and vessels are highly variable between cases. However, vessels are curvilinear and tumors generally round.

The graph cuts segmentation in our approach incorporates constraints for vasculature high enhancement, tumor opacity, and a Hessian-based shape condition to emphasize thin elongated vessels and rounder tumors at multiple scales σ. The eigenvalues of the Hessian ($\lambda_1 > \lambda_2 > \lambda_3$) at point p define unique shape constraints to optimize the segmentation of vessels and reduce tumor false positives [16,18]. The following energy terms are incorporated in the graph-cut definition

$$E_{vesselness} = -\ln \max_{\sigma}(\sigma^2 v(p,\sigma)); \text{ with } v = \begin{cases} |\lambda_2| + \lambda_1 & ,if \lambda_1 < 0 \\ |\lambda_2| - \lambda_1/4, if \lambda_2 & <0< \lambda_1 < 4|\lambda_2| \end{cases};$$

$$E_{blobness} = -\ln \max_{\sigma}(w); \text{ with } \lambda_3 > 0; \text{ and } w = e^{-\left(\lambda_1/\lambda_3 - 1\right)}.$$

Enhanced hepatic vessels were removed prior to tumor segmentation to reduce the false positive detections of tumors. The total volume of tumors was computed for each patient and normalized by the total liver volume to compute tumor burden and monitor cases with metastatic hepatic cancer.

3   Results

The preliminary segmentation technique was less accurate than previously reported [12] due to the presence of tumors and artifacts in our data, and an inconsistent acquisition of contrast-enhanced images. Quantitative results from applying our method to the automated segmentation of the liver are shown in Table 1 before and after the segmentation correction. The use of liver-to-liver shape parameterization coupled with geodesic active contour reduced the percentage of volume error significantly for both cases of severe segmentation failure and cases in need of only minor adjustments. Fig. 2 presents an example of segmentation from a case with artifacts and without contrast-enhancement, a moderately inaccurate segmentation, and a severe segmentation failure with their corresponding shape images and final corrected outputs. Our technique improved significantly the segmentation of cases with large tumors, while avoiding the creation of errors in well-segmented livers. There was no statistical difference in the segmentation of the MICCAI livers after the initial and   final segmentation.

Table 1. Volume Error (VER) for liver segmentation from data of 5mm slice thickness. Initial automatic segmentation results are compared to results following shape analysis and corrected (final) segmentation; p-values were calculated via the Wilcoxon rank sum test. Variability in initial VER ranged from <2% to >50%, therefore cases were separated into severe errors (VER>10%) and small/moderate errors (VER<10%). Cases with small errors, large errors and hepatic tumors are shown separately along with results on the MICCAI dataset.

Group/VER (%)	Initial Segmentation	Final Segmentation	p-value
Small Error (n=31)	5.3±2.4	2.9±2.2	<0.001
Severe Error (n=19)	28.9±14.3	6.6±7.3	<0.001
Tumors (n=22)	17.0±15.8	5.2±6.9	<0.001
MICCAI (n=20)	2.9±2.2	2.8±2.3	0.6

The results of the detection and segmentation of hepatic tumors are presented in Table 2. All tumors were correctly identified. False positives occurred generally near the porta hepatis and coronary ligaments, where there is lack of enhancement and high curvatures, and liver surface. Fig. 3 illustrates the manual and automatic segmentation of hepatic tumors for two patients, each at two time points. Table 2 also presents quantitative results of the MICCAI liver data; the average score was 69 [8].

The average liver tumor burden for the 14 cases with manual segmentations was 6.6±9.0% and 7.1±8.1% according to the manual and automated segmentations respectively. There was no significant difference between the measurements (p>0.6 from the Wilcoxon rank sum test). In Fig. 4, the change over time in liver and tumor volume, and tumor burden is presented for several patients.

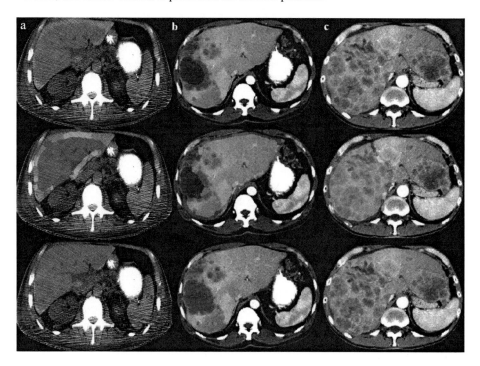

Fig. 2. Examples of liver segmentation (overlayed in green on axial views of 3D CT data) of a case without contrast enhancement and with motion artifacts (a), a moderately inaccurate segmentation (b), and a severe segmentation failure (c). Initial segmentation are in the top row and corresponding shape images in the middle row. Shape ambiguities are shown in a cold (low) to hot (high) colormap. The corrected liver segmentations are shown in the bottom row.

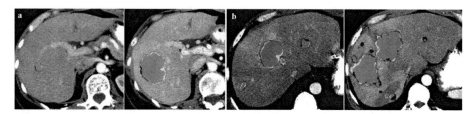

Fig. 3. Examples of hepatic tumor segmentation: manual (blue), automated (yellow) and their overlaps in green overlayed on axial views of 3D CT of two patients (a) and (b), each at two time points. False positives from automated segmentation are displayed in red.

Table 2. True Positives Fraction (TPF) and false positives (FP)/case are reported for the detection of hepatic tumors. Automated and manual segmentations of tumors were compared and we present Dice Overlaps, Volume Errors (VER) and Average Surface Distances (ASD). The Tumor Burden Error (TBE) is the difference between manually and automatically measured tumor burden. Overlaps, VER and ASD are also reported for the MICCAI livers.

Group	TPF (%)	FP/case	Overlap (%)	VER (%)	ASD (mm)	TBE (%)
79 tumors (n=14)	100.0	3.1	74.1±16.9	12.4±12.0	1.6±1.5	0.9±1.0
MICCAI livers (n=20)	--	--	95.7±0.9	2.8±2.3	1.5±0.5	--

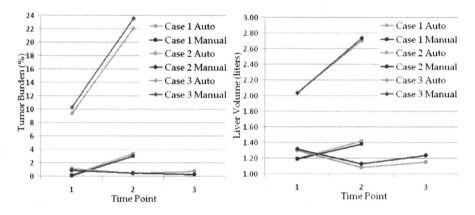

Fig. 4. Change over in tumor burden and liver volume for three cases with small (red), moderate (green) and large (blue) tumors. Manual and automated estimation are presented for comparison. Image data for Cases 1 and 3 are shown in Fig. 3(a) and 3(b) respectively.

4   Discussion

The focus of this method is on the segmentation and analysis of diseased livers from inconsistent data, as existing techniques often fail when the liver is abnormal and imaging conditions are not ideal. CT data were acquired at a slice thickness of 5 mm from a cohort of patients with metastatic liver cancer with highly variable contrast enhancement. Imaging and movement artifacts were also present in the database. It can be noted both visually and from Table 1 that livers in our dataset originate from diseased patients with very complex diseases and images difficult to process.

A novel method for comparing local shape across organs was employed to detect areas of shape ambiguity from a set of training shapes. Livers were represented as planary-convex, a characteristic used to generate an effective parameterization of the surface of organs. This parameterization technique effectively avoids problems with concave object and allows point-to-point comparison of local shapes from an affine invariant shape feature. From areas of ambiguity, liver segmentations were iteratively corrected using geodesic active contours. While active contours are ineffective to segment entire abdominal organs, especially unusual and difficult cases, they are used in our method only locally for corrections in areas of high contrast and gradients.

Comparative results before and after shape correction show significant improvements on the accuracy of liver segmentation in even the most severe cancerous cases. Hepatic tumor segmentation is also demonstrated via optimized graph cuts and allowed to compute the liver tumor burden, estimated with an error of 1%. The method shows very promising results for monitoring the evolution of patients with liver cancer under typical clinical conditions, which include poor imaging quality and unusual livers. In the future, tumor feature extraction and selection will be combined with a classifier to reduce the tumor false positives.

Acknowledgments. This work was supported by the Intramural Research Program of the National Institutes of Health, Clinical Center.

References

1. Boykov, Y., Kolmogorov, V.: An Experimental Comparison of Min-Cut/Max-Flow Algorithms for Energy Minimization in Vision. IEEE Trans. Pattern Anal. Mach. Intell. 26(9), 1124–1137 (2004)
2. Brechbuhler, C., Gerig, G., Kubler, O.: Parameterization of Closed Surfaces for 3D Shape Descriptor. Computer Vision and Image Understanding 61(2), 154–170 (1995)
3. Caselles, V., Kimmel, R., Sapiro, G.: Geodesic Active Contours. International Journal on Computer Vision 22(1), 61–97 (1997)
4. Deng, X., Du, G.: Editorial: 3D Segmentation in the Clinic: A Grand Challenge II - Liver Tumor Segmentation. In: MICCAI Workshop (2008)
5. Ellert, J., Kreel, L.: The Role of Computed Tomography in the Initial Staging and Subsequent Management of the Lymphomas. J. Comput. Assist. Tomogr. 4(3), 368–391 (1980)
6. Floater, M.S., Hormann, K.: Surface Parameterization: a Tutorial and Survey. In: Advances in Multiresolution for Geometric Modeling, pp. 157–186. Springer, Heidelberg (2005)
7. Gonsalves, C.F., et al.: Radioembolization as Salvage Therapy for Hepatic Metastasis of Uveal Melanoma: A Single-Institution Experience. Am. J. Roentgenol. 196(2), 468–473 (2011)
8. Heimann, T., et al.: Comparison and Evaluation of Methods for Liver Segmentation from CT Datasets. IEEE Trans. Med. Imaging 28(8), 1251–1265 (2009)
9. Huang, H., Shen, L., Zhang, R., Makedon, F.S., Hettleman, B., Pearlman, J.D.: Surface Alignment of 3D Spherical Harmonic Models: Application to Cardiac MRI Analysis. In: Duncan, J.S., Gerig, G. (eds.) MICCAI 2005. LNCS, vol. 3749, pp. 67–74. Springer, Heidelberg (2005)
10. Kolmogorov, V., Boykov, Y.: What Metrics Can Be Approximated by Geo-Cuts, or Global Optimization of Length/Area and Flux. In: IEEE Int. Conf. Computer Vision, pp. 564–571 (2005)
11. Lamecker, H., Lange, T., Seebass, M.: A Statistical Shape Model for the Liver. In: Dohi, T., Kikinis, R. (eds.) MICCAI 2002. LNCS, vol. 2489, pp. 421–427. Springer, Heidelberg (2002)

12. Linguraru, M.G., et al.: Atlas-Based Automated Segmentation of Spleen and Liver Using Adaptive Enhancement Estimation. Med. Phys. 37(2), 771–783 (2010)
13. Linguraru, M.G., Pura, J.A., Chowdhury, A.S., Summers, R.M.: Multi-Organ Segmentation from Multi-phase Abdominal CT via 4D Graphs Using Enhancement, Shape and Location Optimization. In: Jiang, T., Navab, N., Pluim, J.P.W., Viergever, M.A. (eds.) MICCAI 2010 Part III. LNCS, vol. 6363, pp. 89–96. Springer, Heidelberg (2010)
14. Manay, S., et al.: Integral Invariants for Shape Matching. IEEE Trans. Pattern Anal. Mach. Intell. 28(10), 1602–1620 (2006)
15. Muller, M.A., Marincek, B., Frauenfelder, I.: State of the Art 3D Imaging of Abdominal Organs. JBR–BTR 90, 467–474 (2007)
16. Pamulapati, V., Wood, B.J., Linguraru, M.G.: Intra-Hepatic Vessel Segmentation and Classification in Multi-Phase CT Using Optimized Graph Cuts. In: ISBI, pp. 1982–1985 (2011)
17. Peterhans, A., et al.: A Navigation System for Open Liver Surgery: Design, Workflow and First Clinical Applications. Int. J. Med. Robotics Comput. Assist. Surg. (2010)
18. Sato, Y., et al.: 3D Multi-Scale Line Filter for Segmentation and Visualization of Curvilinear Structures in Medical Images. In: Troccaz, J., Mösges, R., Grimson, W.E.L. (eds.) CVRMed-MRCAS 1997, CVRMed 1997, and MRCAS 1997. LNCS, vol. 1205, pp. 213–222. Springer, Heidelberg (1997)
19. Sethian, J.A.: Level Set Methods and Fast Marching Methods. Cambridge Univ. Press (1999)
20. Shevchenko, N., et al.: MiMed Liver: A Planning System for Liver Surgery. In: IEEE EMBS, pp. 1882–1885 (2010)
21. Watt, J., Linguraru, M.G., Summers, R.M.: Affine Invariant Shape Parameterization to Assess Local 3D Shape in Abdominal Organs. In: SPIE Medical Imaging (2011)
22. Wimmer, A., Soza, G., Hornegger, J.: A Generic Probabilistic Active Shape Model for Organ Segmentation. In: Yang, G.-Z., Hawkes, D., Rueckert, D., Noble, A., Taylor, C. (eds.) MICCAI 2009, Part II. LNCS, vol. 5762, pp. 26–33. Springer, Heidelberg (2009)

A Bayesian Framework
for Estimating Respiratory Liver Motion
from Sparse Measurements

Frank Preiswerk, Patrik Arnold, Beat Fasel, and Philippe C. Cattin

Medical Image Analysis Center, University of Basel, Switzerland
{frank.preiswerk,philippe.cattin}@unibas.ch

Abstract. In this paper, we present an approach for modelling and predicting organ motion from partial information. We used 4D-MRI sequences of 12 subjects to build a statistical population model for respiratory motion of the liver. Using a Bayesian reconstruction approach, a pre-operative CT scan and a few known surrogate markers, we are able to accurately predict the position of the entire liver at all times. The surrogates may, for example, come from ultrasound, portal images captured during radiotherapy or from implanted electromagnetic beacons. In leave-one-out experiments, we achieve an average prediction error of 1.2 mm over sequences of 20 min with only three surrogates. Our model is accurate enough for clinically relevant treatment intervals and has the potential to be used for adapting the gating window in tumour therapy or even for tracking a tumour continuously during irradiation.

Keywords: respiratory motion, statistical model, prediction, tumour therapy, liver.

1 Introduction

Respiratory organ motion is a complicating factor in the treatment of liver tumours. Besides the superior/inferior (SI) motion caused by the diaphragm, there are secondary modes due to cardiac cycle motion, digestive activity, gravity and muscle relaxation, some of them causing a drift of the organ [10]. Non-rigid deformation during breathing introduces a significant amount of uncertainty in location during irradiation of a tumour. Studies have shown that 4-dimensional treatment planning is important for improved precision in radiotherapy [7], though not much work has been done in the field of precise liver motion estimation for non-invasive treatment of tumours. Rohlfing *et al.* [5] acquired 3D-MRI liver data of exhalation, inhalation and eight time steps in-between. Deformation fields among them were obtained using non-rigid registration. These transformations were then applied to the vertex coordinates of geometrical models derived from the exhalation reference. More recently, He et al. [4] modeled 4D motion of lungs using Kernel PCA. They trained a support vector machine to model the relation between motion of fiducial markers on the lower abdomen/chest and the coefficients of the K-PCA. However, with the latter method, a correlation

H. Yoshida et al. (Eds.): Abdominal Imaging 2011, LNCS 7029, pp. 207–214, 2012.

between organ motion and the motion of an external surrogate may become unreliable over time in presence of organ drift [10]. Their approach is computationally involved and might therefore be inadequate for real-time reconstruction and tracking. Their reported average accuracy was 1.63 mm. Ehrhardt et al. [3] used diffeomorphic nonlinear intensity-based registration and the Log-Euclidean framework to build a motion model from thoracic 4D-CT lung data sets of 17 patients. The chosen approach is mathematically well formulated but it requires quite a few assumptions about breathing-depth and voxel intensities. Furthermore, the respiratory cycle is discretised to only four states and 4D-CT images of the patient are required for estimating a scaling factor for breathing depth. A prediction accuracy of 3.3 mm on average was achieved.

Most importantly, both previous and most other methods established intersubject correspondence implicitly by co-registering all samples to a reference image, thereby relying on a correlation between shape and respiratory motion. Our approach, on the other hand, relies on mechanically corresponding points (*i.e.* points that move similarly), thus precisely focuses our analyis on the type of motion we wish to model. We capture this motion information by learning a PCA model of the deviation from exhalation position during quiet breathing. Thanks to the large amount of data used to learn our model and the applied prediction scheme, we achieve an average prediction error of only 1.2 mm.

This paper is organised as follows. In the next two sections we introduce the correspondence scheme and the statistical population model for respiratory organ motion, which is a generalisation of the statistical population-based model of intrafraction drift by von Siebenthal *et al.* [9]. We then describe the reconstruction approach used to predict the motion of a novel liver from only three known surrogates. Finally, our approach is evaluated using a series of leave-one-out experiments on 4D-MRI data.

2   Materials and Methods

2.1   Data Acquisition and Establishment of Correspondence

For this study, we used 4D-MRI sequences [8] of the liver from 12 healthy subjects (6 female, 6 male, average age 30, ranged 17-75). The in-plane resolution is 1.8 mm × 1.8 mm and the slice thickness is 3-4 mm. The data was acquired over roughly one hour on 22 to 30 sagittal slices and a temporal resolution of 2.6-2.8 Hz. We extracted the deformation fields for each subject using the B-spline based non-rigid registration method proposed by Rueckert [6]. This process involved the manual segmentation of the liver in one master exhalation stack for each subject and results in dense deformation fields between this exhalation master and all respiratory states. In order to build a statistical model from this data, inter subject correspondence had to be established. We used an approach similar to [11] that relies on mechanically corresponding points. Four landmark points were manually selected on each sagittal slice of the exhalation master, namely the delineations between the superior, anterior, posterior and inferior surfaces, see Fig. 1(a). The left liver lobe was kept out of the analysis because it is heavily

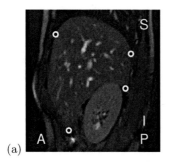 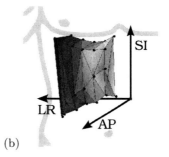

(a) (b)

Fig. 1. (a) The location of a point relative to the liver surface is relevant for mechanical considerations. The white dots mark the delineations between the superior, anterior, posterior and inferior surfaces. (b) A coordinate system was chosen such that the LR-direction is perpendicular to the sagittal plane of the body and the AP-direction is aligned perpendicular to planes fitted to the anterior and posterior pairs of landmarks.

influenced by the motion of the heart, a factor that is not in the scope of this study. These points constituted a prototype shape for each subject, see Fig. 1(b). The prototypes were aligned inside the manually segmented master shape and the edges of the triangulation were projected onto the high resolution surface. That way, the master segmentations were remeshed and inter-subject correspondence of the surface was established. The total number of surface points after this step was 345 per liver. In order to establish correspondence for points within the liver, an isotropic grid with 10 mm resolution was placed in the average liver and then transformed to each of the remeshed surfaces using the Delaunay tetrahedrisation approach in [1], see Fig. 2. This finally gave a set of 12 topologically equivalent 3D liver volumes as well as dense spatio-temporal motion fields for each grid point.

2.2   Statistical Model

A liver instance is represented by a $3n$-dimensional vector $\mathbf{v} = (x_1, y_1, z_1, \dots , x_n, y_n, z_n)$, where n corresponds to the number of vertices. To build a statistical model, 9 respiratory cycles were taken from each of the 12 subjects: 3 cycles from the beginning, middle and end of the acquisition session, respectively. The total number of volumes (12 subjects, 9 cycles, 8-20 steps per cycle) is $m=1312$. By distributing the selection of cycles all along the acquisition session, deformations of the liver due to organ drift over time are better represented. As our aim was to model organ motion and not organ shape, we removed the shape by taking the vector-field difference between each respiratory state and the subject's exhalation master state: $\mathbf{x} = \mathbf{v} - \check{\mathbf{v}}$. Principal Component Analysis (PCA) was then performed on the matrix of shape-neutralised offsets $\mathbf{X} = (\mathbf{x}_1, \dots , \mathbf{x}_m)$. This yields the orthonormal matrix of principal components $\mathbf{U} = (\mathbf{u}_1, \dots , \mathbf{u}_{m-1})$ and their corresponding eigenvalues $\lambda_1, \dots , \lambda_{m-1}$ that give the standard deviation σ_i of the principal components in descending order ($\sqrt{\lambda_i} = \sigma_i$).

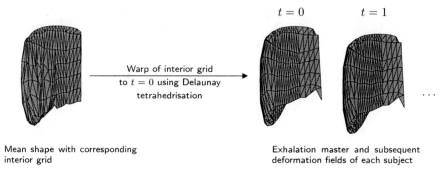

$t = 0$ $t = 1$

Warp of interior grid
to $t = 0$ using Delaunay
tetrahedrisation

Mean shape with corresponding
interior grid

Exhalation master and subsequent
deformation fields of each subject

Fig. 2. An isotropic grid is positioned inside the mean shape and warped to the exhalation master shape $\check{\mathbf{v}}$ at $t = 0$ of each subject. From $t = 0$ to all forthcoming time steps, the deformation field is used to further warp the grid to any of the subsequent respiratory steps. This results in dense intra- and inter-subject correspondence.

We can transform (and thus decorrelate) the data by subtracting the mean offset vector $\mu = \frac{1}{m} \sum \mathbf{x}_i$, followed by a projection into model space:

$$\mathbf{c} = \mathrm{diag}(\sigma_i^{-1})\mathbf{U}^T(\mathbf{x} - \mu) , \tag{1}$$

The deviation of a liver shape from its exhalation position during respiration can now be described in terms of our model,

$$\mathbf{v} = \check{\mathbf{v}} + \mathrm{diag}(\sigma_i)\mathbf{U}\mathbf{c} + \mu . \tag{2}$$

From the observed partial information, we have to estimate a suitable $\mathbf{c}$ that represents the motion information of the whole liver. In the next section, we will explain how this can be done.

2.3   Bayesian Motion Prediction from Sparse Measurements

We would like to use our model to predict the full motion of a liver based on only a few observed surrogate markers. In practice, these points may come, for example, from structures tracked in ultrasound images or from implanted electromagnetic beacons. We use the approach described in [2] to solve this problem. The partial observations are given by the vector $\mathbf{r} = \mathbf{L}(\mathbf{v} - \check{\mathbf{v}} - \mu)$, with a mapping $\mathbf{L} : \mathbb{R}^n \to \mathbb{R}^l, l < n$. Our aim is to find the model coefficient $\mathbf{c}$ for the full vector $\mathbf{x}$ that describes our partial measurement $\mathbf{r} = \mathbf{L}\mathbf{x}$. As we cannot expect to find an exact solution, we define the best reconstruction to be the one with minimal Mahalanobis distance $||\mathbf{c}||^2$, i.e. the one with highest prior probability. This can be formulated as a minimisation problem with regard to the model coefficients,

$$E = ||\mathbf{Q}\mathbf{c} - \mathbf{r}||^2 + \eta \cdot ||\mathbf{c}||^2 , \tag{3}$$

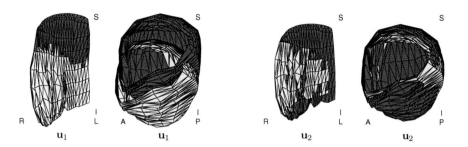

Fig. 3. Coronal and sagittal views of the mean liver shape deformed in direction of the first principal component $\mathbf{u}_1$ (*left*) and the second principal component $\mathbf{u}_2$ (*right*) of our respiratory model. The white and gray surfaces represent deformations of plus and minus $3\sigma_i$, respectively.

with $\mathbf{Q} = \mathbf{LU} \cdot \mathrm{diag}(\sigma_i)$. The regularisation factor η allows to trade off matching quality against prior probability. From the singular value decomposition $\mathbf{Q} = \overline{\mathbf{V}}\mathbf{W}\mathbf{V}^T$ we can calculate the most probable coefficients in a Bayesian sense,

$$\mathbf{c} = \mathbf{V}\,\mathrm{diag}(\frac{w_i}{w_i^2 + \eta})\,\overline{\mathbf{V}}^T\,\mathbf{r}\,. \tag{4}$$

The final shape can then be computed by projecting the model coefficient $\mathbf{c}$ back into spatial domain according to Eq. (2). Note that $\mathbf{Q}$ is of size $l \times \hat{m}$, with $\hat{m} \ll m$ the number of principal components used for reconstruction. Therefore, Eq. 4 can be easily solved in real-time.

3   Results

Figure 3 shows the mean and the variation of the first two principal components of our model. It can be seen that the first component clearly models SI motion. The additional deformation encoded by higher components quickly becomes very small. We further evaluated the quality and robustness of the model by measuring *expressiveness, compactness* and *generalisation*.

Compactness: Figure 4(a) shows a plot of the cumulative variance. The first 8 components already contain 98% of the total variability. It is desirable to have as much information as possible in the first modes, as this is a measure for the quality of the correspondence scheme. Also, a compact model suggests that the model is well suited to represent the specific class knowledge for which it was designed for.

Expressiveness: We computed leave-one-out models for all 12 subjects to evaluate the expressiveness of our model. For each model we projected the full shape of the unseen liver at inhalation into the model. This shows how well the model is able to describe (not predict) the most extreme respiratory state if it is entirely

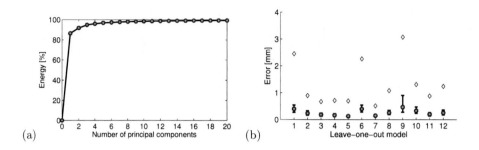

Fig. 4. (a) Cumulative energy plot of the statistical population model for the liver. (b) Median, 25th and 75th percentiles and maximum (diamond) of the projection error at inhalation.

known, and therefore gives an upper bound for model expressiveness, see Fig. 4(b). The lower and upper borders of the bar represent the 25th and the 75th error percentile, respectively, and the bar in between marks the median. The diamonds mark the maximum. Most grid points can be described with an error below 0.5 mm. On the other hand, some regions cannot be explained that accurately. However, as we look at the inhalation state, this is an upper bound for the projection error as the deviation from exhalation position is at its maximum.

Generalisation: We predicted the motion of 12 unseen livers in leave-one-out experiments. For all experiments, we assumed that a static exhalation shape of the left-out subject is given, *i.e.* a pre-operative CT scan. The prediction was based on only three surrogate markers for which we assume that we can track their deviation from exhalation position accurately. These points were selected at the inferior tip of Couinaud segment VI, at the diaphragm and near the center of the right liver lobe, in order to capture both the cyclic respiratory motion as well as organ drift that occurs mostly in the inferior part of the organ. We evaluated our method on a sequence of 20 min of motion data for each subject. A regularisation factor of $\eta = 2$ was chosen to avoid overfitting. As the error does not follow a Gaussian distribution, we give mean and maximum values as well as the 25th, 50th (median) and 95th percentile of the error evaluated at all 1326 grid points and over all respiratory states, see Tab. 1. The resulting average error over all experiments was 1.2 mm. For all subjects, the mean error was below 2 mm and for subjects 4, 5 and 7 it was significantly below 1 mm.

The used reconstruction method is a global optimisation and may not be optimal for single points, as can be seen in the 95th percentile that shows errors up to 5.6 mm. The maximum errors are outliers that originate from erroneous deformation fields in the ground truth data and had only a minor effect on the mean error. Furthermore, if all three surrogate markers are located in the proximity of the tumour, the prediction accuracy will be more stable in the region of the lesion, thus significantly lower maximum errors can be expected.

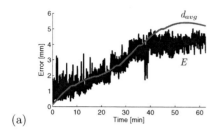
(a)

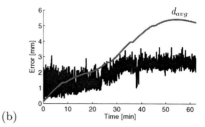
(b)

Fig. 5. Mean prediction error for a 60 min sequence (subject 12) that is subject to organ drift of up to $d_{avg} = 5.6\ mm$ (averaged over the entire liver). (a) Prediction with drift model that only contains states from the beginning of the acquisition session. (b) Prediction with model described in section 2.2.

Table 1. Motion prediction results obtained from leave-one-out experiments over 20 min of respiration and $\eta = 2$

	Prediction errors in [mm] per subject											
	1	**2**	**3**	**4**	**5**	**6**	**7**	**8**	**9**	**10**	**11**	**12**
Mean error	1.4	1.1	1.0	0.8	0.8	2.0	0.8	1.0	1.3	1.9	1.1	1.2
25th **perc.**	0.7	0.7	0.6	0.5	0.5	0.8	0.5	0.6	0.7	0.8	0.6	0.6
50th **perc.**	1.1	1.0	0.9	0.7	0.7	1.4	0.7	0.9	1.2	1.4	1.0	1.0
95th **perc.**	3.5	2.3	2.1	1.6	1.5	5.6	1.8	2.1	2.9	5.0	2.4	2.6
Max error	8.4	11.4	5.1	12.0	12.6	14.7	4.6	8.1	12.0	11.3	6.0	7.5

As some livers are subject to organ drift, their exhalation positions deform over time. In this case, they do not match the exhalation masters anymore which leads to higher prediction errors even at exhalation, see Fig. 5(a). However, since the model includes cycles from all over the acquisition session, most of the drift can be compensated, as Fig. 5(b) nicely shows.

4   Conclusions

We presented a generic statistictal framework for the prediction of organ positions under respiratory motion from sparse measurements and demonstrated it for human livers. Our method accurately predicts the full respiratory motion over 20 min from very few observed points and also compensates for organ drift. The average error for each subject is between 0.8 mm and 2 mm and the average errror over all experiments is 1.2 mm. With our population based approach, no time-consuming pre-computation (*e.g.* 3D image registration) is necessary to apply it to a novel patient, as it is the case for most subject-specific methods reported in the literature. Our method helps to significantly extend the gating window or even to irradiate a tumour continuously, allowing for more efficient and safer treatment. In forthcoming studies, we will increase the number of subjects to further generalise our model and enhance its expressiveness. Also, we plan to relax the constraints on the surrogate markers, *e.g.* for tracking using implanted beads in portal images where one dimension is lost, or with ultrasound, where noisy measurements are expected. A further aspect in the clinical evaluation of our approach that has to be investigated, is the application to cancerous livers. The influence of a tumour on the elasticity and the deformation characteristics is not yet well understood.

Acknowledgement. This work was funded by the Swiss National Science Foundation (SNSF), project CRSII2_127549.

References

1. Barber, C.B., Dobkin, D.P., Huhdanpaa, H.: The quickhull algorithm for convex hulls. ACM T. Math. Software 22(4), 469–483 (1996)
2. Blanz, V., Vetter, T.: Reconstructing the complete 3D shape of faces from partial information. Informationstechnik und Technische Informatik 44(6), 295–302 (2002)
3. Ehrhardt, J., Werner, R., Schmidt-Richberg, A., Handels, H.: Statistical modeling of 4d respiratory lung motion using diffeomorphic image registration. IEEE Transactions on Medical Imaging 30(2), 251–265 (2011)
4. He, T., Xue, Z., Xie, W., Wong, S.T.C.: Online 4-D CT Estimation for Patient-Specific Respiratory Motion Based on Real-Time Breathing Signals. In: Jiang, T., Navab, N., Pluim, J.P.W., Viergever, M.A. (eds.) MICCAI 2010 Part III. LNCS, vol. 6363, pp. 392–399. Springer, Heidelberg (2010)
5. Rohlfing, T., Maurer Jr., C.R., O'Dell, W.G., Zhong, J.: Modeling liver motion and deformation during the respiratory cycle using intensity-based nonrigid registration of gated MR images. Med. Phys. 31(3), 427–432 (2004)
6. Rueckert, D., Sonoda, L.I., Hayes, C., Hill, D.L.G., Leach, M.O., Hawkes, D.J.: Nonrigid registration using free-form deformations: application to breast MR images. IEEE T. Med. Imag. 18(8), 712–721 (1999)
7. Shirato, H., Seppenwoolde, Y., Kitamura, K., Onimura, R., Shimizu, S.: Intrafractional tumor motion: lung and liver. Semin. Radiat. Oncol. 14(1), 10–18 (2004)
8. von Siebenthal, M., Cattin, P.C., Gamper, U., Lomax, A., Székely, G.: 4D MR Imaging Using Internal Respiratory Gating. In: Duncan, J.S., Gerig, G. (eds.) MICCAI 2005. LNCS, vol. 3750, pp. 336–343. Springer, Heidelberg (2005)
9. von Siebenthal, M., Székely, G., Lomax, A., Cattin, P.: Inter-Subject Modelling of Liver Deformation During Radiation Therapy. In: Ayache, N., Ourselin, S., Maeder, A. (eds.) MICCAI 2007, Part I. LNCS, vol. 4791, pp. 659–666. Springer, Heidelberg (2007)
10. von Siebenthal, M., Székely, G., Lomax, A., Cattin, P.: Systematic errors in respiratory gating due to intrafraction deformations of the liver. Med. Phys. 34(9), 3620–3629 (2007)
11. Zsemlye, G.: Shape Prediction from Partial Information. Ph.D. thesis, ETH Zurich (2005)

Semi–automated Subcutaneous and Visceral Adipose Tissue Quantification in Computed Tomography

Marcel Koek[1], Frederico Bastos Goncalves[2], Don Poldermans[2],
Wiro Niessen[1,3], and Rashindra Manniesing[1,4]

[1] Biomedical Imaging Group Rotterdam,
Departments of Radiology & Medical Informatics,
Erasmus MC, Rotterdam, The Netherlands
[2] Department of Vascular Surgery, Erasmus MC, Rotterdam, The Netherlands
[3] Imaging Science & Technology, Department of Applied Sciences,
Delft University of Technology, Delft, The Netherlands
[4] Diagnostic Image Analysis Group, Department of Radiology, RUNMC, Nijmegen,
The Netherlands
m.koek@erasmusmc.nl

Abstract. In this study we propose a novel method for semi–automated 3D quantification of subcutaneous and visceral adipose tissue from CTA data. The method differentiates between subcutaneous and visceral adipose tissue by using gradient based deformable models using simplex meshes. The performance of the method is evaluated against a reference standard containing 27 manually annotated CTA scans made by expert observers. The quality of the reference standard is assessed by intra- and interobserver variability. The performance of the semi–automated method is evaluated against the reference standard by Pearson linear correlation and Bland and Altman analysis.

Keywords: adiposity, quantitative imaging.

1 Introduction

According to the World Health Organisation (WHO), obesity has reached a global epidemic form with approximately 2 billion adults being classified as obese or overweight [1,16,14,11] and this number is ever increasing. Excess weight is associated with Cardiovascular Disease (CVD) [7,10], diabetes and various forms of cancer [3,13,20].

Currently the general measure of adiposity in clinical practice is the Body Mass Index (BMI) proposed by Keys et al. [12] in 1972. Although BMI is easy to calculate and adequate for large epidemiological studies, the measure has a more limited value for individual risk assesment. Most importantly, the measure does not take into account the distribution of the the Adipose Tissue (AT) over the body. Waist Circumference and Waist-to-Hip ratio, which provide indirect measures of central adiposity, demonstrate incremental prognostic value

H. Yoshida et al. (Eds.): Abdominal Imaging 2011, LNCS 7029, pp. 215–222, 2012.

compared to BMI alone [4]. But also these latter methods assessing central adiposity cannot differentiate between Visceral AT (VAT) and Subcutaneous AT (SAT). It has been shown that the different types of AT, play different roles in the pathophysiology of various diseases [8,9,18,19].

Most previously proposed studies for SAT and VAT quantification from CT data do not measure all AT in the complete abdominal region, but they measure only on one or a set of axial slices [15,17,5]. All previous studies to our knowledge evaluate the data in a 2D slice-by-slice fashion [15,17,5,22]. The method we present evaluates the scans in 3D and measures the SAT and VAT in the complete abdominal region. This provides valuable insight in the distribution of the SAT and VAT and presents an opportunity to perform clinical correlation studies and test the performance and validity of the currently used measures for assessing adiposity.

2   Materials and Methods

2.1   Region of Interest

The abdominal region is defined as a 3D volume enclosed by the diaphragm, muscle wall surrounding the abdominal cavity, the vertebral column, the pubic symphysis and the pelvic cavity (see Fig. 1).

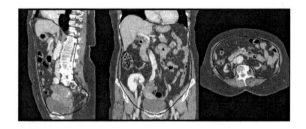

Fig. 1. Dividing surface between VAT and SAT

2.2   Preprocessing

The 3D imaging data is pre-processed by extracting the complete body contour from the imaging data, by intensity thresholding and connected component analysis. This step also removes the possible presence of the CT table and other medical equipments from the image.

2.3   Deformable Model

In order to differentiate between SAT and VAT, a 3D dividing surface is determined (See Fig. 1). This dividing surface mostly runs through regions of muscle and bone tissue, and separates exterior tissue (SAT and lungs) from interior tissue (which includes VAT). Due to the higher CT intensities of bone and muscle compared to both lungs and AT, a gradient–based deformable model can be used for locating the dividing boundary between SAT and VAT. In this study, a simplex mesh is used for representing the model. Simplex mesh based deformable models offer control over the topology, the regularity and the rigidity of the surface [6]. The deformation of the mesh is accomplished by considering the vertices as masses which depend on the Newtonian law of motion (1).

$$m\frac{d^2 P_i}{dt^2} = -\gamma\frac{dP_i}{dt} + \mathbf{F}_{int} + \mathbf{F}_{ext} \tag{1}$$

The internal force ($\mathbf{F}_{int}$) controls the rigidity and the regularity of the simplex mesh. The external force ($\mathbf{F}_{ext}$) depends on image features. This force field consists of vectors pointing towards the dividing surface between SAT and VAT. As stated earlier in this paragraph, the 3D dividing surface consist mainly of transitions between muscle or bone tissue and lung or adipose tissue. Therefore we select $\mathbf{F}_{ext}$ as the gradient of the gradient magnitude of the CT intensities (2). This results in a force field with the forces directed towards the edges of intensity transitions.

$$\mathbf{F}_{ext} = \nabla\|\nabla I\| \tag{2}$$

Figure 2(a) shows an example of an image from which the external force is calculated. Figure 2(c) gives an example of a force field.

The region of interest has the same topology as an ellipsoidal surface. The surface is therefore initialised as an ellipsoid surrounding the body (see Fig. 2(b)). During deformation the topology is preserved. When the summed deformation of the entire mesh drops below a set value, the deformation is stopped. The result is a dividing boundary between the subcutaneous and the visceral region (see Fig. 2(d)).

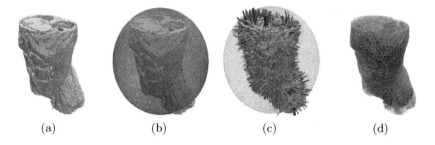

(a)   (b)   (c)   (d)

Fig. 2. (a) 3D rendering of the extracted muscle tissue.(b) 3D rendering of the initialization of the simplex mesh. (c) 3D rendering of the calculated forces which act on the vertices of the simplex mesh. (d) 3D rendering of the resulting mesh after propagating the vertices following (1).

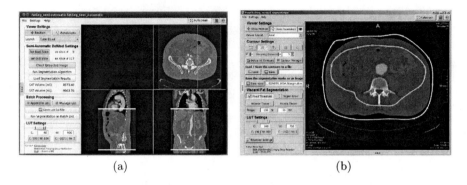

(a)   (b)

Fig. 3. (a) Software tool that is used to indicate the upper and lower boundaries in a scan. (b) Screenshot of the software tool used for annotating the CTA scans.

2.4   Adipose Tissue Classification

The voxels are classified as AT by using the HU range for fat as defined by Yoshizumi et. al. [21]. Voxels enclosed by the surface resulting from the deformable model method are classified as VAT, whereas voxels located outside the deformable model are classified as SAT.

2.5   Semi–automated

The scans included in this study are not all scanned with the same protocol, resulting in differences in the field of view. To analyse the same region of interest in all scans, the upper and lower boundary are indicated by an expert in a specially developed software tool (see Fig. 3(a)). The knowledge of the upper and lower boundaries is used to initialize the simplex mesh resulting in more reliable outcomes. This is the only user interaction required.

3   Experiments and Results

3.1   Reference Standard

To validate the performance of the segmentation method, a reference standard was obtained through manually annoting axial slices. This was performed by 3 expert observers to determine the inter-observer variability. One of the observers annotated the same image set twice at different points in time to estimate the intra-observer variability. A total of 27 abdomino-pelvic CTA scans were selected with a wide range of BMI in both genders. All included scans are from patients submitted to elective abdominal aortic aneurysm repair from 2004 to 2010.

Per subject 5 axial slices were annotated. The slices were selected based on cardiovascular anatomical features, covers the extents of the entire abdominal region and are not overlapping. SAT and VAT are annotated by drawing contours and thresholding on the HU range for AT using a specially developed tool (see Fig. 3(b)).

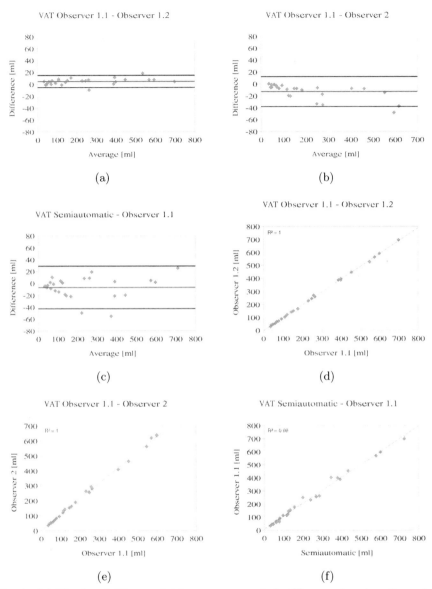

Fig. 4. (a) Bland and Altman plot for measurements by Observer 1 on two timepoints $(4.61\,ml \pm 10.10\,ml)$. (b) Bland and Altman plot for measurements by Observer 1 on timepoint 1 and Observer 2 $(-12.98\,ml \pm 25.07\,ml)$. (c) Bland and Altman plot for measurements by the method and Observer 1 on timepoint 1 $(-6.94\,ml \pm 35.68\,ml)$. (d) Scatterplot showing the linear correlation of measurements of VAT by Observer 1 on different time points $(r = 0.9997, p < 0.001)$. (e) Scatterplot showing the linear correlation of measurements of VAT between Observer 1 on timepoint 1 and Observer 2 $(r = 0.9986, p < 0.001)$. (f) Scatterplot showing the linear correlation of measurements of VAT by the method and Observer 1 on timepoint 1 $(r = 0.9941, p < 0.001)$. Difference plots show the mean difference (red line) and the limits of agreement (blue lines).

Table 1. The mean differences μ_d and the limits of agreement $\pm 1.96\,\sigma_d$

	SAT	VAT	Total AT
	$(\mu_d \pm 1.96\,\sigma_d)\,[ml]$	$(\mu_d \pm 1.96\,\sigma_d)\,[ml]$	$(\mu_d \pm 1.96\,\sigma_d)\,[ml]$
Method – O1.1	1.7 ±28.2	-6.9 ±35.7	-5.2 ±24.9
Method – O1.2	-2.4 ±26.4	-2.9 ±34.9	-5.3 ±24.5
Method – O2	15.8 ±33.2	-21.6 ±34.0	-5.8 ±22.9
Method – O3	11.4 ±31.8	-19.2 ±32.5	-7.8 ±29.9
Intra-observer	-4.6 ±10.2	4.6 ±10.1	-0.02 ±2.3
O1.1 – O2	12.8 ±24.6	-13.0 ±25.1	-0.2 ±0.8
O1.1 – O3	10.2 ±23.5	-12.8 ±24.1	-2.6 ±14.7
O2 – O3	-4.5 ±11.9	1.9 ±16.3	-2.6 ±15.3

Table 2. Pearson correlation coefficients ($p < 0.001$ for all correlations)

	r_{SAT}	r_{VAT}	r_{Total}
Method – O1.1	0.9969	0.9941	0.9993
Method – O1.2	0.9970	0.9942	0.9993
Method – O2	0.9944	0.9967	0.9993
Method – O3	0.9973	0.9954	0.9990
Intra-observer	0.9997	0.9997	1.0000
O1.1 – O2	0.9978	0.9986	1.0000
O1.1 – O3	0.9986	0.9984	0.9997
O2 – O3	0.9995	0.9992	0.9997

3.2   Validation

The agreement between the method and the manually obtained reference standard as well as the inter- and intra-observer variability are assessed according to the method by Bland and Altman [2] and Pearson linear regression analysis. In the analysis VAT, SAT and Total AT are assessed individually. The results of the Bland and Altman analysis are given in Table 1. In Figures 4(d),4(e) and 4(f) Bland and Plots show the agreement between the measurements of VAT. The Pearson correlation coefficients are given in Table 2. Figures 4(d),4(e) and 4(f) show the linear correlation between the measurements of VAT in scatter plots.

The reproducability of the manual annotations is high because the intra-observer correlation is good as well as the intra-observer agreement. Comparable results were found for inter-observer correlation and agreement. Based on the intra- and inter-observervariability we can state that the quality of the reference standard is high.

The correlation between the method and the reference standard is high and comparable to the intra- and inter-observer correlations. Although the limits of agreement for the method and the reference standard are slightly larger than the intra- and inter-observer agreements, the reference standard is still in agreement with the method.

4 Conclusion

In this paper a novel method for quantifying SAT and VAT from CT images is proposed. The method measures the total SAT and VAT in the complete abdominal region in a semi–automated fashion. The differentiation of SAT and VAT is based on a gradient based deformable model using simplex meshes. The performance of the method is evaluated against 27 manually annotated CT scans (5 slices in each scan) which are made by expert observers. The manual annotations and the semi–automated method are positively correlated. The limits of agreement in the differences between method and observers are acceptable. This method is potentially useful for use in clinical correlation studies involving adipose tissue.

References

1. Who obesity and overweight, fact sheet n 311 (2006),
   http://www.who.int/mediacentre/factsheets/fs311/en/index.html
2. Bland, J., Altman, D.: Statistical methods for assessing agreement between two methods of clinical measurement. Lancet (1986)
3. Calle, E.E., Rodriguez, C., Walker-Thurmond, K., Thun, M.J.: Overweight, obesity, and mortality from cancer in a prospectively studied cohort of u.s. adults. The New England Journal of Medicine 348, 1625–1638 (2003)
4. Chan, D., Watts, G., Barrett, P., Burke, V.: Waist circumference, waist-to-hip ratio and body mass index as predicators of adipose tissue compartments in men. QJM 96(6), 441–447 (2003), http://www.biomedsearch.com/nih/Waist-circumference-waist-to-hip/12788963.html
5. Chung, H., Cobzas, D., Lieffers, J., Birdsel, L., Baracos, V.: Automated segmentation of muscle and adipose tissue on ct images for human body composition analysis. In: Medical Imaging: Image Processing. Proc. SPIE, vol. 7261 (2009)
6. Delingette, H.: General object reconstruction based on simplex meshes. International Journal of Computer Vision 32, 111–142 (1999)
7. Ditomasso, D., Carnethon, M., Wright, C., Allison, M.: The associations between visceral fat and calcified atherosclerosis are stronger in women than men. Atherosclerosis (2009)
8. Fontana, L., Eagon, C.J., Trujillo, M.E., Scherer, P.E., Klein, S.: Visceral fat adipokine secretion is associated with systemic inflammation in obese humans. Diabetes 56(4), 1010–1013 (2007), http://dx.doi.org/10.2337/db06-1656
9. Fox, C.S., Massaro, J.M., Hoffmann, U., Pou, K.M., Maurovich-Horvat, P., Lui, C.: Abdominal visceral and subcutaneous adipose tissue compartments:association with metabolic risk factors in the framingham heart study. Circulation 116, 39–48 (2007)
10. Grundy, S.M.: Metabolic syndrome: Connecting and reconciling cardiovascular anddiabetis worlds. Journal of the American College of Cardiology 47(6), 1093–1100 (2006)
11. James, P.T.: Obesity: The worldwide epidemic. Clinics in Dermatology 22(4), 276–280 (2004), http://www.sciencedirect.com/science/article/B6T5G-4DGM0SS-2/2/8fd222f34f92e929a93767214d650880
12. Keys, A., Fidanza, F., Karvonen, M., Kimura, N., Taylor, H.: Indices of relative weight and obesity. Journal of Chronic Disease 25(6), 329–343 (1972)

13. Kort, E., Sevensma, E., Fitzgerald, T.: Trends in esophageal cancer and body mass index by race and gender in the state of michigan. BMC Gastroenterology 9(1), 47 (2009), http://www.biomedcentral.com/1471-230X/9/47
14. McLellan, F.: Obesity rising to alarming levels around the world. The Lancet 259(9315), 1412 (2002)
15. Pednekar, A., Bandekar, A.N., Kakadiaris, I.A., Naghavi, M.: Automatic segmentation of abdominal fat from ct data. In: IEEE Workshop on Applications of Computer Vision and the IEEE Workshop on Motion and Video Computing, vol. 1, pp. 308–315 (2005)
16. Popkin, B., Doak, C.M.: The obesity epidemic is a worldwide phenomenon. Nutrition Reviews 56(4 pt1), 106–114 (1998)
17. Romero, D., Ramirez, J., Marmol, A.: Quanification of subcutaneous and visceral adipose tissue using ct. In: IEEE International Workshop on Medical Measurement and Applications, MeMea 2006, pp. 128–133 (April 2006)
18. Scaglione, R., Chiara, T.D., Cariello, T., Licata, G.: Visceral obesity and metabolic syndrome: Two faces of the same medal? Internal and Emergency Medicine, 111–119 (2009)
19. Taksali, S.E., Caprio, S., Dziura, J., Dufour, S., Cal, A.M., Goodman, T.R., Papademetris, X., Burgert, T.S., Pierpont, B.M., Savoye, M., Shaw, M., Seyal, A.A., Weiss, R.: High Visceral and Low Abdominal Subcutaneous Fat Stores in the Obese Adolescent. Diabetes 57(2), 367–371 (2008), http://diabetes.diabetesjournals.org/content/57/2/367.abstract
20. Tanaka, K., Yano, M., Motoori, M., Kishi, K., Miyashiro, I., Yamada, T., Ohue, M., Ohigashi, H., Ishikawa, O., Imaoka, S.: Excess visceral fat accumulation is a risk factor for postoperative systemic inflammatory response syndrome in patients with esophageal cancer. Esophagus 5(2), 78–80 (2008), http://www.springerlink.com/content/0044h186t3163237/
21. Yoshizumi, T., Nakamura, T., Yamane, M., Islam, A.H.M.W., Menju, M., Yamasaki, K., Arai, T., Kotani, K., Funahashi, T., Yamashita, S., Matsuzawa, Y.: Abdominal fat: Standardized technique for measurement at ct. Radiology 211, 283–286 (1999)
22. Zhao, B., Colville, J., Kalaigian, J., Curran, S., Jiang, L., Kijewski, P., Schwartz, L.H.: Automated quantification of body fat distribution on volumetric computed tomography. Journal of Computer Assisted Tomography 30(5), 777–783 (2006)

Computation and Evaluation of Medial Surfaces for Shape Representation of Abdominal Organs

Sergio Vera[1,2], Debora Gil[1], Agnès Borràs[1], Xavi Sánchez[1], Frederic Pérez[2], Marius George Linguraru[3], and Miguel A. González Ballester[2]

[1] Computer Vision Center, Computer Science Dept., Universitat Autònoma de Barcelona, Spain
[2] Alma IT Systems, Barcelona, Spain
[3] Radiology and Imaging Sciences Dept., Clinical Center, National Institutes of Health, Bethesda, USA
sergio.vera@alma3d.com

Abstract. Medial representations are powerful tools for describing and parameterizing the volumetric shape of anatomical structures. Existing methods show excellent results when applied to 2D objects, but their quality drops across dimensions. This paper contributes to the computation of medial manifolds in two aspects. First, we provide a standard scheme for the computation of medial manifolds that avoid degenerated medial axis segments; second, we introduce an energy based method which performs independently of the dimension. We evaluate quantitatively the performance of our method with respect to existing approaches, by applying them to synthetic shapes of known medial geometry. Finally, we show results on shape representation of multiple abdominal organs, exploring the use of medial manifolds for the representation of multi-organ relations.

Keywords: medial manifolds, abdomen.

1 Introduction

Abdominal diagnosis relies on the comprehensive analysis of groups of organs [10]. Besides the organ appearance and size, the shapes of the organs can be indicators of disorders. Abdominal organs follow global shape constraints, which have proved exceptionally useful to guide segmentation algorithms, for example for the liver [8]. Although local shape differences are key to diagnosis, they are difficult to model without an adequate shape representation [14].

Medial manifolds of organs have proved robust and accurate to study group differences in the brain [4,17]. In the abdomen, shape-based modeling could reveal biomarkers for diagnosis by identifying unusual anatomy and its relation to neighboring organs. Additionally, organ locations, generally defined by centroids [19], and more recently by pose [11], can be more comprehensively characterized by medial manifolds, more intuitive and easily interpretable representations of complex organs.

In order to provide accurate meshes of anatomical geometry, the extraction of medial manifolds should satisfy three main conditions [13]: *homotopy* (mantain the same topology of the original shape), *thinness* (the resulting medial shape should be one pixel wide, taking into account the specific choice of connectivity), and *medialness* (the medial structure should lie as close as possible to the center of the original object). Most

H. Yoshida et al. (Eds.): Abdominal Imaging 2011, LNCS 7029, pp. 223–230, 2012.

methods for medial surface computation are based on morphological thinning operations on binary segmentations. Such methods require the definition of a neighborhood
set and conditions for the removal of *simple voxels*, i.e. voxels that can be removed
without changing the topology of the object. These definitions are trivial in 2D, but
their complexity increases exponentially with the dimension of the embedding space
[9]. Further, simplicity tests alone only produce (1D) medial axis so additional tests are
needed to know if a voxel lies in a surface and thus cannot be deleted even if it is simple [13]. Moreover, surface tests might introduce medial axis segments in the medial
surface, which is against the mathematical definition of manifold and that may require
further pruning [13,1].

Alternative methods rely on an energy map to ensure medialness on the manifold.
Often, this energy image is the distance map of the object [13] or another energy derived
from it, like the average outward flux [16,4], level set [15,18] or ridges of the distance
map [6]. However, to obtain a manifold from the energy image, most methods rely on
morphological thinning, in a two step process [4,13,16], thus inheriting the weak points
of morphological methods.

The contribution of this paper is a two step method for medial surface computation
based on the ridges of the distance map. Firstly, as energy image we propose the ridges
of the distance map, based on a normalized ridge operator. Secondly, our binarization
step is free of topology rules, as it is based on Non-Maxima Suppression (NMS) [5].
Given that, regardless of the space dimension, NMS only requires 1 direction to be
defined, our method scales well with dimension. Quantitative evaluation of our method
in comparison with existing approaches is shown on synthetic shapes of known medial
geometry. Finally, results are shown on sets of segmented livers obtained from [8], as
well as multi-organ datasets [14].

2   Extracting Anatomical Medial Surfaces

The computation of medial manifolds from a segmented volume may be split into two
main steps: computation of a medial map from the original volume and binarization of
such map. Medial maps should achieve a discriminant value on the shape central voxels. Meanwhile, the binarization step should ensure that the resulting medial structures
fulfill the three conditions: medialness, thinness and homotopy.

Distance transforms are the basis for obtaining medial manifolds in any dimension.
The distance map is generated by computing the Euclidean distance transform of the
binary mask representing the volumetric shape. By definition, the maximum values of
the distance map are located at the center of the shape at voxels corresponding to the
medial structure. It follows that the medial surface could be extracted from the raw
distance map by an iterative thinning process [13]. Two alternative binarizations that
scale well with dimension are thresholding and NMS. Thresholding keeps pixels with
medial map energy above a given value. Therefore, it requires that the medial map is
constant along the medial surface. Non-Maxima Suppression keeps only those pixels
attaining a local maximum of the medial map in a given direction. Unless the medial
map maxima are flat, NMS also produces one pixel-wide surfaces.

Further examination of the distance map shows that its central maximal voxels are connected and constitute a ridge surface of the distance map. We propose using a normalized ridge map with NMS-based binarization for computing medial surfaces.

2.1 Normalized Medial Map

Ridges/valleys in a digital N-Dimensional image are defined as the set of points that are extrema (minima for ridges and maxima for valleys) in the direction of greatest magnitude of the second order directional derivative [7]. From the available operators for ridge detection, we chose the creaseness measure described in [12] because it provides (normalized) values in the range $[-N, N]$. The ridgeness operator is computed by the structure tensor of the distance map as follows.

Let D denote the distance map to the shape and let its gradient, ∇D, be computed by convolution with partial derivatives of a Gaussian kernel:

$$\nabla D = (\partial_x D_\sigma, \partial_y D_\sigma, \partial_z D_\sigma) = (\partial_x g_\sigma * D, \partial_y g_\sigma * D, \partial_z g_\sigma * D)$$

being g_σ a Gaussian kernel of variance σ and ∂_x, ∂_y and ∂_z partial derivative operators. The structure tensor or second order matrix [2] is given by averaging the projection matrices onto the distance map gradient:

$$ST_{\rho,\sigma}(D) = \begin{pmatrix} g_\rho * \partial_x D_\sigma^2 & g_\rho * \partial_x D_\sigma \partial_y D_\sigma & g_\rho * \partial_x D_\sigma \partial_z D_\sigma \\ g_\rho * \partial_x D_\sigma \partial_y D_\sigma & g_\rho * \partial_y D_\sigma^2 & g_\rho * \partial_y D_\sigma \partial_z D_\sigma \\ g_\rho * \partial_x D_\sigma \partial_z D_\sigma & g_\rho * \partial_y D_\sigma \partial_z D_\sigma & g_\rho * \partial_z D_\sigma^2 \end{pmatrix} \quad (1)$$

for g_ρ a Gaussian kernel of variance ρ. Let V be the eigenvector of principal eigenvalue of $ST_{\rho,\sigma}(D)$ and consider its reorientation along the distance gradient, $\tilde{V} = (P, Q, R)$, given as:

$$V = \text{sign}(< \tilde{V} \cdot \nabla D >) \cdot \tilde{V}$$

for $< \cdot >$ the scalar product. The ridgeness measure [12] is given by the divergence:

$$\mathcal{R} := \text{div}(\tilde{V}) = \partial_x P + \partial_y Q + \partial_z R \quad (2)$$

The above operator assigns positive values to ridge pixels and negative values to valley ones. The more positive the value is, the stronger the ridge patterns are. A main advantage over other operators (such as second order oriented Gaussian derivatives) is that $\mathcal{R} \in [-N, N]$ for N the dimension of the volume. In this way, it is possible to set a threshold, τ, common to any volume for detecting significant ridges and, thus, points highly likely to belong to the medial surface.

2.2 Non-maxima Suppression Binarization

We use NMS to obtain the voxels with higher ridgeness value and obtain a thin, one pixel wide medial surface. NMS consists in checking the two neighbors of a pixel in a specific direction, V, and delete pixels if their value is not the maximum one:

$$NMS(x, y, z) = \begin{cases} \mathcal{R}(x, y, z) & \text{if } \mathcal{R}(x, y, z) > \max(\mathcal{R}_{V+}(x, y, z), \mathcal{R}_{V-}(x, y, z)) \\ 0 & \text{otherwise} \end{cases}$$

for $\mathcal{R}_{V+} = \mathcal{R}(x + V_x, y + V_y, z + V_z)$ and $\mathcal{R}_{V-} = \mathcal{R}(x - V_x, y - V_y, z - V_z)$.

A main requirement is identifying the local-maxima direction from the medial map derivatives. The search direction for local maxima is obtained from the structure tensor of the ridge map, $ST_{\rho,\sigma}(\mathcal{R})$. The eigenvector of greatest eigenvalue of the structure tensor indicates the direction of highest variation of the ridge image. In order to overcome small glitches due to discretization of the direction, NMS is computed using interpolation along the search direction.

One drawback of the ridge operator is that anywhere the structure tensor does not have a clear predominant direction, the creaseness response decreases. This may happen at points where two medial manifolds join and can introduce holes on the medial surface that violate the homotopy principle. Such holes are exclusively localized at self-intersections, and are removed by means of a closing operator.

3   Validation Experiments

As multiple algorithms generate different surfaces, we are interested in finding a way to evaluate the quality of the generated manifold as a tool to recover the original shape. We propose a benchmark for medial surface quality evaluation that starts from known medial surfaces, that we consider as ground truth, and generates objects from them. The medial surface obtained from the newly created object is then compared against the ground truth surface. We have applied our NMS using $\sigma = 0.5$, $\rho = 1$ for both $ST_{\rho,\sigma}(D)$ and $ST_{\rho,\sigma}(\mathcal{R})$. In order to compare to morphological methods, we also applied an ordered thinning using a 6-connected neighborhood (labeled Thin6C) described in [3], a 26-connected neighborhood (labeled Thin26C) described in [13] and a pruning of the 26-connected neighborhood (labeled Thin26CP).

The quality of medial surfaces has been assessed by comparing them to ground truth surfaces in terms of surface distance [8]. The distance of a voxel y to a surface X is given by: $d_X(y) = \min_{x \in X} \|y - x\|$, for $\| \cdot \|$ the Euclidean norm. If we denote by X the reference surface and Y the computed one, the scores considered are:

1. *Standard Surface Distances*:

$$AvD = \frac{1}{|Y|} \left(\sum_{y \in Y} d_X(y) \right) \qquad MxD = \max_{y \in Y}(d_X(y))$$

2. *Symmetric Surface Distances*:

$$AvSD = \frac{1}{|X| + |Y|} \left(\sum_{x \in X} d_Y(x) + \sum_{y \in Y} d_X(y) \right)$$

$$MxSD = \max \left(\max_{x \in X}(d_Y(x)), \max_{y \in Y}(d_X(y)) \right)$$

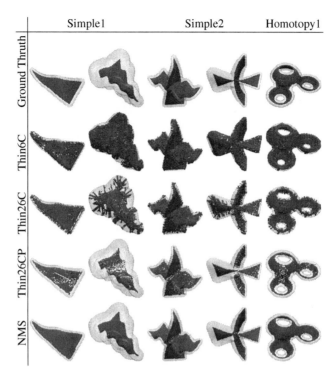

Fig. 1. Synthetic Volume examples. Each row corresponds to a compared method, while columns exemplify the different objects families tested: one and two foil surfaces, with constant (1st and 3rd columns) or variable distance (2nd and 4th columns), and with holes (last column).

Standard distances measure deviation from medialness, while differences between standard and symmetric distances indicate homotopy artifacts. Thinness has been visually assessed.

The ground truth medial surfaces cover 3 types: non-intersecting trivial homotopy (denoted Simple1), intersecting trivial homotopy (denoted Simple2) and non-trivial (homeomorphic to the circle) homotopy group (denoted Homotopy1). Thirty volumes having the synthetic surfaces as medial manifolds have been generated by thresholding the distance map to the synthetic surface. We have considered constant (denoted UnifDist) and varying (denoted VarDist) thresholds.

Figure 1 shows an example of the synthetic volumes in the first row and results in the remaining rows. The shape of surfaces produced using morphological thinning strongly depends on the connectivity rule used. In the absence of pruning, surfaces, in addition, have extra medial axes attached. On the contrary, NMS medial surfaces have a well defined shape matching the original synthetic surface.

Table 1 reports error ranges for the four methods and the different types of synthetic volumes. For all methods, there are not significant differences between standard and symmetric distances for a given volume. This indicates a good preservation of homotopy. Thinning without pruning has significant geometric artifacts (maximum distances increase) and might drop its performance for variable distance volumes due to a different ordering for pixel removal. The performance of NMS presents high stability across volume geometries and produces accurate surfaces matching synthetic shapes. These results show that our approach has better reconstruction power.

Table 1. Error ranges for the Synthetic Volumes

		Simple1		Simple2		Homotopy1
		UnifDist	VarDist	UnifDist	VarDist	
NMS	AvD	0.218 ± 0.034	0.245 ± 0.052	0.279 ± 0.103	0.270 ± 0.058	0.175 ± 0.085
	MxD	2.608 ± 0.660	2.676 ± 2.001	3.000 ± 0.000	3.000 ± 0.000	2.873 ± 0.229
	AvSD	0.209 ± 0.059	0.250 ± 0.075	0.243 ± 0.085	0.273 ± 0.053	0.171 ± 0.045
	MxSD	2.745 ± 0.394	2.813 ± 1.924	2.873 ± 0.312	3.281 ± 0.562	2.873 ± 0.229
Thin6C	AvD	1.853 ± 0.237	6.523 ± 0.162	1.843 ± 0.266	3.128 ± 0.860	2.801 ± 0.661
	MxD	6.946 ± 1.377	23.293 ± 1.869	7.995 ± 1.052	12.868 ± 1.598	9.749 ± 0.718
	AvSD	1.582 ± 0.188	5.922 ± 0.195	1.897 ± 0.674	2.695 ± 0.805	2.451 ± 0.645
	MxSD	6.946 ± 1.377	23.293 ± 1.869	8.926 ± 1.730	12.868 ± 1.598	9.749 ± 0.718
Thin26C	AvD	1.466 ± 0.102	5.523 ± 0.341	1.527 ± 0.187	2.679 ± 0.472	2.610 ± 0.735
	MxD	6.918 ± 1.537	21.807 ± 2.477	7.973 ± 1.256	12.702 ± 1.697	9.519 ± 0.810
	AvSD	1.226 ± 0.124	4.868 ± 0.349	1.222 ± 0.153	2.251 ± 0.450	2.282 ± 0.717
	MxSD	6.918 ± 1.537	21.807 ± 2.477	7.973 ± 1.256	12.702 ± 1.697	9.519 ± 0.810
Thin26CP	AvD	0.771 ± 0.110	0.686 ± 0.135	0.755 ± 0.118	0.865 ± 0.150	0.748 ± 0.064
	MxD	2.544 ± 0.797	2.440 ± 0.676	2.864 ± 0.632	7.220 ± 3.239	2.782 ± 0.254
	AvSD	0.664 ± 0.158	0.566 ± 0.184	1.039 ± 0.695	0.961 ± 0.384	0.567 ± 0.048
	MxSD	2.544 ± 0.797	2.676 ± 0.779	5.289 ± 3.291	9.860 ± 3.962	2.782 ± 0.254

4   Application to Abdominal Organs

Our method was applied to sets of manually segmented livers selected from a public database[1] of CT volumes [8]. CT images were acquired with scanners from different manufacturers (4, 16 and 64 detector rows), a pixel spacing between 0.55 and 0.80mm and inter-slice distance from 1 to 3mm. Figure 2 shows medial surfaces for two livers. The extracted medial surfaces show the robustness of our approach. The images in the bottom row show a liver with a remarkably prominent right lobe in its superior aspect, which is captured by our medial representation.

Our next experiment focuses on the representation of multi-organ datasets [14]. Initial results on the medial representation of multiple abdominal organs are shown in Fig. 3. It can be observed that medial representations of neighboring organs contain information about shape and topology that can be exploited for the description of organ shape and configuration.

---

[1] Collected from sliver07 competition hosted at MICCAI07 and available at sliver07.isi.uu.nl.

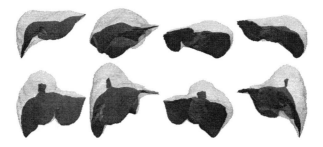

Fig. 2. Medial surfaces from livers. Upper row, normal liver. Bottom, protruding superior lobe.

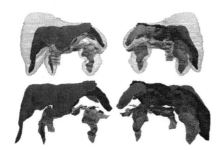

Fig. 3. Abdominal set of organs and surfaces: liver (red), kidneys (blue), pancreas (yellow), spleen (purple), and stomach (green).

5   Conclusions and Discussion

Medial manifolds are powerful descriptors of anatomical shapes. The method presented in this paper overcomes the limitations of existing morphological methods: it extracts medial surfaces without medial axis segments, and the binarization scales well with increasing dimension. Additionally, we have presented a quantitative comparison study to evaluate the performance of medial surface calculation methods and calculate their deviation from an ideal medial surface. Finally, we have shown the performance of our method for the analysis of multiple abdominal organs.

Future work includes the use of the medial surfaces computed using our methods as basis for shape parameterization [20], in order to construct anatomy-based reference systems for implicit registration and localization of pathologies. Further, we will explore correspondences between medial representations of neighboring organs to define inter-organ relations in a more exhaustive way than simply using centroid and pose parameters [10,11,19].

Acknowledgements. This work was supported by the Spanish projects TIN2009-13618, CSD2007-00018, 2009-TEM-00007, PI071188 and NIH Clinical Center Intramural Program. The 2nd author has been supported by the Ramon y Cajal Program.

References

1. Amenta, N., Choi, S., Kolluri, R.: The power crust, unions of balls, and the medial axis transform. Computational Geometry: Theory and Applications 19(2-3), 127–153 (2001)
2. Bigun, J., Granlund, G.H.: Optimal orientation detection of linear symmetry. In: ICCV, pp. 433–438 (1987)
3. Bouix, S., Siddiqi, K.: Divergence-Based Medial Surfaces. In: Vernon, D. (ed.) ECCV 2000. LNCS, vol. 1842, pp. 603–618. Springer, Heidelberg (2000)
4. Bouix, S., Siddiqi, K., Tannenbaum, A.: Flux driven automatic centerline extraction. Med. Imag. Ana. 9(3), 209–221 (2005)
5. Canny, J.: A computational approach to edge detection. IEEE Trans. Pat. Ana. Mach. Intel. 8, 679–698 (1986)
6. Chang, S.: Extracting skeletons from distance maps. Int. J. Comp. Sci. Net. Sec. 7(7) (2007)
7. Haralick, R.: Ridges and valleys on digital images. Comput. Vision Graph. Image Process. 22(10), 28–38 (1983)
8. Heimann, T., van Ginneken, B., Styner, M., Arzhaeva, Y., Aurich, V., et al.: Comparison and evaluation of methods for liver segmentation from CT datasets. IEEE Trans. Med. Imag. 28(8), 1251–1265 (2009)
9. Lee, T.C., Kashyap, R.L., Chu, C.N.: Building skeleton models via 3-D medial surface axis thinning algorithms. Grap. Mod. Imag. Process 56(6), 462–478 (1994)
10. Linguraru, M.G., Pura, J.A., Chowdhury, A.S., Summers, R.M.: Multi-organ Segmentation from Multi-phase Abdominal CT via 4D Graphs Using Enhancement, Shape and Location Optimization. In: Jiang, T., Navab, N., Pluim, J.P.W., Viergever, M.A. (eds.) MICCAI 2010, Part III. LNCS, vol. 6363, pp. 89–96. Springer, Heidelberg (2010)
11. Liu, X., Linguraru, M.G., Yao, J., Summers, R.M.: Organ Pose Distribution Model and an MAP Framework for Automated Abdominal Multi-Organ Localization. In: Liao, H., Edwards, P.J., Pan, X., Fan, Y., Yang, G.-Z. (eds.) MIAR 2010. LNCS, vol. 6326, pp. 393–402. Springer, Heidelberg (2010)
12. Lopez, A., Lumbreras, F., Serrat, J., Villanueva, J.: Evaluation of methods for ridge and valley detection. IEEE Trans. Pat. Ana. Mach. Intel. 21(4), 327–335 (1999)
13. Pudney, C.: Distance-ordered homotopic thinning: A skeletonization algorithm for 3D digital images. Comp. Vis. Imag. Underst. 72(2), 404–413 (1998)
14. Reyes, M., González Ballester, M., Li, Z., Kozic, N., Chin, S., Summers, R., Linguraru, M.: Anatomical variability of organs via principal factor analysis from the construction of an abdominal probabilistic atlas. In: IEEE Int. Symp. Biomed. Imaging, pp. 682–685 (2009)
15. Sabry, H.M., Farag, A.A.: Robust skeletonization using the fast marching method. In: IEEE Int. Conf. on Image Processing, vol. (2), pp. 437–440 (2005)
16. Siddiqi, K., Bouix, S., Tannenbaum, A., Zucker, S.W.: Hamilton-Jacobi skeletons. Int. J. Comp. Vis. 48(3), 215–231 (2002)
17. Styner, M., Lieberman, J.A., Pantazis, D., Gerig, G.: Boundary and medial shape analysis of the hippocampus in schizophrenia. Medical Image Analysis 8(3), 197–203 (2004)
18. Telea, A., van Wijk, J.J.: An augmented fast marching method for computing skeletons and centerlines. In: Symposium on Data Visualisation, VISSYM 2002, pp. 251–259. Eurographics Association (2002)
19. Yao, J., Summers, R.M.: Statistical Location Model for Abdominal Organ Localization. In: Yang, G.-Z., Hawkes, D., Rueckert, D., Noble, A., Taylor, C. (eds.) MICCAI 2009, Part II. LNCS, vol. 5762, pp. 9–17. Springer, Heidelberg (2009)
20. Yushkevich, P., Zhang, H., Gee, J.: Continuous medial representation for anatomical structures. IEEE Trans. Medical Imaging 25(12), 1547–1564 (2006)

Discontinuity Preserving Registration of Abdominal MR Images with Apparent Sliding Organ Motion

Silja Kiriyanthan, Ketut Fundana, and Philippe C. Cattin

Medical Image Analysis Center, University of Basel, Switzerland
silja.kiriyanthan@stud.unibas.ch
{ketut.fundana,philippe.cattin}@unibas.ch

Abstract. Discontinuous displacement fields are quite common in the medical field, in particular at organ boundaries with breathing induced organ motion. The sliding motion of the liver along the abdominal wall clearly causes a discontinuous displacement field. Today's common medical image registration methods, however, cannot properly deal with this kind of motion as their regularisation term enforces a smooth displacement field. Since these motion discontinuities appear at organ boundaries, motion segmentation could play an important guiding role during registration. In this paper we propose a novel method that integrates registration and globally optimal motion segmentation in a variational framework. The energy functional is formulated such that the segmentation, via continuous cuts, supports the computation of discontinuous displacement fields. The proposed energy functional is then minimised in a coarse-to-fine strategy by using a fast dual method for motion segmentation and a fixed point iteration scheme for motion estimation. Experimental results are shown for synthetic and real MR images of breathing induced liver motion.

Keywords: liver, motion analysis.

1   Introduction

Image registration is an essential tool for many medical applications. Registration is a yet powerful but also very challenging task as it is generally an ill-posed problem. A good survey on the state-of-the-art in image registration can be found in [13]. Although today's image registration methods can handle rigid and non-rigid motion nicely, they have difficulties dealing with discontinuous motion fields. These discontinuities occur for example when organs, such as the liver, are sliding along the abdominal wall during the breathing cycle. Whereas the organs are moving mainly in superior-inferior direction, the abdominal wall is moving anterior-posteriorly. The regularisation constraints of the state-of-the-art registration methods, however, enforce a smooth displacement field along these discontinuities yielding inaccurate motion information.

Although the problem of discontinuities has been a topic of research in image segmentation and classical optical flow for some decades, its influence on

H. Yoshida et al. (Eds.): Abdominal Imaging 2011, LNCS 7029, pp. 231–239, 2012.

medical image registration was neglected. Mumford and Shah for example introduced in their pioneering work [8] from 1989 a functional, that avoids spatial smoothing on a certain set of the image and therefore preserves the discontinuities there. Several methods were proposed to solve the Mumford and Shah minimisation problem. One such approach is the widely used method proposed by Vese and Chan [12]. They reformulated the Mumford-Shah functional in a level set framework to perform piecewise constant and piecewise smooth segmentation of an image. Another seminal approach, which is known to preserve discontinuities and is based on the total variation norm, was proposed by Rudin et al. [10] for image denoising. The beneficial behaviour of the total variation norm was also exploited in image registration and optical flow, see e.g. [9] and [2]. Recently, Schmidt-Richberg et al. [11] introduced a direction-dependent regularisation method to preserve discontinuities in the displacement field. This regularisation method, however, depends on the calculation of the normals at the object boundaries and therefore a rather good manual segmentation has to be provided in advance.

Since motion discontinuities appear in particular at object boundaries, motion segmentation can influence the registration process positively. More specifically, it is a chicken-and-egg problem. By providing a good motion segmentation, a proper discontinuous displacement field can be estimated and vice versa. In fact, motion estimation and motion segmentation can benefit from each other. One method that combines optical flow computation with motion segmentation was proposed by Amiaz et al. [1]. They embedded the optical flow method of Brox et al. [2] into the level set framework of Vese and Chan [12]. A drawback of the level set formulation is, that it is non-convex and therefore is fraught with the risk of getting stuck in local minima during optimisation of the energy functional.

In this paper we propose a variational elastic registration approach able to properly handle discontinuities. To guarantee a globally optimal motion segmentation, we will make use of the approach of Chan et al. [5], also called "continuous cuts" in [7]. Instead of formulating a level set function, we define a binary function and extend it to a continuous function. The resulting minimisation problem then becomes convex with respect to this continuous function and the globally optimal motion segmentation is gained by a threshold, which can be interpreted as a cut. Although motion segmentation turns into a convex problem, motion estimation still remains a non-convex optimisation task and will be solved similar to [2] and [1] through fixed point iterations.

2 Method

In this section we describe the proposed registration method which integrates the accurate optical flow estimation of Brox et al. [2] into the convex segmentation method of Chan et al. [5], in order to find smooth displacement fields whilst preserving the discontinuities. The generalisation of the method from 2D to higher dimensional images is straightforward.

2.1 Registration and Motion Segmentation Framework

Optical Flow-Based Registration. Let $\Omega \subset \mathbb{R}^2$ be the domain of the pixel positions $\boldsymbol{x} = (x, y)$. We then define by the functions $R : \Omega \to \mathbb{R}$ and $T : \Omega \to \mathbb{R}$ our reference and target image. The aim of image registration is to find a transformation $\Phi(\boldsymbol{x}) := \boldsymbol{x} + \boldsymbol{w}(\boldsymbol{x})$ such that the identity $T \circ \Phi \approx R$ holds. The function

$$\boldsymbol{w} : \begin{cases} \Omega \to \mathbb{R}^2 \\ \boldsymbol{x} \mapsto \boldsymbol{w}(\boldsymbol{x}) := (u(\boldsymbol{x}), v(\boldsymbol{x})) \, , \end{cases}$$

with $u, v : \Omega \to \mathbb{R}$, describes the displacement field and will be the intrinsic function we investigate. For convenience we will use the abbreviations $\boldsymbol{w}$, u and v for $\boldsymbol{w}(\boldsymbol{x})$, $u(\boldsymbol{x})$ and $v(\boldsymbol{x})$.

To solve a non-rigid registration problem with expected discontinuities in the displacement field, we adopt the method proposed by Brox et al. [2], that has been proven to be highly accurate for optical flow estimation. They define the energy functional as

$$E_{Brox}(\boldsymbol{w}) = \int_\Omega f(\boldsymbol{w}) + \mu \, s(\boldsymbol{w}) \, d\boldsymbol{x} \, , \tag{1}$$

where $\mu \in \mathbb{R}^+$ is a weighting parameter, f and s are the fidelity term and the smoothness term, respectively, which are defined as

$$f(\boldsymbol{w}) = f(u, v) := \Psi \left(|T(\boldsymbol{x} + \boldsymbol{w}) - R(\boldsymbol{x})|^2 + \gamma |\nabla T(\boldsymbol{x} + \boldsymbol{w}) - \nabla R(\boldsymbol{x})|^2 \right) \text{ and}$$

$$s(\boldsymbol{w}) = s(u, v) := \Psi \left(|\nabla u|^2 + |\nabla v|^2 \right) .$$

The function $\Psi(s^2) = \sqrt{s^2 + \epsilon^2}$, with $\epsilon \in \mathbb{R}^+$ small, is an approximation of the L^1 norm and is therefore robust against outliers. The fidelity term f incorporates the gradient constancy constraint to complement the grey value constancy, which is weighted by a parameter $\gamma \in \mathbb{R}_0^+$.

Motion Segmentation. Now we would like to integrate the optical flow estimation into the convex segmentation model of Chan et al. in [5]. Instead of using the level set function $\phi : \Omega \to \mathbb{R}$ and the Heaviside function $H : \mathbb{R} \to \{0, 1\}$ to differentiate the displacement field $\boldsymbol{w}$ into $\boldsymbol{w}^+$ and $\boldsymbol{w}^-$ as proposed by Amiaz et al. [1], we choose a binary function

$$\tilde{u} : \begin{cases} \mathbb{R}^2 \to \{0, 1\} \\ \boldsymbol{x} \mapsto \tilde{u}(\boldsymbol{x}) := \mathbf{1}_\Sigma(\boldsymbol{x}) \, , \end{cases}$$

where $\Sigma \subseteq \Omega \subseteq \mathbb{R}^2$, with $\Sigma := \{ \boldsymbol{x} \in \Omega \, | \, \tilde{u}(\boldsymbol{x}) = 1 \}$. By defining $D(\boldsymbol{w}) := f(\boldsymbol{w}) + \mu \, s(\boldsymbol{w})$ as a data term, we formulate our energy functional as

$$E(\boldsymbol{w}^+, \boldsymbol{w}^-, \tilde{u}) = \lambda \int_\Omega D(\boldsymbol{w}^+) \, \tilde{u}(\boldsymbol{x}) \, d\boldsymbol{x} + \lambda \int_\Omega D(\boldsymbol{w}^-) \, (1 - \tilde{u}(\boldsymbol{x})) \, d\boldsymbol{x}$$

$$+ \int_\Omega |\nabla \tilde{u}(\boldsymbol{x})| \, d\boldsymbol{x} \, , \tag{2}$$

where the last term of the above energy is a regularisation defined by the total variation (TV) norm, and $\lambda \in \mathbb{R}^+$ is a weighting parameter to control the weighting of the fidelity and smoothness term in D with respect to the TV norm of $\tilde{u}$. As pointed out by Chan et al. in [5], (2) is strongly related to the Mumford-Shah functional [8] and can be written as

$$\widetilde{E}(\boldsymbol{w}^+, \boldsymbol{w}^-, \Sigma) = \lambda \int_\Sigma D(\boldsymbol{w}^+) \, d\boldsymbol{x} + \lambda \int_{\Omega \setminus \Sigma} D(\boldsymbol{w}^-) \, d\boldsymbol{x} + \mathrm{Per}(\Sigma; \Omega), \quad (3)$$

where $\mathrm{Per}(\Sigma; \Omega)$ denotes the perimeter of the set $\Sigma \subseteq \Omega$. In order to find a global minimiser Σ_{min} of $\widetilde{E}(\boldsymbol{w}^+, \boldsymbol{w}^-, \cdot)$, we arrive at the proposition below.

Proposition 1. *For any fixed $\boldsymbol{w}^+, \boldsymbol{w}^- : \Omega \to \mathbb{R}^2$, a global minimiser for $\widetilde{E}(\boldsymbol{w}^+, \boldsymbol{w}^-, \cdot)$ can be found by solving the convex problem*

$$\min_{0 \leq \tilde{u} \leq 1} E(\boldsymbol{w}^+, \boldsymbol{w}^-, \tilde{u})$$

and finally setting

$$\Sigma = \Sigma(\eta) := \{\boldsymbol{x} \in \Omega \mid \tilde{u}(\boldsymbol{x}) \geq \eta\} \text{ for almost every } \eta \text{ with } \eta \in [0, 1].$$

Proof. The proof can be carried out similar to the one in [5] with the help of the layer cake representation and the coarea formula. □

Note, that the set of functions, over which minimisation is performed, is not restricted to binary functions $\tilde{u}$ anymore. To achieve a convex problem the feasible set allows for functions that take values between 0 and 1. We refer the reader to [5] for further exploration. To this end, by having the globally optimal motion segmentation we obtain the final displacement field $\boldsymbol{w} := \boldsymbol{w}^+ \tilde{u} + \boldsymbol{w}^- (1 - \tilde{u})$.

To illustrate our method we show a synthetic example in Fig. 1. The motion segmentation function $\tilde{u}$ splits the displacement field $\boldsymbol{w}$ into the parts $\boldsymbol{w}^+$ and $\boldsymbol{w}^-$. The function $\tilde{u}$ is close to a binary function, although we perform minimisation over non-binary functions. This property was also pointed out in [5].

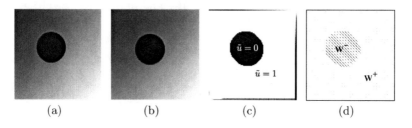

(a)   (b)   (c)   (d)

Fig. 1. The template image (a), the reference image (b), the motion segmentation function $\tilde{u}$ (c) and the displacement field $\boldsymbol{w}$ (d)

2.2   Minimisation

To minimise our energy functional in (2) with respect to $\tilde{u}$ in a fast and efficient way, we follow an approach similar to Pock *et al.* in [9], which allows us to exploit the powerful work of Chambolle [3]. We introduce a new variable $\tilde{v}$ and consider the energy functional

$$\widehat{E}(\boldsymbol{w}^+, \boldsymbol{w}^-, \tilde{u}, \tilde{v}) = \int_\Omega |\nabla \tilde{u}(\boldsymbol{x})| \, d\boldsymbol{x} + \frac{1}{2\theta} \int_\Omega (\tilde{u}(\boldsymbol{x}) - \tilde{v}(\boldsymbol{x}))^2 \, d\boldsymbol{x}$$

$$+ \lambda \int_\Omega D(\boldsymbol{w}^+) \, \tilde{v}(\boldsymbol{x}) \, d\boldsymbol{x} + \lambda \int_\Omega D(\boldsymbol{w}^-) \, (1 - \tilde{v}(\boldsymbol{x})) \, d\boldsymbol{x} \,. \quad (4)$$

For a small $\theta \in \mathbb{R}^+$ the minimisation of (4) with respect to $\tilde{u}$ and $\tilde{v}$ leads to $\tilde{u} \approx \tilde{v}$ and therefore approximates the energy functional E in (2). We propose the following iterative scheme to minimise the energy functional $\widehat{E}$ with respect to $\boldsymbol{w}^+$, $\boldsymbol{w}^-$, $\tilde{u}$ and $\tilde{v}$:

1. For fixed $\boldsymbol{w}^+$, $\boldsymbol{w}^-$ and $\tilde{v}$, solve

$$\min_{\tilde{u}} \left\{ \int_\Omega |\nabla \tilde{u}(\boldsymbol{x})| \, d\boldsymbol{x} + \frac{1}{2\theta} \int_\Omega (\tilde{u}(\boldsymbol{x}) - \tilde{v}(\boldsymbol{x}))^2 \, d\boldsymbol{x} \right\} \,. \quad (5)$$

2. For fixed $\boldsymbol{w}^-$, $\tilde{u}$ and $\tilde{v}$, solve

$$\min_{\boldsymbol{w}^+} \left\{ \int_\Omega D(\boldsymbol{w}^+) \, \tilde{v}(\boldsymbol{x}) \, d\boldsymbol{x} \right\} \,. \quad (6)$$

3. For fixed $\boldsymbol{w}^+$, $\tilde{u}$ and $\tilde{v}$, solve

$$\min_{\boldsymbol{w}^-} \left\{ \int_\Omega D(\boldsymbol{w}^-) \, (1 - v(\boldsymbol{x})) \, d\boldsymbol{x} \right\} \,. \quad (7)$$

4. For fixed $\boldsymbol{w}^+$, $\boldsymbol{w}^-$ and $\tilde{u}$, solve

$$\min_{\tilde{v} \in [0,1]} \left\{ \frac{1}{2\theta} \int_\Omega (\tilde{u}(\boldsymbol{x}) - \tilde{v}(\boldsymbol{x}))^2 \, d\boldsymbol{x} \right.$$

$$\left. + \lambda \int_\Omega D(\boldsymbol{w}^+) \, \tilde{v}(\boldsymbol{x}) \, d\boldsymbol{x} + \lambda \int_\Omega D(\boldsymbol{w}^-) \, (1 - \tilde{v}(\boldsymbol{x})) \, d\boldsymbol{x} \right\} \,. \quad (8)$$

The minimisation problem (5) is basically the denoising problem of the Rudin, Osher and Fatemi (ROF) model [10], and can be solved by the fast dual method of Chambolle [3]. The resulting Euler-Lagrange equations for (6) and (7) are similar to the ones in [1], and can be solved by the fixed point iteration scheme as described there. For the minimisation problem (8), the explicit solution can be derived from the corresponding Euler-Lagrange equation and is given by

$$\tilde{v}(\boldsymbol{x}) = \min \left\{ \max \left\{ \tilde{u}(\boldsymbol{x}) - \theta \lambda \left(D(\boldsymbol{w}^+) - D(\boldsymbol{w}^-) \right), 0 \right\}, 1 \right\} \,. \quad (9)$$

2.3   Implementation

Although, we have a convex minimisation problem with respect to the functions $\tilde{u}$ and $\tilde{v}$, the ones with respect to the displacement fields w^+ and w^- are still non-convex. To avoid the risk of getting stuck in a local minimum during the optimisation of the displacement fields, we wrap the iterative minimisation procedure in a coarse-to-fine framework. By choosing a minimal size n_{min} of the images at the coarsest level, we calculate the number of levels with the help of a certain scaling factor ξ. In our experiments we set $n_{min} = 32$ and $\xi = 0.9$. The coarse-to-fine strategy has also the advantage, that we can use trivial initialisations for the displacement fields. In contrary, Amiaz et. al. [1] had to use additional methods to initialise the displacement fields. At the coarsest level we therefore initialise the displacement fields w^+ and w^- with $\mathbf{0}$.

Because of Proposition 1 the choice of the initialisation for the function $\tilde{u}$ is irrelevant. Whatever initialisation we choose, the global minimiser will be the same for fixed w^+ and w^-. This property has been also exploited during the experiments, by choosing a random initialisation for $\tilde{u}$. Again, this is a great advantage of our method in contrast to the one in [1], where the initialisation for the level set function ϕ was also dependent on additional methods.

Our final iteration scheme consist of two loops. The outer loop iterates over the pyramid levels. In each level an inner loop updates the values for $\tilde{u}$, w^+, w^- and $\tilde{v}$, following steps _1 - 4_ in Section 2.2. Thus, in each iteration of this inner loop one step of Chambolle's method [3] is performed to update $\tilde{u}$. To achieve a better convergence of $\tilde{u}$ we update w^+ and w^- only each 10th iteration by executing one step of the inner fixed point iteration as described in [2] and [1]. To obtain the motion segmentation Σ we choose $\eta = 0.5$ and set $\Sigma = \Sigma(\eta) := \{x \in \Omega \,|\, \tilde{u}(x) \geq \eta\}$ (see Proposition 1). Finally, $\tilde{v}$ is updated according to the explicit solution given in (9).

As soon as the finest level is reached, the inner loop is executed until a certain tolerance or the maximum number of iterations is reached. The final displacement field is then obtained by setting

$$w(x) = \begin{cases} w^+(x) & \text{if } x \in \Sigma, \\ w^-(x) & \text{if } x \in \Omega \setminus \Sigma, \end{cases}$$

and we use bicubic interpolation to calculate the images $T(x + w^\pm)$ during the iterations and to obtain the final registered image $T(x + w)$.

3   Results

In this section we give a qualitative and quantitative evaluation of the proposed method on MR images of the liver, where the liver is sliding along the chest wall. In particular we compare our method to the demon algorithm with anisotropic diffusion filtering [6] and the registration algorithm of Brox et al. [2], which are known to preserve discontinuities in the displacement field.

In Fig. 2 a qualitative result is given comparing the various methods. One can clearly see, that a discontinuous motion field is achieved by our method and compared to the demon algorithm with anisotropic diffusion filtering and the registration algorithm of Brox *et al.* these discontinuities are more defined. The proposed approach managed to nicely separate the motion of the abdominal wall and the motion of the internal organs.

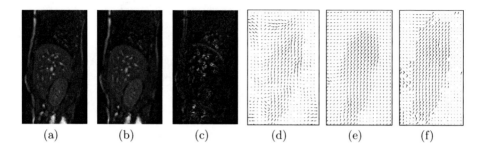

(a)   (b)   (c)   (d)   (e)   (f)

Fig. 2. The template image (a), the reference image (b) and the difference image (c). The displacement field for the demon algorithm with anisotropic diffusion filtering is shown in (d), the one for the registration algorithm of Brox *et al.* in (e) and finally the one of our method in (f).

In Fig. 3 a quantitative evaluation is shown for 22 different liver image pairs. We chose the parameters for all the three methods by optimising them with respect to these image pairs. The parameters of our method were set to $\gamma = 0.4$, $\mu = 0.05$, $\lambda = 0.05$, $\theta = 4$ and $\epsilon = 0.00001$. For the demon algorithm with anisotropic diffusion filtering we could use the suggested parameters and for Brox *et al.*'s method we used $\gamma = 5$, $\alpha = 80$ and $\sigma = 0.9$. The registration results were compared by calculating the mean squared error (MSE) and the normalised mutual information (NMI), where the grey values were scaled from 0 to 1. For all examples the proposed method performed better than the demon algorithm with anisotropic diffusion filtering. Compared to the method of Brox *et al.*, our approach provided better results except for the mean squared error in example 15.

Using the R software package (Version 2.10.1), we used the Kolmogorov-Smirnov test to check the normal distribution of the results. Assuming a significance level of 0.05, the t-tests showed that the proposed method performed significantly better than the demon algorithm with anisotropic diffusion filtering and the method of Brox *et al.* for MSE and NMI with both $p < 0.05$.

4   Conclusion

In this paper we presented a novel discontinuity preserving non-rigid registration method, which uses the advantage of the continuous cuts framework. We introduced a Proposition, which shows that a globally optimal motion segmentation can be found for fixed displacement fields w^+ and w^-. During motion estimation the so gained motion segmentation plays an aiding role. The minimisation of the energy functional is implemented in a coarse-to-fine strategy and

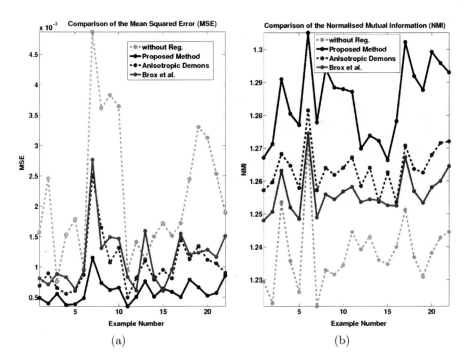

Fig. 3. Quantitative evaluation for 22 pairs of liver images with a discontinuous displacement field. Comparison of the MSE (a) and NMI (b).

exploits the rapidity of the dual method of Chambolle [3] and the accuracy of Brox *et al.*'s optical flow method. Our experimental results demonstrated desirable performance of the proposed method in comparison with those of the demon algorithm with anisotropic diffusion filtering and the registration algorithm of Brox *et al.*

Currently, we are working on a fast primal-dual method [4] based on the pure L^1 norm to improve the efficiency and accuracy of the method. We also plan to investigate the use of multi-label functions $\tilde{u}$ in order to capture more complex piecewise smooth displacement fields.

Acknowledgement. This work has been funded by Dr. Hansjörg Wyss.

References

1. Amiaz, T., Kiryati, N.: Piecewise-Smooth Dense Optical Flow via Level Sets. International Journal of Computer Vision 68(2), 111–124 (2006)
2. Brox, T., Bruhn, A., Papenberg, N., Weickert, J.: High Accuracy Optical Flow Estimation Based on a Theory for Warping. In: Pajdla, T., Matas, J. (eds.) ECCV 2004. LNCS, vol. 3024, pp. 25–36. Springer, Heidelberg (2004)
3. Chambolle, A.: An Algorithm for Total Variation Minimization and Applications. Journal of Mathematical Imaging and Vision 20(1-2), 89–97 (2004)

4. Chambolle, A., Pock, T.: A First-Order Primal-Dual Algorithm for Convex Problems with Applications to Imaging. Journal of Mathematical Imaging and Vision 40(1), 120–145 (2011)
5. Chan, T.F., Esedoglu, S., Nikolova, M.: Algorithms for Finding Global Minimizers of Image Segmentation and Denoising Models. Siam Journal on Applied Mathematics 66(5), 1632–1648 (2006)
6. Demirovic, D., Serifovic, A., Cattin, P.C.: An anisotropic diffusion regularized demons for improved registration of sliding organs. In: 18th International Electrotechnical and Computer Science Conference, ERK (2009)
7. Fundana, K., Heyden, A., Gosch, C., Schnörr, C.: Continuous Graph Cuts for Prior-Based Object Segmentation. In: 19th International Conference on Pattern Recognition, vol. 1-6, pp. 34–37 (2008)
8. Mumford, D., Shah, J.: Optimal Approximations by Piecewise Smooth Functions and Associated Variational-Problems. Communications on Pure and Applied Mathematics 42(5), 577–685 (1989)
9. Pock, T., Urschler, M., Zach, C., Beichel, R.R., Bischof, H.: A Duality Based Algorithm for TV-L^1-Optical-Flow Image Registration. In: Ayache, N., Ourselin, S., Maeder, A. (eds.) MICCAI 2007, Part II. LNCS, vol. 4792, pp. 511–518. Springer, Heidelberg (2007)
10. Rudin, L.I., Osher, S., Fatemi, E.: Nonlinear Total Variation Based Noise Removal Algorithms. Physica D 60(1-4), 259–268 (1992)
11. Schmidt-Richberg, A., Ehrhardt, J., Werner, R., Handels, H.: Slipping Objects in Image Registration: Improved Motion Field Estimation with Direction-Dependent Regularization. In: Yang, G.-Z., Hawkes, D., Rueckert, D., Noble, A., Taylor, C. (eds.) MICCAI 2009, Part I. LNCS, vol. 5761, pp. 755–762. Springer, Heidelberg (2009)
12. Vese, L.A., Chan, T.F.: A Multiphase Level Set Framework for Image Segmentation Using the Mumford and Shah Model. J. of Computer Vision 50(3), 271–293 (2002)
13. Zitova, B., Flusser, J.: Image registration methods: a survey. Elsevier, Image and Vision Computing 21(11), 977–1000 (2003)

Segmentation of Cervical Images by Inter-subject Registration with a Statistical Organ Model

Floris F. Berendsen[1], Uulke A. van der Heide[2], Thomas R. Langerak[1], Alexis N.T.J. Kotte[2], and Josien P.W. Pluim[1]

[1] Image Sciences Institute
[2] Department of Radiotherapy,
University Medical Center Utrecht, P.O. Box 85500,
3508 GA, Utrecht, The Netherlands
floris@isi.uu.nl

Abstract. For radiation therapy of cervical cancer, segmentation of the cervix and the surrounding organs are needed. The aim is to develop a fully automatic method for the segmentation of all relevant organs. Our approach is an atlas-based segmentation, with a registration scheme that is aided by statistical knowledge of the deformations that are to be expected. A statistical model that acts on the boundary of an organ is included as a soft constraint in a free-form registration framework. As a first evaluation of our approach, we apply it to the segmentation of the bladder. Statistical models for the bladder were trained on a set of manual delineations. Experiments on a leave-one-patient-out basis were performed, with the quality defined as the Dice similarity to the manual segmentations. Compared to a registration without the use of statistical knowledge, the segmentations are slightly, but significantly improved.

Keywords: Cervical cancer, radiation therapy.

1 Introduction

In radiation therapy for cancer, delineations of organs and the target volume are required to plan the treatment. While the tumor should receive a high dose, the neighboring organs should receive a dose as low as possible. For the treatment of cervical cancer, segmentations are made for the cervix, bladder, rectum, sigmoid and bowel. The organs are manually delineated in MR images, which is a time-consuming task.

Segmentation by registration is an automatic method that may be used for organ delineation. Registration finds topological relation between the target image and an atlas image. This topological relation is used to propagate the segmentations of the atlas to the target. Registration of cervical images of two different subjects is not described in literature. Only intra-subject registration, using contrast enhanced CT images [2] and MR images [5] has been reported.

H. Yoshida et al. (Eds.): Abdominal Imaging 2011, LNCS 7029, pp. 240–247, 2012.

Large and complex deformations due to differences in rectum and bladder fillings as well as sliding organ interfaces make these registrations a challenging task. Additionally, the MR images for cervical cancer treatment have thick transversal slices, showing only little detail in the out-of-plane direction.

Registration schemes that have to deal with large and complex deformations, normally demand a transformation model with a huge number of parameters. Even if coarse-to-fine approaches are applied, the registration can easily end up in a wrong, local minimum. To guide registration to deformations that are likely, prior shape knowledge is incorporated. Where the image data give a strong, but false, similarity (for instance, an edge in a neighboring structure), a shape model can restrain deformations into the false edge, when it is confident that these parts of the organ hardly have to deform. For parts of the organ where the image data give no clear evidence for correspondence, the model drives the organ into a shape (and position) that is likely given the population.

Rueckert et al. [4], for instance, use statistical deformation models (SDMs) that model all the control points of the B-spline deformation grid in a statistical way. Deformations are limited to the space spanned by a trained deformation model.

To not restrict the target deformation space spanned by the training data, the model could be used as a soft constraint in registration. This is done in [1], where the span of the model is increased to all the degrees of freedom of the transformation, by regularization called shrinkage estimation. However, registration examples of 2D images are shown only.

In our approach, we use a B-spline deformation grid, but apply a model on a certain set of displacement vectors only. This results in a deformation model that acts as a soft constraint, like in [1], but that is feasible for 3D image registration. We limit the model to the set of vectors that describe the deformations of the boundaries of a certain organ.

In the following, the framework for inter-subject registration and the inclusion of a statistical model are explained. The algorithm is implemented as an additional module in the registration toolbox Elastix [3]. As a first evaluation of our approach, we apply it to segmentation of the bladder, because the bladder has the best contrast. The Results section shows the segmentation performance compared to a registration without modeling shapes. Finally, in the last section, the conclusions and discussion are presented.

2   Method

2.1   Data

The data used, comprises MR images of 17 patients. Five images are available for each patient, acquired in five consecutive weeks, except for one patient who was scanned four times. In the first week a CT scan was made also.

The T2-weighted MR images were acquired with a 1.5 T scanner (Gyroscan NT Intera; Philips Medical Systems, Best, The Netherlands). The scans were made in the transversal direction. The image dimensions are $512 \times 512 \times 30$ voxels, with a voxel size of $0.625\,\mathrm{mm}\times0.625\,\mathrm{mm}\times4.5\,\mathrm{mm}$. The CT images (Aura; Philips Medical Systems, Best, The Netherlands) have a dimension of $512 \times 512 \times 118$ voxels. The voxel size is $0.885\,\mathrm{mm}\times0.885\,\mathrm{mm}\times3\,\mathrm{mm}$.

Manual delineations of the bladder and clinical target volume (CTV), which mainly contains the cervix, are available for each MR image. The delineations were made for clinical purposes by a radiation oncologist and approved by a radiologist. The rigid transform parameters that map MR coordinates to CT, were provided. Figure 1 gives examples of the MR images.

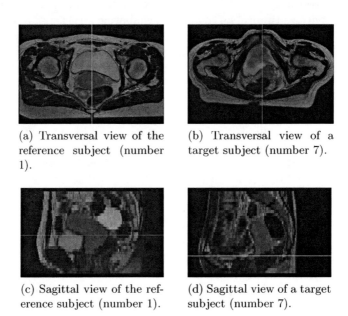

(a) Transversal view of the reference subject (number 1).

(b) Transversal view of a target subject (number 7).

(c) Sagittal view of the reference subject (number 1).

(d) Sagittal view of a target subject (number 7).

Fig. 1. MR images of two subjects. The bladder is shown with a blue and the CTV with a green overlay. The yellow lines denote the crossings of the viewing planes.

2.2   Registration Framework

In order to propagate the segmentations of an atlas image I_{ref} to any other subject image I_{target} a spatial transformation that relates both images is obtained by registration. The registration of the cervical images is split into two parts, a global and a local part. The global transform T_{global} serves as an alignment in location, orientation and scale of the two subjects. It is found by registration of the bone structures in the CT image

As an affine transform is not sufficient to model global differences between subjects, a course B-spline registration with a grid spacing of 80 mm is additionally performed. To remove the influence of the soft tissue (including the contours of the body), the images are preprocessed by replacing all voxels that are not part of the bone structures with a neutral value. The global transform is the composition of respectively a rigid (MR to CT), a bone-to-bone and a rigid (CT to MR) transform.

The other part is the local registration, which deals with the highly flexible organ deformations. For this registration, a model is added that statistically describes the deformations of an object boundary to the boundaries of the corresponding objects of all other atlases.

Because the statistical model will be defined in the coordinates of the reference image, the target I_{target} is transformed to the reference space using T_{global}, resulting in I'_{target}. The residual transform between I'_{target} and I_{ref} is called T_{local}.

Registration can be expressed as a minimization of a cost function $\mathcal{C}$:

$$\hat{\mu} = \arg\min_{\mu} \mathcal{C}(T_{\mu}; I_{ref}, I'_{target}) \tag{1}$$

with μ the vector of parameters of the transformation. The cost function in this registration scheme consists of an image similarity measure $\mathcal{S}$ and penalty function $\mathcal{P}$:

$$\mathcal{C} = -\mathcal{S} + \alpha\mathcal{P}. \tag{2}$$

The similarity function can be any image similarity. The statistical model defines the penalty term $\mathcal{P}(T_{\mu}; p_{ref})$, with p_{ref} denoting the boundary in the reference image. A weighting factor α is used to bring the metrics in the same scale and to control their influences.

2.3   Statistical Model

Deformations of the reference shape are evaluated by the model and its result acts as a penalty term in the registration process. The model is based on a point distribution model that is made from the collection of meshes. In this application, the delineations of the atlas data are converted into the meshes. Corresponding mesh samples are obtained by registering the binary images of the delineations.

For registration a kappa statistics metric is used, which maximizes overlap of binaries. The transformation model is a 3-level pyramid of B-splines with grid a spacing schedule of 40-20-10 mm.

The M vertices of an atlas mesh are concatenated into an atlas shape vector:

$$p_{atlas} = [x_1, y_1, z_1, \ldots, x_M, y_M, z_M]^{T} \tag{3}$$

The space of all atlas shape vectors is characterized by a multivariate normal distribution defined by its mean $\bar{p}$ and covariance Σ. The mean and the covariance of the distribution are estimated by the arithmetic mean and the sample covariance.

Especially in cases where the number of vectors is smaller than the dimensionality of these vectors, this distribution is supported only in a subspace of possible shapes. To compute the penalty an arbitrarily deformed reference shape, the inverse of the covariance matrix is needed, which does not exist in these cases.

This inversion problem is circumvented by a shrinkage estimator, like is done in [1]. The modified covariance matrix Σ' is a mixture of the estimated covariance matrix and a diagonal matrix:

$$\Sigma' = (1 - \beta)\Sigma + \beta\sigma_0^2 I, \tag{4}$$

with $0 < \beta < 1$ the shrinkage intensity and σ_0^2 an assumed variance. By this manipulation, the multivariate normal distribution will have a variance of at least $\beta\sigma_0^2$ in all directions. The matrix $\sigma_0^2 I$ is the assumed covariance matrix that defines the normal distribution if there was no knowledge available, except for the mean $\bar{p}$. If the number of samples is large enough to have a reliable estimate, the shrinkage intensity should approach to zero.

2.4 Penalty

With the estimated distribution, deformations of the reference mesh p_{ref} can be evaluated by means of the Mahalanobis distance, which will be used as the penalty term. The penalty value is the distance of the deformed reference mesh to the mean mesh $\bar{p}$, taking into account that modes of deformations that are common in the population are regarded as less distant.

In registration it is beneficial to use gradient based optimizers. Consequently, the derivatives of the penalty term with respect to the transform parameters are required. For the analytical derivative of the penalty function, the Mahalanobis distance to the mean of the distribution, is expressed as a function of the transform parameters. Firstly, the mean mesh vector is subtracted from the transformed mesh vector.

$$p(\mu) = T\left(\mu; p_{\text{ref}}\right) - \bar{p} \tag{5}$$

The difference mesh vector $p(\mu)$ is now a function of the transform parameters. By including the difference vector, the Mahalanobis distance can be expressed as:

$$M(\mu) = \sqrt{p^{\text{T}}(\mu)\Sigma'^{-1}p(\mu)} \tag{6}$$

The partial derivatives with respect to the transform parameters are:

$$\frac{\partial M}{\partial \mu} = \frac{1}{M}p^{\text{T}}(\mu)\Sigma'^{-1}\frac{\partial p(\mu)}{\partial \mu} \tag{7}$$

Given 5, it is easy to see that $\frac{\partial p(\mu)}{\partial \mu} = \frac{\partial T}{\partial \mu}\left(p_{\text{ref}}\right)$, where $\frac{\partial T}{\partial \mu}\left(p_{\text{ref}}\right)$ is a concatenation of the spatial derivatives at the locations of the vertices of the mesh p_{ref}. These spatial derivatives with respect to the transform parameters are available in the registration package Elastix.

3 Experiments

The model as described in this paper was implemented as a module in the registration package Elastix. Although the idea is to apply this method on the different types of organs in the subject eventually, we chose to experiment with one organ, i.e. the bladder, first. Registration is restricted to a masked area, with the mask created from the manual delineation with an extra margin of 4.5 mm.

For all experiments normalized cross correlation was used as image similarity measure. The transformation was parameterized with a 3-level pyramid of B-splines with grid a spacing schedule of 40-20-10 mm. The adaptive stochastic gradient descent optimizer was used with 5000 randomly selected samples for 300 iterations each level.

One patient was chosen as the reference image, the others functioned either as a target or as an atlas image. The experiments were done in a leave-one-patient-out fashion. Each patient's first week scan served as a target image once and the data of the other 15 patients (i.e. excluding the target and the reference patient) constituted the atlas. This resulted in 74 atlas images. The bladder meshes were generated with 84 vertices. The weight α of the penalty in (2) is set such that the influence on the cost function matches the influence of the image similarity metric. With $\alpha = 0.01$ the gradient magnitude of the penalty metric is scaled to the same order of magnitude as the gradient magnitude of the normalized cross correlation, during optimization.

Empirical testing showed that a suitable value for the shrinkage intensity is $\beta = 0.2$ and for the assumed variance it is $\sigma_0^2 = 1000$. The volume of the bladder of the reference image is similar to the average bladder volume of all subjects. The quality of segmentation is measured with the Dice similarity coefficient in the target domain. A segmentation in the target image is obtained by applying respectively the local and global transform to a densely triangulated reference shape and converting it to a binary image.

The baseline of the experiments is the Dice score of the initial overlap after global registration. For comparison, the scores of registration without the enhancement of a model (effectively setting $\alpha = 0$) are also reported. The starting point for this, so-called conventional registration, is the same initial transformation as used for the model-enhanced registration.

4   Results

The overlap scores of the experiments performed for all target subjects are shown in Fig. 2. The initial Dice similarity coefficient, i.e. after global alignment, is on average 0.50 When additionally performing a conventional registration, the average score is improved to 0.63. The registration enhanced by the model, performed after the initial alignment, gives an average Dice score of 0.67. The improvement over the conventional registration is found to be significant ($p = 0.022$), using a two-sided paired t-test.

5   Discussion

The results of the experiments show that the inclusion of the statistical model significantly improves atlas registration. However the average Dice score increased

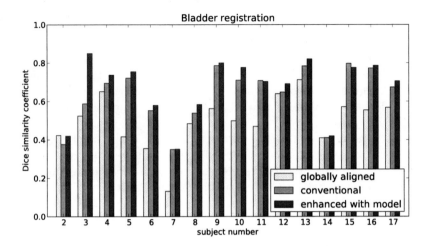

Fig. 2. Bladder overlap scores for leave-patient-out registration experiments with subject 1 as reference image

by only 0.04 points to 0.67, which leaves the quality of the segmentation too low for clinical use. The quality is not yet at the level of *intra-patient* registration, of which a median Dice similarity coefficient of 0.8 for bladder alignment was reported [5].

As mentioned before, the segmentations are made for clinical purposes. This may not always be a good gold standard. As can be seen in Fig. 1, the segmentation of the bladder in the reference does not cover the edges exactly. These inaccuracies can reduce the apparent quality of the registration results.

For the results shown in Fig. 2, it seems that when conventional registration obtains low scores, the inclusion of the model does not improve things. When looking into the individual scores, this is the case for subjects 2 and 7, who happen to have very small bladders and for subject 14, who has a very big bladder. When inspecting the relation with volume size, as shown in Fig. 3a, there appears to be a trend toward a decreasing Dice overlap for bladder volumes that have larger difference with the reference volume. Too severe expansion and compression create discrepancies, for instance the blurring or sharpening of edges, which hamper registration.

An effect, imposed by the model, is that all target shapes that are on the periphery of the distribution will be harder to register correctly, since there is a constant pull toward the average shape. To have an idea what the penalty term would be in case of a correct registration, the delineation of a target is directly evaluated by the model. This is the Mahalanobis distance to the mean, based on the same leave one patient out training as is used for registration. To investigate the effect on the quality of registration, the obtained Dice score is plotted against the target penalty (Fig. 3b). The target shapes that have a low

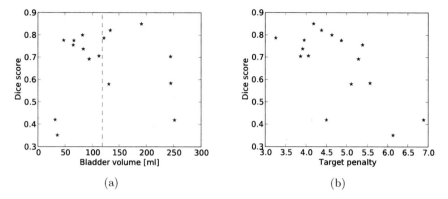

(a)   (b)

Fig. 3. The obtained Dice score after registration with the model is plotted against (a) the target bladder volume, with the dashed line denoting the volume of the bladder in the reference and (b) the target penalty

penalty term will generally have higher overlap scores after registration. The linear way of describing the distribution by the model can be too harsh for describing all shapes in the population at once.

The effect of mismatch of bladder volumes could be countered by selecting a more suitable reference image. The negative effect of the model for valid shapes that deviate too much from average shape, could be decreased by selecting the right training shapes. However, since it is difficult to predict what these selections should be for an arbitrary target image, multi-atlas registration can be employed for a number of settings. The challenge is to find the right combinations of training sets and reference images that effectively cover the population.

Although the registration method presented, does not yet solve the clinical problem of organ segmentation, atlas-based segmentation is improved. An overall higher quality of segmentations is beneficial for multi-atlas fusion methods.

References

1. Albrecht, T., Luthi, M., Vetter, T.: A statistical deformation prior for non-rigid image and shape registration. In: IEEE Conference on CVPR, pp. 1–8 (2008)
2. Bondar, L., Hoogeman, M.S., Vasquez Osorio, E.M., Heijmen, B.J.: A symmetric nonrigid registration method to handle large organ deformations in cervical cancer patients. Med. Phys. 37, 3760–3772 (2010)
3. Klein, S., Staring, M., Murphy, K., Viergever, M.A., Pluim, J.P.W.: elastix: A toolbox for intensity-based medical image registration. IEEE Trans. Med. Imaging 29, 196–205 (2010)
4. Rueckert, D., Frangi, A.F., Schnabel, J.A.: Automatic construction of 3D statistical deformation models using non-rigid registration. IEEE Trans. Med. Imaging 22, 77–84 (2003)
5. Staring, M., van der Heide, U.A., Klein, S., Viergever, M.A., Pluim, J.P.W.: Registration of cervical MRI using multifeature mutual information. IEEE Trans. Med. Imaging 28, 1412–1421 (2009)

A New Method for Contour Determination of the Prostate in Ultrasound Images

Farhang Sahba

Toronto, ON, Canada
farhang@ieee.org

Abstract. In this paper a method for prostate segmentation in ultrasound images is presented. This method contains several tasks including edge enhancement, edge-preserving smoothing filter, speckle reduction, local contrast adaptation, and Canny edge detector to extract the final boundary. The proposed method is relatively easy to implement with some degree of adaptivity with respect to the image characteristics. Experimental results show the performance for some cases.

Keywords: prostate segmentation, ultrasound.

1 Introduction

Prostate cancer is one of the most frequently diagnosed forms of cancer in the male population and ultrasound imaging is one of the most widely used technologies for diagnosing of this cancer. The accurate detection of the prostate boundary in these images is crucial for automatic cancer diagnosis/classification. However, in ultrasound images the contrast is usually low and the boundaries between the prostate and background are fuzzy. Also speckle noise and weak edges make the ultrasound images inherently difficult to segment. Furthermore, the quality of the image depends on the type and particular settings of the machine. Despite of these challenging factors, ultrasound imaging remains an important modality for prostate cancer detection where the automatic segmentation is highly desirable. Currently, in most applications the prostate boundaries are manually extracted from ultrasound images which have a very low signal-to-noise ratio. Consequently, some methods have been introduced to facilitate more accurate automatic or semi-automatic segmentation of the prostate boundaries from the ultrasound images [1–5, 8, 9]. In spite of all these researches, prostate segmentation in ultrasound images has still remained a very challenging problem. Due to some limitations, most of the existing methods can deliver acceptable results in regular cases while they may have some difficulties with other ones where the segmentation error may increase.

The aim of this work is to introduce an approach to deal with this problem for some cases. The method presented in this paper rely on edge information as an important features in such images.

H. Yoshida et al. (Eds.): Abdominal Imaging 2011, LNCS 7029, pp. 248–255, 2012.
© Springer-Verlag Berlin Heidelberg 2012

2   Methodology

In the proposed approach there are some major stages explained in the following sections.

2.1   Edge Enhancement and Bilateral Filtering

Considering the shape of the prostate and to enhance its edges a special type of gradient, called *radial gradient* for each pixel is computed. The radial gradient is the image gradient along the radial direction relating to a center point at (x_C, y_C). The radial gradient at each pixel (x, y) can be determined as [6]:

$$\phi_r^{\tilde{I}}(x, y) = \left| \left[\partial \tilde{I}/\partial x, \partial \tilde{I}/\partial y \right]' . r(x, y) \right| / \left| r(x, y) \right| \qquad (1)$$

where $r(x, y) = [x - x_C, y - y_C]'$. We suppose that the center point, (x_C, y_C), is a point around the central area of the prostate in the original image and is provided by the user as an input. This gives an image I_g with the same size of the original image having high values in the areas of the prostate edges. By adding the absolute values of the radial gradient image $| I_g |$ to the original image I an image I_e with more emphasis on the prostate edges is created $((I_e = I_g + I))$. A sample prostate image, the result of the radial gradient values, and the image with more emphasis on the prostate edges are shown in Fig.1 (a), (b), and (c), respectively. Then by applying a bilateral filter, which uses both spatial and intensity values, edges are preserved while noise is filtered out (Fig.1 (d)).

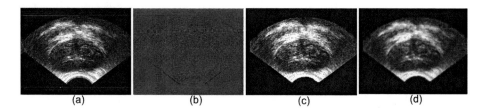

Fig. 1. (a) Sample prostate ultrasound image. Results of: (b) Radial gradient, (c) Edge enhanced image, (d) Bilateral filtering.

2.2   Speckle Reduction

Ultrasound images have low signal-to-noise ratio (SNR). This is especially because of the speckle noise which has nonzero correlation over the large distances. Direct applying of an edge-detection algorithm to these images results in a number of false edges. To reduce this noise, conventional low-pass filters are generally not usable due to the loss of detail in low-contrast border regions. An alternative method is to use sticks to reduce speckle noise. This filter, called stick filter, can reduce the speckle noise by modelling edges in ultrasound images as a line process. This filter can suppress speckle without losing edge detail. Fig 2 (a) shows the result of applying stick filter to the output of the bilateral filter. It demonstrates increasing the contrast near the prostate borders, while reducing speckle noise. According to our dataset we have selected a midway stick length of 15 to reduce the speckle while improving the contrast of the image [4].

2.3   Fuzzy Contrast Adaptation

After enhancement using stick filter, additional contrast enhancement is required before the prostate boundary can be reliably delineated. Therefore, the contrast of the image is further enhanced via an algorithm whose aim is to construct a locally-adaptive contrast adaptation function being well fit to the image characteristics [7]. This technique helps to achieve better detection of the prostate edges by performing a contrast adaptation method. In this method an image I is considered as an array of fuzzy singletons, each having a value denoting its degree of membership to a property of image. If we denote the intensity property of mn^{th} pixel by g_{mn} and membership function μ_{mn} , we can represent it in fuzzy notation as follow [7]:

$$I = \bigcup_{m} \bigcup_{n} \mu_{mn}/g_{mn} \quad m, n \in Area\ Of\ Interest \tag{2}$$

The main idea is that, we find the local maximum and minimum gray levels for some supporting points and then interpolate these values to obtain corresponding values for each pixel [7].

First, the image is divided into M_S rows and N_S columns (as the number of steps in y and x directions, respectively). This leads to $M_S \times N_S$ sub-images. The central point of each sub-image is used as the location of a supporting point. A window around each supporting point is then considered to find the local minimum $(g_{min,local})$ and maximum $(g_{max,local})$ gray levels for that point. To avoid loss of information during the interpolation, the size of windows are chosen to have at least 50% overlap with each other. Fig. 2(b) schematically shows how this technique works [7].

Next, spatial parameters of local minimum gray level $(g_{min,local})$ and local maximum gray level $(g_{max,local})$ inside these windows are calculated. After finding $M_S \times N_S$ sets of local minimum and maximum values, a 2-D interpolation function is applied to obtain corresponding interpolated values $g_{min,intp}$ and $g_{max,intp}$ for each pixel. Then we use this information to calculate a new membership function over the whole image as:

$$\mu(g_{mn}) = \frac{(g_{mn} - g_{min,intp})}{(g_{max,intp} - g_{min,intp})} \tag{3}$$

Next we employ a fuzzy intensification operator to modify the membership values [7]. This operator reduce the fuzziness of the image resulting in an increase in image contrast.

$$\mu'_{mn} = \begin{cases} 2[\mu_{mn}]^2 & 0 \le \mu_{mn} \le 0.5, \\ 1 - 2[1 - \mu_{mn}]^2 & 0.5 \le \mu_{mn} \le 1, \end{cases} \tag{4}$$

where μ and μ' indicate the inside membership before and after the enhancement, respectively. The result of applying the above method on the gray levels of a prostate image is shown in Fig.2 (c).

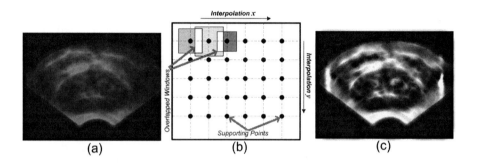

Fig. 2. (a) Result of stick filter, (b) contrast adaptation technique: supporting points and their adaptive windows for calculation of local minimum and maximum gray level values for each of them and then interpolation of these values. (c) result of applying contrast adaptation technique.

The main advantage of applying this method is that the bright areas around the prostate edges get large gray level intensities in comparison to their neighbors. It is interesting to note that this step has the capability to best suit to local image characteristics. To apply this method in our case we have used a maximum window size and a minimum window size. The algorithm calculates the proper window size using fuzzy rules.

2.4   Multi-scale Canny Edge Detection

An important aspect of segmentation techniques is to focus on the relevant edge information and eliminate unrelated edges created by noise or irrelevant small image detail. The Canny edge detector is widely used in computer vision applications to find object boundaries in an image [11]. The reputation of the Canny edge detector is because of its optimality with respect to the three criteria: good detection, good localization, and low spurious response.

-*Extracting the major edges:* In the majority of cases, the prostate has two parts of boundaries, the upper boundary and the lower boundary that can be identified as a dark-to-light transition of intensities from the inside of the prostate to its outside [5]. Due to the strong intensity transition, these two parts can be revealed using a Canny edge detector with large scale and deliver the Major edges of the prostate.

-*Extracting the minor edges:* Due to the poor signal to noise ratio in ultrasound images, some important edges on the prostate boundary are missed. It is because that when the direction of gradient at a ridge point is not normal to the ridge contour, the point is not classified as an edge and removed. As a result the Canny edge detector cannot detect some important branching edges. To overcome this problem, we use some properties of the concept of minor edges. It marks a pixel as a minor edge if the gradient magnitude of that pixel is larger than those adjacent to it but not necessarily in the gradient direction. The minor edge contours are traced and only the correct parts of the contours that are connected to the major edges are kept. This repeats intentionally. To keep away from formation of false loops, the minor edge contours are partitioned and those that do not contain any major edges are removed. Then the portions enclosed by the new major edges are indicated to be used in the procedure.

Fig 3 (a), (b), (c), and (d) show the results of applying Canny edge detector for large and small scales.

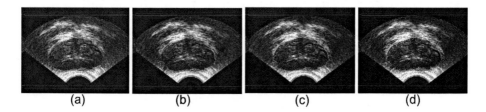

Fig. 3. Canny detection for four different scales, (a) scale 4, (b) scale 3, (c) scale 2, and (d) scale 1

2.5 Contour Tracing

After finding the new edge map from the previous stage, there are still some missed parts on the prostate boundary. These parts usually located at the right and left sides of the prostate and caused by shadowing effect. To find these parts and complete the border, the existing edge pieces can be traced. For this purpose, we can use an edge tracing method to complete the segmentation. By employing this strategy, the missed parts on the boundary can be estimated.

3   Results and Discussions

We have selected and examined forty five ultrasound images of prostate. The images were noisy, with low contrast and shadow effects. The results of the proposed method have been evaluated by comparing the algorithm-based segmentation and the manual segmentation (gold standards) and are shown in Fig. 4

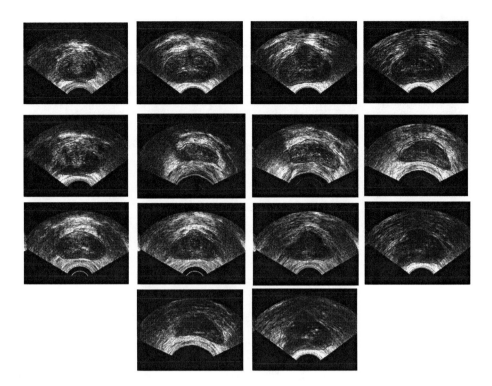

Fig. 4. Automatic and manual boundaries for some sample cases. Red lines and blue lines show manually segmented and algorithm-base segmentation, respectively.

for sample images. From the experiments, it can be seen that for these cases the difference between two contours is acceptable and the proposed method is able to deliver good results.

For quantitative evaluation, we have used the following error measures between the algorithm-based and manual-based segmentations to validate the performance of the proposed method compared to the manual segmentation performed by a radiologist [10]:

δ = Average distance (in pixels),
E_A = Area error, and
AO = Area Overlap.

Table 1 and 2 summarize these results.

Comparing to some other approaches the proposed method can work better in terms of accuracy. In terms of running time, using the MATLAB code on average it took 12s to process an image. This time can be even better by optimization of the code.

Table 1. Quantitatively Evaluation of Proposed Algorithm in Comparison with Manual Segmentation for regular cases

	Aver Dist. (Pixels)	Area Err. (%)	Area Overlap (%)
Mean	3.07	5.24	91.26
Var	1.65	3.94	2.84

Table 2. Quantitatively Evaluation of Proposed Algorithm in Comparison with Manual Segmentation for some more difficult cases

	Aver Dist. (Pixels)	Area Err. (%)	Area Overlap (%)
Mean	4.79	13.79	82.87
Var	1.81	7.96	4.47

4   Conclusion

A method for prostate segmentation in transrectal ultrasound images using an edge-based method was presented in this paper. In this method, the different processing steps are arranged to best suit the studied cases such that the prostate edge can be detected. The algorithm uses a suitable form of modification as well as parameter selection based on local information. The proposed method is relatively easy to implement with a degree of adaptivity with respect to the image characteristics. The processing time is also acceptable compare to some statistical methods. Preliminary experiments showed some improvements in the results, although it needs to be explored much more thoroughly in future works.

References

1. Knoll, C., Alcaniz, M., Grau, V., Monserrat, C., Juan, M.C.: Outlining of the prostate using snakes with shape restrictions based on the wavelet transform. Pattern Recognit 32, 1767–1781 (1999)
2. Ladak, H.M., Mao, F., Wang, Y., Downey, D.B., Steinman, D.A., Fenster, A.: Prostate boundary segmentation from 2D ultrasound images. Med. Phys. 27, 1777–1788 (2000)
3. Ghanei, A., Soltanian-Zadeh, H., Ratkesicz, A., Yin, F.: A three-dimensional deformable model for segmentation of human prostate from ultrasound image. Med. Phys. 28, 2147–2153 (2001)
4. Pathak, S.D., Chalana, V., Haynor, D.R., Kim, Y.: Edge-guided boundary delineation in prostate ultrasound images. IEEE Transactions on Medical Imaging 19, 1211–1219 (2000)
5. Shen, D., Zhan, Y., Davatzikos, C.: Segmentation of Prostate Boundaries From Ultrasound Images Using Statistical Shape Model. IEEE Transactions on Medical Imaging 22(4) (2003)

6. Zheng, Y., Yu, J., Bing Kang, S., Lin, S., Kambhamettu, C.: Single-Image Vignetting Correction Using Radial Gradient Symmetry. In: IEEE Computer Society Conference on Computer Vision and Pattern Recognition (CVPR 2008), pp. 24–26 (2008)
7. Tizhoosh, H.R., Krell, G., Muchaelis, B.: Locally Adaptive Fuzzy Image Enhancement. In: Reusch, B. (ed.) Fuzzy Days 1997. LNCS, vol. 1226, pp. 272–276. Springer, Heidelberg (1997)
8. Shen, D., Herskovits, E.H., Davatzikos, C.: An adaptive-focus statistical shape model for segmentation and shape modeling of 3D brain structures. IEEE Trans. Med. Imag. 20, 257–270 (2001)
9. Fenster, A., Downey, D.: Three-dimensional ultrasound imaging. In: SPIE: Med. Phys., vol. 3659, pp. 2–11 (1999)
10. Nanayakkara, N.D., Samarabandu, J., Fenster, A.: Prostate segmentation by feature enhancement using domain knowledge and adaptive region based operations. Physics in Medicine and Biology 51, 1831–1848 (2006)
11. Canny, J.: A Computational Approach To Edge Detection. IEEE Trans. Pattern Analysis and Machine Intelligence 8(6), 679–698 (1986)

Analyses of Missing Organs
in Abdominal Multi-Organ Segmentation

Miyuki Suzuki[1], Marius George Linguraru[2,3],
Ronald M. Summers[2], and Kazunori Okada[1]

[1] Department of Computer Science
San Francisco State University
{miyukis,kazokada}@sfsu.edu
[2] Radiology and Imaging Sciences
National Institutes of Health Clinical Center
{lingurarum,rsummers}@mail.nih.gov
[3] Sheikh Zayed Institute for Pediatric Surgical Innovation
Children's National Medical Center

Abstract. Current methods for abdominal multi-organ segmentation
(MOS) in CT can fail to handle clinical patient population with missing
organs due to surgical removal. In order to enable the state-of-the-art
atlas-guided MOS for these clinical cases, we propose 1) statistical organ
location models of 10 abdominal organs, 2) organ shift models that capture organ shifts due to specific surgical procedures, and 3) data-driven
algorithms to detect missing organs by using a normality test of organ
centers and a texture difference in intensity entropy. The proposed methods are validated with 34 contrast-enhanced abdominal CT scans, resulting in 80% detection rate at 15% false positive rate for missing organ
detection. Additionally, the method allows the detection/segmentation
of abdominal organs from difficult diseased cases with missing organs.

Keywords: multi-organ segmentation, contrast-enhanced CT.

1 Introduction

Segmentation of abdominal organs is a crucial building block for computer-aided
diagnosis (CAD) of various diseases in CT and also a major technical challenge
due to similar intensity of neighboring organs and high inter subject variability of organ's geometry [4]. Addressing this challenge, multi-organ segmentation
(MOS) approach has recently become popular toward improving overall segmentation accuracy and enabling comprehensive analysis of multi-focal abdominal
diseases [10, 15, 13, 9, 12, 14, 6–8].

In this paper, we investigate how such MOS can be extended to a patient population with missing organs. Without considering this population, MOS cannot
be applied to a number of important clinical applications such as follow up studies of surgical treatment and cancer recurrence in abdomen. Despite this clinical
importance, however, the literature discussing how MOS performs with data
from such population is lacking. Current MOS solutions are also not designed
to handle irregular anatomy cases. A common process in various MOS methods

H. Yoshida et al. (Eds.): Abdominal Imaging 2011, LNCS 7029, pp. 256–263, 2012.

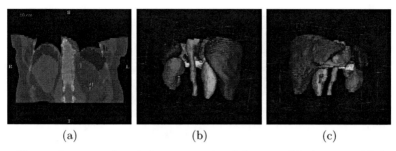

(a)   (b)   (c)

Fig. 1. Illustrative examples of a) segmentation failures and b,c) ten modeled organs. Red: liver, blue: spleen, cyan: r-kidney, magenta: l-kidney, yellow: pancreas, orange: aorta, dark green: gall bladder, purple: l-adrenal, lavender: r-adrenal, green: stomach.

is to fit an atlas of normal organ anatomy to an image to be analyzed. When analyzing a case with missing organs, regardless of atlas formats (i.e., static [15], probabilistic [10, 13, 9, 6, 7], or geometric [13, 12, 14, 6, 8]), MOS can fail to segment other intact organs because of 1) post-surgical organ shifts and 2) mis-match of the atlas' part corresponding to the missing organs to nearby non-targets. As a result, these MOS methods applied to missing organ cases can underperform organ-specific segmentation schemes. Fig.1(a) illustrates such a case with a missing right kidney (cyan) where the liver (red) shifted downward into the cavity caused by the removed kidney and a part of the liver was identified as kidney. The main contribution of this paper is two-fold. First, surgical procedure-specific organ shift models are proposed and built using nine clinical cases of nephrectomy (kidney removal) and splenectomy (spleen removal). 3D centers of ten abdominal organs are first estimated by a geometric Gaussian mixture model (GMM) then statistically modeled with respect to normal organ locations. Second, two new features for data-driven missing organ detection are proposed. As a base MOS, the atlas-guided MAP algorithm proposed in [13] is used, which fits a GMM with a probabilistic atlas constructed from ten normal organ cases. One feature characterizes the probability of each segmented organ being normal by using statistical organ location models, while the other feature examines the intensity entropy under an atlas mask and compares it against normal anatomical organs. The automatic missing organ detection allows us to handle clinical scan data more robustly even when previous medical history information is missing or corrupted in patient record or DICOM tag [2]. The proposed method is related to a multi-organ identification framework [3, 5, 14] such as the spine-based statistical location model (SLM) proposed by Yao and Summers [14]. This paper focuses on applying the SLM approach to the missing organ cases as a pre-step of MOS.

2 Method

2.1 Atlas-guided MAP Multi-Organ Segmentation

We follow Shimizu et al. [13] as our base atlas-guided MOS method. The MAP estimation of organ label $l \in \{1, .., L\}$ over 4D spatiointensity feature vector $\mathbf{v} =$

$(x, y, z, I(x, y, z))$ is employed: $\hat{l} = \text{argmax}_l p(\mathbf{v}|l)p(l)$. A standard probabilistic atlas [10, 7] is built by registering K training cases of normal anatomy to a fixed reference volume I_R then computing a probability map for each of L modeled organs by counting manually segmented organs. The prior $p(l)$ is modeled by this atlas. For each organ l, a normal spatiointensity model $(\mathbf{u}_{\mathbf{v}l}, \mathbf{\Sigma}_{\mathbf{v}l})$ is also computed where $\mathbf{u}_{\mathbf{v}l}$ and $\mathbf{\Sigma}_{\mathbf{v}l}$ are the mean and covariance of feature vectors of the organ l from the K training cases. The likelihood $p(\mathbf{v}|l)$ is modeled by an extended GMM $p(\mathbf{v}) = \sum_{l=1}^{L} \left(\frac{1}{N} \sum_{n=1}^{N} \alpha_l(n) \right) N(\mathbf{v}; \mathbf{u}_l, \mathbf{\Sigma}_l)$ where N denotes the number of voxels and the mixing weights $\alpha_l(n)$ are defined over each voxel n. To segment L organs in a test case I_{te}, I_{te} is first registered to I_R using affine transformation followed by B-spline non-rigid registration [11]. Then the GMM is initialized by the normal spatiointensity model and fit to I_{te} using the EM-algorithm [1].

2.2   Organ Location and Shift Models

Geometry of abdominal organs varies due to a) inter-subject variation, b) post-surgical organ shifts, c) postures and d) pathology. Focusing on modeling the first two factors, we prepare a set $\{I_m^{na}|m = 1, .., M_{na}\}$ with L normal anatomy and a set $\{I_{m'}^{mo}|m' = 1, .., M_{mo}\}$ with one or two organs missing. After registering all cases to I_R, each organ's location is modeled by the point distribution density of organ centers $\mathbf{x}_{lm}$, each of which is given by either the segmented organ's median coordinate or expert's manual estimation. Organ location models (OLMs) for normal anatomy (NA) and for missing organs (MO) are built as a set of normal densities over M_{na} NA and M_{mo} MO cases, respectively

$$NA = \{NA_l\} = \{N(\mathbf{x}; \mu_l, \mathbf{\Sigma}_l)|l = 1, .., L\} \tag{1}$$

$$MO = \{MO_l\} = \{N(\mathbf{x}; \mu_l', \mathbf{\Sigma}_l')|l = 1, .., L\} \tag{2}$$

where $\mu_l = 1/M_{na} \sum_m \mathbf{x}_{lm}$, $\mu_l' = 1/(M_{mo} - \#MO_l) \sum_{m'} \mathbf{x}_{lm'}$, $\#MO_l$ denotes the number of missing cases for organ l, and $\mathbf{\Sigma}_l$ and $\mathbf{\Sigma}_l'$ are covariance matrices corresponding to μ_l and μ_l', respectively.

While both NA and MO model the inter-subject variation of organ locations, MO is also influenced by the post-surgical organ shifts. Organ shift model (OSM) is then designed by a set of normal point-difference distributions $\{\mathbf{y}_{lm} = \mathbf{x}_{lm} - \mu_l\}_l$ in a local frame centered at μ_l for each organ l

$$OS = \{OS_l\} = \{N(\mathbf{y}_l; \mu_l' - \mu_l, \mathbf{\Sigma}_l')|l = 1, .., L\} \tag{3}$$

Surgical procedure-specific organ shift models $\{OS_t|t = 1, .., T\}$ where T is the number of organ-specific missing cases are modeled by computing an OSM in Eq.(3) with a subset of the MO cases specific to a surgical procedure such as nephrectomy and splenectomy. OSM can take two different variations according to their purposes: anatomical and detectional OSM. Anatomical OSM is created by manually estimated organ centers which visualize true post-surgical organ shifts. Whereas detectional OSM applies centers estimated by EM algorithm which detects the failure of EM algorithm for missing organs and this used as a part of our missing organ detection method.

2.3 Missing Organ Detection

When fitting the GMM $p(\mathbf{v})$ described in Sec 2.1 to a missing organ case I^{mo}, a normal model corresponding to a missing organ will be fitted to arbitrary non-target organ(s) located nearby. Data-driven detection of such missing organs can therefore be used to mitigate this EM estimation error. Each organ in the atlas is first linearly translated to the center estimated by EM algorithm for each NA and MO cases resulting in organ-specific binary atlas masks $B_l(\mathbf{x})$.

The first indicator feature F_l of missing organ l is the probability of estimated organ centers by EM being abnormal with respect to estimated organ centers of NA,

$$F_l = 1 - p(x|\theta_l) = 1 - N(x; \mu_l, \boldsymbol{\Sigma}_l) \tag{4}$$

where $\theta_l = (\mu_l, \boldsymbol{\Sigma}_l)$.

The second indicator feature G_l examines the difference in texture pattern under the atlas mask $B_l(\mathbf{x})$ comparing entropies of MO to NA and scales it to the same range as F_l,

$$G_l = 1 - e^{-|E_l - E_l^{NA}|} \tag{5}$$

where E_l and E_l^{NA} denote intensity entropy computed with the MO case I^{mo} and with the NA cases $\{I_m^{na}\}$ masked by $B_l(\mathbf{x})$, respectively.

3 Experiments

3.1 Data

Nine MO (M_{mo}=9) and twenty five NA (M_{na}=25) cases, totaling 34 contrast-enhanced diseased abdominal CT scans, are used in this study. Each scan consists of $512 \times 512 \times 50$ voxel slices with 5mm thickness stored in Mayo analyze format. CT scanners from various manufacturers are used to acquire this dataset with the ISOVUE 300 contrast agent. The MO dataset contains three different types of surgical organ removal: i) 5 splenectomy cases (spleen removed), ii) 3 nephrectomy cases (right kidney removed), and iii) 1 splenectomy and nephrectomy case (spleen and left kidney removed). Ten abdominal organs ($L = 10$) are considered in this study: aorta (AO), gallbladder (GB), left/right adrenal glands (LA,RA), liver (LV), left/right kidney (LK,RK), pancreas (PN), spleen (SP), and stomach (ST). For validation, segmentation ground-truth is generated for 9 NA and 9 MO cases with ITK-Snap tool. Fig.1(b,c) illustrate the examples of the segmentation ground-truth. The probabilistic atlas is built with ten ($K = 10$) abdominal thin-slice CT scans of normal anatomy delineated by expert radiologists.

3.2 Results

We first evaluate OLMs and OSMs that are built by using our data. To estimate each organ center, we use 3D center of gravity of B_l computed by our base MOS. Fig.2(a) shows an example view of the constructed NA in Eq(1). Fig.2(b)

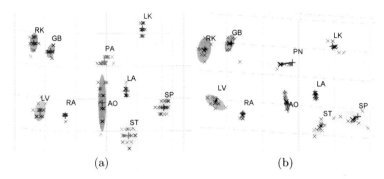

Fig. 2. OLM and OSM. (a) NA with 10 organs. Estimated organ and model centers are denoted by blue 'x' and red '+', respectively. An ellipse shows an iso-contour of the 3D covariance multiplied by two for each organ. (b) Detectional OS with the organ shift vectors shown in indigo arrows. MO's and NA's centers are denoted by black 'x' and red '+', respectively.

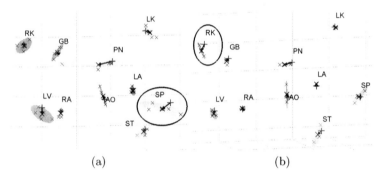

Fig. 3. Detectional OS_t for splenectomy and nephrectomy. (a) With five splenectomy cases. (b) With three nephrectomy cases. Blue ellipses show removed organs for respective procedures.

illustrates a similar example view of the detectional OS in Eq.(3). Next the surgical procedure-specific detectional OSMs are evaluated. Fig.3(a,b) show detectional OS_t for splenectomy and nephrectomy in the same format of Fig.2. Larger shifts are observed by the removed organs indicated by ellipses.

Quantitative analyses of constructed OLMs and detectional OSMs are evaluated in Fig.4. Fig.4(a) summarizes the variance of OLMs for each organ. The trace of a covariance matrix is equivalent to the sum of eigenvalues thus proportional to the average variance across the three spatial axes. For NA, the covariance trace for the stomach was the largest (92.8) and that for the left kidney was the smallest (1.2). For MO, the trace for the pancreas was the largest (428.7) and that for the left adrenal was the smallest (6.1). The unit of the measures is in voxels. The pancreas exhibited the largest magnitude of the organ shift (16.3), followed by the spleen (8.0), stomach (3.6), and aorta (3.2). Fig.4(b) compares the magnitudes of organ shift vectors $\mathbf{y}_{lm}$ for each organ. Pancreas and

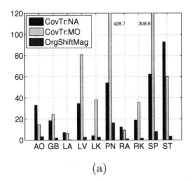
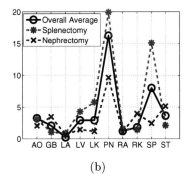

(a)   (b)

Fig. 4. Analyses of organ location variances and organ shift magnitudes. (a) Blue: trace of covariances in NA, green: trace of covariances in MO, magenta: magnitudes of organ shift vectors in voxels. (b) Comparison of magnitudes of organ shift vectors in voxels for the two surgical procedures against the overall average.

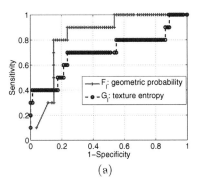
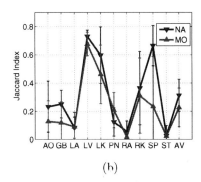

(a)   (b)

Fig. 5. (a) ROC analysis for missing organ detection with F_l and G_l features. (b) Segmentation accuracy in Jaccard index (JI). Blue down-triangles and red up-triangles show organ-wise average JIs for NA and MO cases, respectively. Captions of organs are defined in Sec.3.1. 'AV' indicates the average JI over all organs.

spleen resulted in large organ shifts for both procedures. For splenectomy, pancreas, left kidney, liver and spleen exhibited the shifts larger than average. For nephrectomy, gall bladder, stomach and right kidney exhibited larger shifts. In both cases, organs that were removed (spleen and right kidney) resulted in large shifts, which indicate mismatch to non-target organ(s). Fig. 5(a) summarizes the receiver operating characteristic (ROC) analysis of missing organ detection using F_l in Eq.(4) and G_l in Eq.(5). Both features exhibit positive correlations to the missing organ occurrences. At 3.75% false positive rate (FPR), sensitivity for F_l and G_l are 10% and 40%. At 15% FPR, sensitivity for F_l and G_l are 80% and 40%. The area under the curve (AUC) for F_l and G_l are 0.83 and 0.71, respectively.

Finally, we evaluate the baseline MOS results on our data from the diseased population. Fig. 5(b) shows organ-wise segmentation accuracy in Jaccard index ($JI = \frac{|A \cap B|}{|A \cup B|}$ where A and B are equal-length binary patterns) averaged over

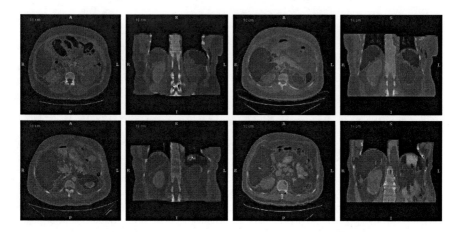

Fig. 6. Illustrative examples of the baseline atlas-guided MOS results. Top row: NA cases. Second row: spleen removed (left), spleen and left kidney removed (right). The same color scheme in Fig.1 is used.

the NA (blue 'V') and MO (red 'A') cases with ground truths. Liver, left kidney and spleen have relatively high accuracy. The accuracy for MO cases is lower than that for NA in general due to difficulties for handling the diseased cases. The accuracy for spleen and left kidney of MO is significantly lowered since MO includes cases missing them. Not only missing organ itself but even neighboring organ, liver, is influenced by right kidney missing such that the bottom of liver is segmented as right kidney that causes the lower accuracy of MO liver. Segmentation of adrenal glands and gall bladder is challenging because they are very small and their shape varies widely. Stomach also yields very low JI because its shape and intensity is extremely various.

Fig. 6 demonstrates four illustrative examples of segmentation results. NA cases shown in the top row indicate successful segmentations of major abdominal organs except for the pancreas in the left case. On the other hand, MO cases shown in the bottom row encountered more issues. On the splenectomy case on the left, the spleen model (blue) was falsely put on the left kidney and missed the aorta. On the splenectomy/nephrectomy case on the right, the spleen and left kidney models are falsely put on the stomach and intestine moved to the cavity vacated by the removed organs. In both cases, liver and right kidney are segmented correctly.

4   Conclusions and Discussion

This paper presented novel methods for modeling abdominal organ shifts due to surgical procedures and for detecting occurrence of missing organs. Our experimental results are promising in that 1) organ shift models depicted different patterns of organ movements for splenectomy and nephrectomy and 2) two features applied for detection exhibited reasonable accuracy with different patterns. Texture entropy performed better in low FPR while geometric probability performed better in higher FPR. Our future work includes building and analyzing

OLMs and OSMs with a larger dataset and exploring a combined feature with the two proposed as well as others. Finally, the resulting missing organ detection will be integrated with our overall MOS scheme in order to improve segmentation accuracy for the targeted diseased population.

References

1. Dempster, A.P., Laird, N.M., Rubin, D.B.: Maximum likelihood from incomplete data via the EM algorithm. J. Roy. Stats. Soc. Series B 39, 1–38 (1977)
2. Guld, M.O., Kohnen, M., Keysers, D., Schubert, H., Wein, B.B., Bredno, J., Lehmann, T.M.: Quality of DICOM header information for image categorization. In: SPIE, vol. 4685, pp. 280–287 (2002)
3. Kobashi, M., Shapiro, L.G.: Knowledge-based organ identification from CT images. Pattern Recognition 28, 475–491 (1995)
4. Kobatake, H.: Future CAD in multi-dimensional medical images - project on multi-organ, multi-disease CAD system. Computerized Medical Imaging and Graphics 31, 258–266 (2007)
5. Lee, C.C., Chung, P.C., Tsai, H.M.: Identifying multiple abdominal organs from CT image series using a multimodule contextual neural network and spatial fuzzy rules. IEEE Trans. Info. Tech. in Biomed. 7, 208–217 (2003)
6. Linguraru, M.G., Pura, J.A., Chowdhury, A.S., Summers, R.M.: Multi-Organ Segmentation from Multi-Phase Abdominal CT via 4D Graphs using Enhancement, Shape and Location Optimization. In: Jiang, T., Navab, N., Pluim, J.P.W., Viergever, M.A. (eds.) MICCAI 2010, Part III. LNCS, vol. 6363, pp. 89–96. Springer, Heidelberg (2010)
7. Linguraru, M.G., Sandberg, J.K., Li, Z., Pura, J.A., Summers, R.M.: Atlas-based automated segmentation of spleen and liver using adaptive enhancement estimation. Medical Physics 37, 771–783 (2010)
8. Liu, X., Linguraru, M.G., Yao, J., Summers, R.M.: Organ pose distribution model and an MAP framework for automated abdominal multi-organ localization. In: Proc. Medical Imaging and Augmented Reality, pp. 393–402 (2011)
9. Okada, T., Yokota, K., Hori, M., Nakamoto, M., Nakamura, H., Sato, Y.: Construction of Hierarchical Multi-Organ Statistical Atlases and their Application to Multi-Organ Segmentation from CT Images. In: Metaxas, D., Axel, L., Fichtinger, G., Székely, G. (eds.) MICCAI 2008, Part I. LNCS, vol. 5241, pp. 502–509. Springer, Heidelberg (2008)
10. Park, H., Bland, P.H., Meyer, C.R.: Construction of an abdominal probabilistic atlas and its application in segmentation. IEEE Trans. Medical Imaging 22, 483–492 (2003)
11. Rueckert, D., Sonoda, L.I., Hayes, C., Hill, D.L.G., Leach, M.O., Hawkes, D.J.: Non-rigid registration using free-form deformations: Application to breast MR images. IEEE Trans. Medical Imaging 18, 712–721 (1999)
12. Seifert, S., Barbu, A., Zhou, S.K., Liu, D., Feulner, J., Huber, M., Suehling, M., Cavallaro, A., Comaniciu, D.: Hierarchical parsing and semantic navigation of full body CT data. In: Proc. SPIE Conf. Medical Imaging (2008)
13. Shimizu, A., Ohno, R., Ikegami, T., Kobatake, H., Nawano, S., Smutek, D.: Segmentation of multiple organs in non-contrast 3D abdominal CT images. Int. J. CARS 2, 135–143 (2007)
14. Yao, J., Summers, R.M.: Statistical Location Model for Abdominal Organ Localization. In: Yang, G.-Z., Hawkes, D., Rueckert, D., Noble, A., Taylor, C. (eds.) MICCAI 2009, Part II. LNCS, vol. 5762, pp. 9–17. Springer, Heidelberg (2009)
15. Zhou, Y., Bai, J.: Multiple abdominal organ segmentation: An atlas-based fuzzy connectedness approach. IEEE Trans. Info. Tech. in Biomed. 11, 348–352 (2007)

Geometric Modelling of Patient-Specific Hepatic Structures Using Cubic Hermite Elements

Harvey Ho[1], Adam Bartlett[2], and Peter Hunter[1]

[1] Bioengineering Institute
[2] Department of Surgery,
University of Auckland, Auckland, New Zealand
{harvey.ho,p.hunter,a.bartlett}@auckland.ac.nz

Abstract. In this paper we use cubic Hermite elements to represent hepatic structures that are digitised from a computed tomography angiography (CTA) image. 1D, 2D and 3D linear elements are first created for hepatic vasculature, surface and parenchyma, respectively. Cubic Hermite elements are then generated by evaluating and updating the nodal derivatives of the corresponding linear elements. We show that the main features of the liver can be captured by a very small number of cubic Hermite elements (e.g., 55 elements for the liver volume), and propose potential applications of these elements in biomechanical modelling of the liver.

1 Introduction

3D reconstruction of the liver plays an important role in pre-operative simulation and virtual resection. It aids surgeons in locating hepatic lesions, constructing virtual segmental lobes, and delineating complex vascular networks, to name a few of its many applications in open and laparosopic surgeries [1–3].

The visualisation and segmentation of liver structures (lobes and blood vessels) have been studied by many research groups, with various algorithms proposed (e.g., see [4, 5]). While most of these studies focused on geometric representation of the liver without considering the physical properties of hepatic tissues (parenchyma and blood vessel), Cotin et al pointed out the importance of simulating soft-tissue deformation in surgical procedures [6]. Besides the conventionally used spring-mass method and Finite Element Method (FEM), they proposed a 'tensor-mass' model to simulate deformations and cutting on complex anatomical structures [6]. The computational volume mesh they used was a tetrahedra mesh, which included 7,039 elements [6]. This could be computationally expensive and a high-end computer was required to simulate surgical procedures in real-time.

In this paper we employ the cubic Hermite elements to model blood vessels, surfaces and parenchyma of the liver. We show that with a much smaller number of elements the main geometric features of a patient-specific liver can be captured. We outline the basic steps used in constructing these element, and also discuss its potential applications in biomechanical modelling.

H. Yoshida et al. (Eds.): Abdominal Imaging 2011, LNCS 7029, pp. 264–271, 2012.
© Springer-Verlag Berlin Heidelberg 2012

2   Method

2.1   Linear and Cubic Hermite Elements

Linear and Cubic Hermite elements are often used in Finite Element Analysis (FEA) which uses basis functions to interpolate physical values at element nodes to other non-nodal points. The most commonly used basis function is the linear Lagrange functions which reserve C^0 continuity across element boundaries. Cubic Hermite basis function further retain C^1 connectivity i.e. the nodal coordinate and derivative continuity.

The imaging and visualization tool, CMGUI, developed by Auckland Bioengineering Institute (ABI), New Zealand, was employed in constructing Hermite elements. The nodal orderings of single 1D, 2D and 3D cubic Hermite elements, following the convention used in [7], are illustrated in Fig. 1.

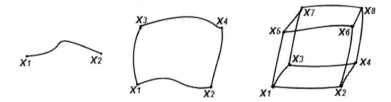

Fig. 1. Node ordering of 1D, 2D and 3D elements used in CMGUI

1D Cubic Hermite Element The interpolation formula for 1D linear mesh is given by:

$$x(\xi) = \xi x_1 + (1 - \xi)x_2 \tag{1}$$

where ξ ranges from $[0, 1]$, x_i are end nodes, $x(\xi)$ represent any points along the 1D mesh. The formula for a 1D Cubic Hermite mesh is given by:

$$x(\xi) = \Psi_1^0(\xi)x_1 + \Psi_1^1(\xi)\left(\frac{dx}{d\xi}\right)_1 + \Psi_2^0(\xi)x_2 + \Psi_2^1\left(\frac{dx}{d\xi}\right)_2 \tag{2}$$

where Ψ are the Hermite basis functions given by:

$$\begin{cases} \Psi_1^0 = 2\xi^3 - 3\xi^2 + 1 \\ \\ \Psi_2^0 = -2\xi^3 + 3\xi^2 \\ \\ \Psi_1^1 = \xi^3 - 2\xi^2 + \xi \\ \\ \Psi_2^1 = \xi^3 - \xi^2 \end{cases} \tag{3}$$

Here Ψ_1^0 and Ψ_2^0 are applied to nodal values, and Ψ_1^1 and Ψ_2^1 are applied to node derivatives so that the curve bends in the desired direction at the start and endpoint.

The derivatives of $x(\xi)$ in Eq. (3) are defined as:

$$\frac{dx}{d\xi} = \left(\frac{dx}{ds}\right) \cdot \left(\frac{ds}{d\xi}\right) \tag{4}$$

where dx/ds is the physical arc length derivative and $ds/d\xi$ is the scale factor that scales dx/ds to the ξ coordinate derivative [7]. The degree of freedom (DoF) of a 1D cubic Hermite node, as defined in Eq. (2), is 4.

2D and 3D Hermite Elements The bicubic Hermite function $x(\xi_1, \xi_2)$ is formed from the tensor product of two 1D cubic Hermite functions (Eq. 2). Note, that both first order derivative $(\partial x/\partial \xi_i)$ and cross-derivatives are present in the bicubic Hermite function. They are evaluated by:

$$\frac{\partial x}{\partial \xi_i} = \left(\frac{\partial x}{\partial s_i}\right) \cdot (S_i) \tag{5}$$

$$\frac{\partial^2 x}{\partial \xi_1 \partial \xi_2} = \left(\frac{\partial x^2}{\partial s_1 \partial s_2}\right) \cdot (S_1) \cdot (S_2) \tag{6}$$

where S_i is the scale factor and $\partial x/\partial s_i$ is the physical arc length derivative. In the same fashion, the 3D tricubic Hermite basis function is the product of three 1D cubic Hermite functions. The aim is to interpolate a function defined on nodes to an arbitrary point in 3D space.

The formulas for 2D and 3D cubic Hermite elements are not listed here due to their lengths. The DoF of a 2D and 3D cubic Hermite elements are 16 and 64, respectively. We refer the interested reader to the literature [7] for more details.

2.2   Medical Imaging and Segmentation

To demonstrate the geometric modelling process, we retrospectively studied a CTA abdominal image (GE Lightspeed VCT, voxel resolution $0.432 \times 0.432 \times 0.625$mm) of Fig. 2. The image was scanned at the arterial phase, i.e., the arteries were enhanced by a contrast agent. The segmentation software used was MIMICS 10 (Materialise, Leuven, Belgium). Manual segmentation was used at locations where the liver border was not distinguishable from other tissues (e.g., point **A** in Fig. 2a). The segmentation result is shown in Fig. 2(b). The liver surface was exported as a stereolithography (STL) file, which yields a dense data cloud of about 83,000 points, as shown in Fig. 2(c). Other abdominal organs i.e. the kidneys, the spleen and the stomach were also segmented to indicate their spatial relationships with the liver.

Extraction of arteries was relatively straightforward due to its enhanced image intensity (e.g., the aorta indicated by the arrow in Fig. 2a). To enable blood flow simulation to be carried out in future work, the connectivity information

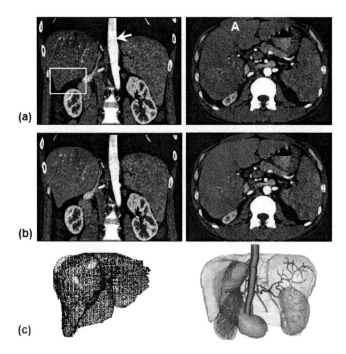

Fig. 2. Liver segmentation: (a) Image processing of the CTA abdominal image: arteries (e.g., aorta indicated by the arrow) were enhanced in the image; at location **A** there were no clear boundary between liver parenchyma and other tissues; region growing algorithm is applied to the rectangular region; (b) the segmentation results; (c) data clouds yielded from the segmented liver surface, and visualization of abdominal organs

between network generations must be explicitly expressed. To that end the arterial tree was reconstructed manually using a 1D cubic Hermite mesh. The detailed procedure is introduced next.

2.3 1D, 2D and 3D Element Mesh Construction

To generate the 1D cubic Hermite mesh, some key points along the centerline of blood vessels, in particular those at bifurcations and vessels with high curvatures, were manually selected as nodes (Fig. 3a), and the radius at each node as its field. These nodes were then connected by linear 1D elements (Fig. 3b). 1D cubic Hermite mesh was generated by updating nodal derivatives and incorporating nodal radius field (Fig. 3c).

The data cloud of Fig. 2c is the basis for 2D and 3D cubic Hermite mesh construction. The actual procedure is illustrated in Fig. 4: in Fig. 4(a), seven data point slices were selected, upon which linear 2D elements were created; in Fig. 4(b), the derivatives of each node were evaluated and updated to form a bicubic Hermite mesh; in Fig. 4(c), each golden point represents the centre of a 3D element, and six 3D elements constitute a slice of liver parenchyma volume.

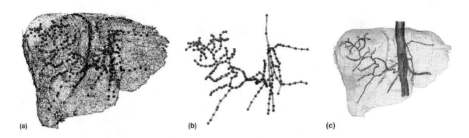

Fig. 3. Creation of 1D elements: (a) Key points (nodes) along vessel centreline were selected; (b) 1D linear elements are created by connecting the nodes; (c) nodal radius incorporated to simulate blood vessels

3   Results

Using the mesh construction techniques introduced above, the hepatic vasculature, surface and parenchyma were represented by a combination of 1D, 2D and 3D cubic Hermite elements. These structures, with three different views, are shown in Fig. 5.

The arterial tree (in red colour) ranges from the aorta (diameter $D \approx 19.0mm$) to the small hepatic arteries ($D \approx 1.1mm$). It consists of 45 segments spanning eleven generations. The right hepatic artery (indicated by arrow 1) stems from the common hepatic artery which bifurcates from the celiac artery. The left hepatic artery (indicated by arrow 2) arises from the gastric artery instead of growing from the common hepatic artery. This anatomical variation occurs in 25% of the population [8].

The reconstructed venous tree (in blue colour) contains the inferior vena cava (IVC), renal veins and the right hepatic vein. The portal system was not segmented and visualised because it was barely visible in the CTA image. Nevertheless, the same vessel delineating technique applies to the portal veins. Note, that the critical topological information i.e. the connectivities between parent and daughter vessels are maintained in generated 1D mesh files.

The liver surface was represented by 130 bicubic Hermite elements. The main geometric features such as the curved lobe surface were shown in the image, as well as the spatial relation between the liver and the blood vessels. However, some fine details such as the gallbladder bed and the complex hilum were not totally reproduced due to the high order nature of cubic Hermite elements. Although this can be improved by using more elements, a tradeoff decision has to be made between geometric realism and computational analysis cost.

The liver volume was represented by 55 tricubic Hermite elements. They are not shown in Fig. 5 but are a smoothed version of the linear elements in Fig. 4c. The number of volume elements used, therefore, is much less than the tetrahedra required (e.g., 7,039 tetrahedra in [6]) for a similar liver model.

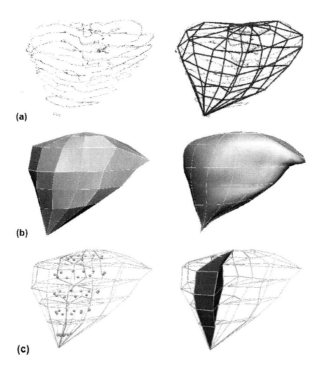

Fig. 4. Creation of 2D and 3D elements: (a) data points were selected from the data cloud of Fig. 2, and 2D linear elements were constructed from selected nodes; (b) a bicubic Hermite mesh was created from the linear mesh to represent liver surface; (c) a volume Hermite mesh was created to represent parenchyma

4   Discussion

In this paper we introduced a geometric modelling technique that employs cubic Hermite elements to represent hepatic structures i.e., the liver surface, parenchyma and blood vessels. This technique is different from previous work (e.g., in [2–4]) in that a much smaller number of elements can be employed to represent similar geometric entities. The cost, however, is that more nodal values (spatial coordinates and derivatives) need to be determined for each node. This difficulty may be solved by using a custom-made FEM software (e.g., CMISS, www.cmiss.org) whereby the nodal derivatives can be generated automatically.

The main purpose of using cubic Hermite elements for hepatic structures is to facilitate our future work in biomechanical analysis for the liver. This includes both hemodynamic and soft-tissue analysis for the hepatic vasculture and parenchyma, respectively. For example, based on a 1D mesh of the arterial tree, the governing equations for the blood flow may be solved using numerical methods. This is illustrated in Fig. 6 where the flow equations (Fig. 6(b))

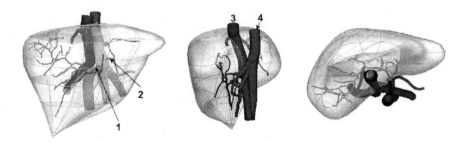

Fig. 5. Representing hepatic structures using cubie Hermite elements: 1. right hepatic artery; 2. left hepatic artery; 3. inferior vena cava; 4. descending aorta

were solved and the computed blood pressure was postprocessed along the tree. Such a method can be readily applied to larger vasculatures, e.g., that of Fig. 5. However, a unique challenge of hemodynamics modelling for the liver is its dual-blood-supply system, and the portal flow and hepatic arterial flow are inter-related. Therefore, a control mechanism will need to be incorporated.

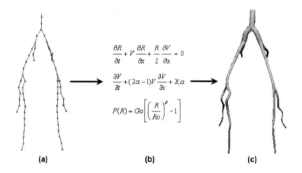

$$\frac{\partial R}{\partial t} + V\frac{\partial R}{\partial x} + \frac{R}{2}\frac{\partial V}{\partial x} = 0$$

$$\frac{\partial V}{\partial t} + (2\alpha - 1)V\frac{\partial V}{\partial x} + 2(\alpha$$

$$P(R) = Go\left[\left(\frac{R}{Ro}\right)^{\beta} - 1\right]$$

(a)   (b)   (c)

Fig. 6. (a) 1D mesh for an arterial tree; (b) governing equations for blood flow; (c) blood pressure postprocessed on the tree

Another example is the analysis of liver deformation due to the effects of heart-beat, ventilation, or laparoscopic insufflation. Such an analysis relies on the determination of mechanical properties of the liver tissue, either from literature data or from in vitro mechanical experiments. The aim is to describe the nonlinear stress-strain relationship of the liver tissue, and to model the large deformation of the liver under different loading conditions. Although the actual biomechanic simulations are yet to be performed, FEA has been carried out for other organs (e.g., for the heart [9]) modeled with similar 3D cubic Hermite mesh.

5   Conclusion

Cubic Hermite elements are used to model the hepatic vasculature, surface and volume in this paper. The resulting mesh has a small number of elements while each node has more nodal values. Using a 3D CT image we demonstrated the workflow of constructing patient-specific hepatic structures. We also discussed potential applications of these elements in biomechanical analysis.

References

1. Mutter, D., Dallemagne, B., Bailey, C., Soler, L., Marescaux, J.: 3D virtual reality and selective vascular control for laparoscopic left hepatic lobectomy. Surgical Endoscopy 23(2), 432–435 (2008)
2. Marescaux, J., Rubino, F., Arenas, M., Mutter, D., Soler, L.: Augmented-Reality-Assisted laparoscopic adrenalectomy. Journal of the American Medical Association 292(18), 2214–2215 (2004)
3. Hansen, C., Wieferich, J., Ritter, F., Rieder, C., Peitgen, H.: Illustrative visualization of 3D planning models for augmented reality in liver surgery. International Journal of Computer Assisted Radiology and Surgery 5(2), 133–141 (2010)
4. Marescaux, J., Clément, J.M., Tassetti, V., Koehl, C., Cotin, S., Russier, Y., Mutter, D., Delingette, H., Ayache, N.: Virtual reality applied to hepatic surgery simulation: the next revolution. Annals of Surgery 228(5), 627–634 (1998)
5. Esneault, S., Lafon, C., Dillenseger, J.: Liver vessels segmentation using a hybrid geometrical moments/graph cuts method. IEEE Transactions on Bio-Medical Engineering 57(2), 276–283 (2010)
6. Cotin, S., Delingette, H., Ayache, N.: A hybrid elastic model for real-time cutting, deformations, and force feedback for surgery training and simulation. The Visual Computer 16(8), 437–452 (2000)
7. Bradley, C., Pullan, A., Hunter, P.: Geometric modeling of the human torso using cubic hermite elements. Annals of Biomedical Engineering 25(1), 96–111 (1997)
8. Tank, P.W.: Grant's Dissector. Lippincott Williams & Wilkins (2008)
9. Nash, M., Hunter, P.: Computational mechanics of the heart. Journal of Elasticity 61, 113–141 (2000)

Author Index